DATE DUE

MAR 1 9 2004	

Allergies
SOURCEBOOK

Second Edition

Health Reference Series

Second Edition

Allergies
SOURCEBOOK

Basic Consumer Health Information *about*
Allergic Disorders, Triggers,
Reactions, and Related Symptoms,
Including Anaphylaxis, Rhinitis, Sinusitis,
Asthma, Dermatitis, Conjunctivitis, and
Multiple Chemical Sensitivity

Along with Tips on Diagnosis, Prevention
and Treatment, Statistical Data, a Glossary,
and a Directory of Sources for Further
Help and Information

Edited by
Annemarie S. Muth

Omnigraphics

615 Griswold Street • Detroit, MI 48226

Bibliographic Note

Because this page cannot legibly accommodate all the copyright notices, the Bibliographic Note portion of the Preface constitutes an extension of the copyright notice.

Each new volume of the *Health Reference Series* is individually titled and called a "First Edition." Subsequent updates will carry sequential edition numbers. To help avoid confusion and to provide maximum flexibility in our ability to respond to informational needs, the practice of consecutively numbering each volume has been discontinued.

Edited by Annemarie S. Muth

Health Reference Series

Peter D. Dresser, *Managing Editor*
Karen Bellenir, *Series Editor*
David A. Cooke, MD, *Medical Consultant*
Maria Franklin, *Permissions Assistant*
Joan Margeson, *Research Associate*
Dawn Matthews, *Verification Assistant*
Carol Munson, *Permissions Assistant*

Omnigraphics, Inc.

Matthew P. Barbour, *Vice President, Operations*
Laurie Lanzen Harris, *Vice President, Editorial Director*
Kevin Hayes, *Production Coordinator*
Thomas J. Murphy, *Vice President, Finance and Controller*
Peter E. Ruffner, *Senior Vice President*
Jane J. Steele, *Marketing Coordinator*

Frederick G. Ruffner, Jr., *Publisher*

© 2002, Omnigraphics, Inc.

Library of Congress Cataloging-in-Publication Data

Allergies sourcebook : basic consumer health information about allergic disorders, triggers, reactions, and related symptoms, including anaphylaxis, rhinitis, sinusitis, asthma, dermatitis, conjunctivitis, and multiple chemical sensitivity; along with tips on diagnosis, prevention and treatment, statistical data, a glossary, and a directory of sources for further help and information / edited by Annemarie S. Muth.--2nd ed.
    p. cm. -- (Health reference series)
    Includes bibliographical references and index.
    ISBN 0-7808-0376-0
    1. Allergy--Popular works. I. Muth, Annemarie. II. Health reference series (Unnumbered)

RC584 .A3443 2001
616.97--dc21

2001054876

∞

This book is printed on acid-free paper meeting the ANSI Z39.48 Standard. The infinity symbol that appears above indicates that the paper in this book meets that standard.

Printed in the United States

Table of Contents

Part IV: Allergy Triggers

Part V: Diagnosis, Treatments, and Aids to Wellness

Part VI: Additional Help and Information

Preface

About This Book

According to statistics compiled by the National Institute of Allergy and Infectious Diseases, nearly 50 million Americans—one in every five—suffer from allergies. The most prevalent, pollen allergies, affect nearly 26 million people and result in 9.2 million office visits to physicians every year. Allergy symptoms can range from mild sniffling and sneezing to serious respiratory diseases and disabling skin conditions. They can even be life threatening. For example, approximately 40 deaths are caused each year as a result of allergic reactions to stinging insects.

This book, *Allergies Sourcebook, Second Edition*, offers a completely revised and updated look at the subject of allergies. It contains basic information for the layperson about common allergies and their triggers, symptoms, treatment, and management. It offers facts about anaphylaxis, rhinitis, sinusitis, asthma, dermatitis, conjunctivitis, and multiple chemical sensitivity. A glossary and resource directories offer additional help and information.

Allergy patients, family members, friends, and the general public will find this volume a good place to begin to understand the complexities of allergic reactions. Some topics related to allergies, however, are covered in more detail in other volumes of the *Health Reference Series*. Readers may wish to also consult:

- *Asthma Sourcebook*
- *Immune System Disorders Sourcebook*

- *Respiratory Diseases and Disorders Sourcebook*
- *Skin Disorders Sourcebook*

How to Use This Book

This book is divided into parts and chapters. Parts focus on broad areas of interest. Chapters are devoted to single topics within a part.

Part I: Allergies: An Overview includes general and statistical information about allergies and their impact on people's lives. A description of the body's allergic response mechanisms and reports on recent research help explain how and why allergies effect human health.

Part II: Allergic Disorders and Related Symptoms provides information about a wide range of symptoms related to allergic disorders, including rhinitis, sinusitis, asthma, dermatitis, conjunctivitis, and anaphylaxis. A chapter on multiple chemical sensitivity, which has also been called "total allergy syndrome," explains the medical controversy surrounding this confusing disorder. A final chapter presents information about the possible link between Ménière's disease, a hearing disorder, and allergies that affect the inner ear.

Part III: Food Allergies and Intolerances explains the differences between food allergies and food intolerances and debunks commonly held myths regarding food allergies. Individual chapters offer detailed information about some of the most common food allergies including peanuts and tree nuts, milk, wheat, soy, and shellfish.

Part IV: Allergy Triggers offers information about non-food allergy triggers including common household irritants, pets and other animals, cockroaches, pollens, molds, insect venom, poison ivy and related plants, medications, latex, cosmetics, fragrances, indoor air pollutants, and exercise.

Part V: Diagnosis, Treatments, and Aids to Wellness explains the tests used to screen for and diagnose allergies. It provides information about various over-the-counter and prescription medications used to prevent and combat allergy symptoms. Other in-home items that may help allergy sufferers are also described.

Part VI: Additional Help and Information includes a glossary of terms, a directory of sources of information about allergies, and a listing of resources for allergy sufferers.

Bibliographic Note

This volume contains documents and excerpts from publications issued by the following government agencies: National Center for Complementary and Alternative Medicine (NCCAM); National Heart, Lung, and Blood Institute (NHLBI); National Institute for Occupational Safety and Health (NIOSH); National Institute of Allergy and Infectious Diseases (NIAID); National Institute of Diabetes and Digestive and Kidney Diseases (NIDDK); National Institute of Environmental Health Sciences (NIEHS); U.S. Environmental Protection Agency (EPA); and the U.S. Food and Drug Administration (FDA).

This volume also contains copyrighted documents produced by the following organizations: about.com; adam.com; Allergy Society of South Africa; American Academy of Family Physicians; American Academy of Otolaryngology–Head Neck Surgery; American Lung Association; Dairy Farmers of Ontario; Health on the Net Foundation; InteliHealth, Inc.; International Food Information Council Foundation; Johns Hopkins Health System; Medical Economics Publishing; National Consumers League; National Jewish Medical and Research Center; P/S/L Consulting Group, Inc.; and the University of Illinois, College of Veterinary Medicine.

In addition, this volume contains copyrighted articles from the following magazines and journals: *American Family Physician; Archives of Environmental Health; Business and Health; Cancer Biotechnology Weekly; Consultant; Consumers' Research Magazine; Countryside and Small Stock Journal; Flower and Garden Magazine; HR Magazine; Medical Sciences Bulletin; Nutrition Research Newsletter; Patient Care; Pediatrics for Parents; The Physician and Sportsmedicine; Skin Care Today for the Health Professional;* and *Today's Homeowner*.

Full citation information is provided on the first page of each chapter. Every effort has been made to secure all necessary rights to reprint the copyrighted material. If any omissions have been made, please contact Omnigraphics to make corrections for future editions.

Acknowledgements

In addition to the many organizations and agencies that contributed the material included in this book, thanks go to Joan Margeson for her tireless efforts in tracking down documents and Dawn Matthews for her verification assistance.

Note from the Editor

This book is part of Omnigraphics' *Health Reference Series*. The series provides basic information about a broad range of medical concerns. It is not intended to serve as a tool for diagnosing illness, in prescribing treatments, or as a substitute for the physician/patient relationship. All persons concerned about medical symptoms or the possibility of disease are encouraged to seek professional care from an appropriate health care provider.

Our Advisory Board

The *Health Reference Series* is reviewed by an Advisory Board comprised of librarians from public, academic, and medical libraries. We would like to thank the following board members for providing guidance to the development of this series:

Dr. Lynda Baker, Associate Professor of Library and Information Science, Wayne State University, Detroit, MI

Nancy Bulgarelli, William Beaumont Hospital Library, Royal Oak, MI

Karen Imarasio, Bloomfield Township Public Library, Bloomfield Township, MI

Karen Morgan, Mardigian Library, University of Michigan-Dearborn, Dearborn, MI

Rosemary Orlando, St. Clair Shores Public Library, St. Clair Shores, MI

Medical Consultant

Medical consultation services are provided to the *Health Reference Series* editors by David A. Cooke, MD. Dr. Cooke is a graduate of Brandeis University, and he received his M.D. degree from the University of Michigan. He completed residency training at the University of Wisconsin Hospital and Clinics and is board-certified in Internal Medicine. Dr. Cooke currently works as part of the University of Michigan Health System and practices in Brighton, MI. In his free time, he enjoys writing, science fiction, and spending time with his family.

Health Reference Series *Update Policy*

The inaugural book in the *Health Reference Series* was the first edition of *Cancer Sourcebook* published in 1992. Since then, the *Series* has been enthusiastically received by librarians and in the medical community. In order to maintain the standard of providing high-quality health information for the layperson the editorial staff at Omnigraphics felt it was necessary to implement a policy of updating volumes when warranted.

Medical researchers have been making tremendous strides, and it is the purpose of the *Health Reference Series* to stay current with the most recent advances. Each decision to update a volume will be made on an individual basis. Some of the considerations will include how much new information is available and the feedback we receive from people who use the books. If there is a topic you would like to see added to the update list, or an area of medical concern you feel has not been adequately addressed, please write to:

Editor
Health Reference Series
Omnigraphics, Inc.
615 Griswold
Detroit, MI 48226

The commitment to providing on-going coverage of important medical developments has also led to some format changes in the *Health Reference Series*. Each new volume on a topic is individually titled and called a "First Edition." Subsequent updates will carry sequential edition numbers. To help avoid confusion and to provide maximum flexibility in our ability to respond to informational needs, the practice of consecutively numbering each volume has been discontinued.

Part One

Allergies: An Overview

Chapter 1

Allergy Fact Sheet

Allergy Statistics

- Estimates from a skin test survey suggest that allergies affect more than 50 million people in the United States.[9]

- Allergy testing accounted for 1.4 million office visits to physicians in 1991.[10]

- Pollen allergy (hay fever or allergic rhinitis) affects an estimated 10% or 26 million Americans, not including those with asthma.[11] Allergic rhinitis is the reason for 9.2 million office visits to physicians yearly.[12]

- The estimated overall costs of allergic rhinitis in the United States in 1996 totaled $6 billion.[13]

- Allergic dermatitis (itchy rash) is the most common skin condition in children younger than 11 years of age.[14] The percentage of American children diagnosed with it has increased from 3 percent in the 1960s to 10 percent in the 1990s.[15]

- Urticaria (hives; raised areas of reddened skin that become itchy) and angioedema (swelling of throat tissues) together affect approximately 15 percent of the U.S. population every year.[15]

From "NIAID Fact Sheet: Asthma and Allergy Statistics," Office of Communications and Public Liaison, National Institute of Allergy and Infectious Diseases (NIAID), National Institutes of Health (NIH), January 2000. Available online at http://www.niaid.nih.gov/factsheets/allergystat.htm.

- More than 1,000 systemic allergic reactions to natural rubber latex, including 15 deaths, were reported to the FDA between 1988 and 1993. Follow ups showed the reactions were caused by residual rubber tree proteins in medical devices such as rubber gloves and catheters. Most (82 percent) allergic reactions to latex are caused by rubber additives.[16]

- Chronic sinusitis affects nearly 35 million people in the United States.[3]

- Allergic drug reactions, commonly caused by antibiotics such as penicillin and cephalosporins, occur in 2 to 3% of hospitalized patients.[17]

- Eight percent of children younger than 6 years old experience food intolerance(s). Researchers estimate that up to 2 to 4 percent of all children under 6 have food allergy.[18]

- A severe allergic reaction known as anaphylaxis occurs in 3.3 percent of the U.S. population as a result of insect stings. At least 40 deaths per year result from insect sting anaphylaxis.[19]

Asthma Statistics

- In 1994, the estimated number of people with self-reported asthma in the United States was 14.6 million. The estimate for 1998 has risen to 17 million.[1,2,3]

- Asthma was diagnosed more often than any other illness of 468,000 U.S. hospital admissions in 1993.[1,3]

- In the United States in 1994, asthma affected an estimated 4.8 million children (under age 18) out of an estimated 68 million children. Asthmatic youngsters under age 15 were hospitalized 159,000 times in 1993, and stayed 3.4 days on average.[1,3]

- Asthma is only slightly more prevalent in African-American children than in white children.[1] African-American children with asthma, however, experience more severe disability and have more frequent hospitalizations than do white children.[4,5]

- Among 5–24-year-olds, the asthma death rate nearly doubled from 1980 to 1993. In 1993, African Americans in this age group were 4 to 6 times more likely to die from asthma than whites; and males were 1.5 times at greater risk than females.[1,7]

- Overall, asthma treatment cost an estimated $6.2 billion in 1990; 43% of that total cost was associated with emergency room use, hospitalization, and death. Loss of school days, alone, caused decreased productivity that cost an estimated $1 billion.[8]

References

1. Centers for Disease Control and Prevention, CDC Surveillance Summaries, *Morbidity and Mortality Weekly Report (MMWR)*, 47(SS-1), April 24, 1998.

2. CDC, Forecasted State-Specific Estimates of Self-Reported Asthma Prevalence—United States, 1998; *MMWR*, 47(47):1022-1025, December 4, 1998.

3. CDC, Vital and Health Statistics, Current Estimates from the National Health Interview Survey, 1994 (U.S. Department of Health and Human Services, Public Health Service, National Center for Health Statistics): DHHS Pub. No. PHS 96-1521, December 1995.

4. CDC; Vital and Health Statistics, National Hospital Discharge Survey: Annual Summary, 1995 (US DHHS, CDC); DHHS Publication No. PHS 98-1794 (Series 13, no. 133), 1998.

5. Taylor, W.R., Newacheck, P.W., Impact of Childhood Asthma on Health, *Pediatrics,* 90(5):657-662, 1992.

6. Evans, R., Asthma among Minority Children: A Growing Problem, *Chest,* 101(6):368S-371S, 1992.

7. CDC, Asthma Mortality and Hospitalization among Children and Young Adults, 1980-1993, *MMWR,* 45(17):350-353, May 3, 1996.

8. Weiss, K.B., Gergen, P.J., Hodgson, T.A., An Economic Evaluation of Asthma in the U.S. *New England Journal of Medicine,* 326:862-6, 1992.

9. Gergen, P.J., Turkeltaub, P.C., Kaovar, M.G., The Prevalence of Allergic Skin Reactivity to Eight Common Allergens in the U.S. Population: Results from the Second National Health and Nutrition Examination Survey, *J Allergy Clinical Immunol,* 800:669-79, 1987.

10. CDC, Vital and Health Statistics, National Ambulatory Medical Care Survey: 1991 Summary (US DHHS, PHS, NCHS); DHHS Publication No. PHS 94 1777. May 1994.

11. CDC, National Health Survey, Series 10, Prevalence of Selected Chronic Conditions: United States, 1990-92, DHHS Pub. No. 97-1522, January 1997.

12. CDC/NCHS Vital Health Statistics, Advanced Data: National Ambulatory Medical Care Summary, 1994, April 1996.

13. Ray, N.F., Baraniuk, J.N., Thamer, M., et al, Healthcare Expenditures for Sinusitis in 1996: Contributions of Asthma, Rhinitis, and Other Airway Disorders. *J Allergy Clin Immunol*, 103(3 Pt 1): 408-514, 1999.

14. Lapidus, C.S., Schwarz, D.F., Honig, P.J., Atopic Dermatitis in Children: Who Cares? Who Pays? *J American Academy of Dermatology*, 28(5):699-703, 1993.

15. Leung, D.Y.M., Diaz, L.A., DeLeo, V., Soter, N.A., Allergic skin disorders and mastocytosis, *J American Medical Association (JAMA)*, 278(22):1914-1923, 1997.

16. Sussman, G.L, Beezhold, D.H., Allergy to Latex Rubber, *Annals Internal Medicine,* 122:43-46, 1995.

17. Adkinson, N.F., Jr., Drug Allergy, in *Allergy, Principles and Practice,* 5th edition, E. Middleton et al., Mosby, St. Louis, p.1212, 1998.

18. James, J.M. and H.A. Sampson, An Overview of Food Hypersensitivity, *Pediatric Allergy Immunology*, 3:67-78, 1992.

19. Valentine, M.D., Anaphylaxis and Stinging Insect Hypersensitivity, *JAMA*, 268:2830-2833, 1992.

About the NIAID

The National Institute of Allergy and Infectious Diseases (NIAID), a component of the National Institutes of Health (NIH), supports research on AIDS, tuberculosis, and other infectious diseases as well as allergies and immunology. NIH is an agency of the U.S. Department of Health and Human Services.

Chapter 2

Allergy Sufferers' Quality of Life Survey

An allergy symptom is not always just a sneeze, a sniff, a teary eye. Allergy symptoms also cause embarrassment, moodiness, and others' misperceptions. A survey probed allergy sufferers to find out what it's really like to suffer from seasonal allergies. The survey found that allergy symptoms make the lives of sufferers more difficult in some unexpected ways. It also found that the medications sufferers take do not always provide the relief they are looking for.

The survey of more than 1,000 allergy sufferers was conducted by Louis Harris and Associates during the spring 1996 allergy season.

More than Annoying Symptoms

The survey asked allergy sufferers to rate the speed of their average allergy sneeze. Forty-six percent compared it to a "gale force wind," 25 percent compared it to a "gentle wind," 16 percent compared it to a "mild breeze," and 11 percent compared it to a "hurricane." A majority of sufferers (59 percent) report that people respond to sneezing with "bless you." But one in four allergy sufferers (26 percent) report that most people say nothing at all. The survey also revealed that seven is the average for the most number of sneezes sneezed in a row, as reported by sufferers.

From "New Survey Takes a Look into Daily Lives of Allergy Sufferers," in *Doctor's Guide to the Internet*, August 20, 1996. ©1999 by P\S\L Consulting Group Inc. Reprinted by permission. *Doctor's Guide to the Internet* is at http:// www.docguide.com.

Allergy attacks can be a source of embarrassment for the sufferer, with nearly one-third (32 percent) saying they "frequently" or "sometimes" find themselves in embarrassing social situations due to their symptoms. For example, 73 percent report that allergies have caused them to sneeze in a place that should be quiet, with 65 percent of those reporting they have sneezed in a church or synagogue.

For many sufferers, mundane, everyday activities such as driving, eating, exercising, and applying makeup have become difficult as a result of allergies. In fact, more than half of the respondents (55 percent) say they have experienced a sneezing fit while driving; have had a hard time enjoying food (56 percent); or have had difficulty in exercising or participating in sporting activities (55 percent). One-third of women indicate that sneezing or watery eyes have caused them to misapply makeup, yet only seven percent of men have cut themselves shaving. And a vast majority (79 percent) indicate that their sleep is hindered by allergies.

Given the difficulties in carrying out daily tasks, it seems natural that allergies would affect a sufferer's general outlook and attitude. In fact, 45 percent of allergy sufferers compare their mood during allergy season to that of a "crawling snail."

Apparently, allergies interfere to the extent that more than half of sufferers would trade their allergies for other common medical conditions. Specifically, 61 percent say they would rather have dandruff than allergies; 43 percent would rather suffer heartburn; and nearly one-third (29 percent) would prefer the flu to allergies.

Perceptions of Suffering

Sufferers compare how watery their eyes get to a "dripping faucet" (80 percent), and also report that runny noses (51 percent) and itchy mouths and throats (50 percent) nag at them almost constantly. Nearly two out of three (66 percent) say that when their allergies are acting up, they "look and feel a little under the weather." Moreover, 13 percent of women and eight percent of men say they feel like a "wreck and in need of serious medical treatment." Only two percent of sufferers report that they look fine during an allergy attack.

Allergy sufferers also believe their allergies affect the way others perceive them. During a typical allergy season, nearly two out of three report hearing "You look tired" (65 percent), or "You don't look well, do you have a cold?" (60 percent). Allergy sufferers say that non-sufferers are unsympathetic to the difficulties caused by allergies. A large majority (72 percent) say "people don't realize how difficult life can be for an allergy sufferer." Additionally, 63 percent report both that "people don't understand how difficult it is to perform at my best when I'm having allergy attacks," and that "people don't understand how bad I feel when I have an allergy attack."

On the other hand, family members at least do appear to be more supportive of allergy sufferers. This could be because most allergy sufferers (62 percent) report another person in their family suffers from allergies. Sixty-two percent of allergy sufferers say their family members are "very understanding" when they are suffering from allergies. However, 31 percent say their families are only "somewhat understanding," and six percent report that their families are "not very" or "not at all understanding."

Anticipation, Preparation, and Medication

Two out of three (64 percent) allergy sufferers report that they can generally anticipate when they are about to have an allergy attack. The most common signs are the onset of sneezing (19 percent), watery eyes (17 percent), and itchy or scratchy eyes (16 percent).

Forty-five percent believe it takes one hour or more for an allergy attack to go from nothing to full-blown, while 47 percent say it takes less than one hour. The onset of an allergy attack can catch many sufferers unprepared. Many sufferers (59 percent) say they wait for symptoms before taking medication. Only 26 percent of those who buy over-the-counter medication use it early to prevent the onset of symptoms, compared to 55 percent who take a prescription medication.

Although 90 percent of allergy sufferers report using some kind of medication, only 22 percent rate their own allergy medication as "excellent." Seventy-nine percent believe that allergy medications in general are effective in stopping symptoms. Fourteen percent rate their medication as "fair" or "poor." People who take a prescription medication (37 percent) are more likely to rate their medication as "excellent" than people who take an over-the-counter medication (21 percent). However, more than 50 percent of sufferers find their current allergy medication takes more than one hour to give them relief. Fast relief is more likely considered by people under 45 years old to be the most important attribute (39 percent) in an ideal medication.

Half of allergy sufferers (51 percent) take a 12-hour medication; only 12 percent take a 24-hour medication. Forty-four percent of those using a 24-hour medication report that when they wake up in the morning, their medication has already worn off.

Drowsiness and overall safety are clearly important concerns of sufferers when choosing an allergy medication. When asked about which side effect is the worst to experience from medication, 44 per cent said drowsiness. Other noted side effects include dry mouth (15 percent), dizziness (13 percent), and nervousness or excitability (11 percent). However, when it comes to choosing the most important attribute of an ideal allergy medication, 41 percent say they choose safety overall. Thirty four percent said they would choose speed of relief, and 23 percent chose an absence of sedative effects.

Survey Methodology

A total of 1,006 American adults (age 18+) who suffer from allergies were interviewed by Louis Harris and Associates between May 16 and May 26, 1996. The survey was funded by Hoechst Marion Roussel.

Chapter 3

The Economics of Allergies

Chapter Contents

Section 3.1

Allergy's Sting: It's Partly Economic

By Marilyn Dix Smith and William F. McGhan, in *Business & Health*,
October 1997, vol. 14, no. 10, p. 47(2); © 1997 Medical Economics Publishing
Company. Reprinted with permission from *Business & Health*, vol. 17, no. 3,
Medical Economics Co., Montvale, N.J.

Allergies—the immune system's overreaction to normally harmless substances—are a major cause of illness and disability in the U.S.,
affecting as many as 40 to 50 million people. Allergic reactions range
from mild to life-threatening. Indeed, a severe reaction to a bee sting
or other toxin can trigger anaphylactic shock—rapid inflammation of
the bronchial tubes, leading to closure of the breathing passages
within minutes.

In an allergic reaction, the body responds to a foreign substance,
or antigen—pollen, insect venom, and food are among the most
common—as it would to a virus or other toxic invader. The immune
system mobilizes for attack by generating large amounts of immunoglobulin E, a type of antibody that subsequently attaches to tissues
and blood cells. Then, the next time the antigen's presence is detected,
the antibody attaches to it, activating the release of powerful inflammatory chemicals such as histamine, prostaglandins, and leukotrienes. The chemicals move into various parts of the body, such as
the respiratory system, and cause allergic symptoms.

Allergies are classified either by the part of the body they affect—
the skin or respiratory system, for instance—or the type of substances
that causes them.

Respiratory

Hay fever, or allergic rhinitis, is one of the most common chronic
diseases. In the course of a year, some 36 million people in this country experience its symptoms, at a direct medical cost of an estimated
$3.4 billion. The annual cost for prescription medications for allergic
rhinitis is estimated at about $910 million. Add to that $1.40 billion
for over-the-counter (OTC) drugs and $1.15 billion in physician costs.

One study projected a $2 billion savings from the use of OTC drugs to alleviate allergy symptoms, based on a comparison of the average cost of an OTC product with the expense of an office visit, prescription drug, and time lost from work to get to the doctor.

Airborne allergens causing allergic rhinitis are pollen, mold and yeast spores, house dust and mites, proteins present on dog and cat fur and chemicals from paint, carpeting, plastics and other substances. The symptoms: sneezing, often accompanied by a runny or clogged nose; coughing and postnasal drip; itchy eyes, nose, and throat; watery eyes; inflammation of the lining of the eyelids, and dark circles under the eyes caused by increased blood flow near the sinuses.

Treatment includes avoidance of the allergen, medication to relieve symptoms and immunotherapy, or allergy shots. Complete avoidance of airborne allergens may not be possible, but decreasing exposure may ameliorate the symptoms. That might mean reducing exposure to pollen by remaining indoors in the morning when pollen is highest or vacationing in a pollen-free environment during high pollen count season at home; reducing exposure to mold by using a dehumidifier to dry a basement, and using a vacuum cleaner with a high-efficiency particulate air filter. Hardwood floors are preferable to carpeting, and dusting with a damp or oiled cloth, washing clothes with hot water, and eliminating house pets and items such as feather pillows are also recommended.

The symptoms of airborne allergies may be treated with non-sedating antihistamines such as clemastine fumarate (OTC), oral prescription drugs such as astemizole and cetirizine and corticosteroid nasal sprays. Immunotherapy, administered in a series of allergy shots, is the only treatment that can reduce rather than alleviate symptoms. Injections of increasing concentrations of a specific allergen—at about $13 per injection—reduce the amount of the immunoglobulin E antibodies and cause the body to create a protective antibody, called immunoglobulin G. About 85 percent of patients with allergic rhinitis experience a significant reduction in symptoms and need for medication within 24 months of immunotherapy.

Skin

Contact dermatitis, the most common skin allergy, is caused by direct exposure to an allergen such as poison ivy, oak, or sumac. The interval between contact and the appearance of the rash and accompanying symptoms varies with the degree of sensitivity, as well as the amount of allergen and the thickness of the skin at the site. Reaction time is usually two to three days. Diluted bleach can deactivate the antigen if applied shortly after contact.

Symptoms include rash, raised fluid filled lesions, and mild to intense itching and burning. Depending on the severity, treatment consists of alleviating the itching with oral antihistamines such as diphenhydramine and topical anti-itching agents like calamine lotion and minimizing the inflammation with topical corticosteroids. In severe cases, an oral corticosteroid such as methylprednisolone may be taken for four to 10 days, with gradually descending daily doses.

Hives (an eruption of itchy, swollen, reddened welts that lasts anywhere from minutes to days) and angioedema (swelling around the eyes and lips) are generally reactions to a food, airborne substance, drug or, bug bite, but may be caused by emotional stress that triggers histamine release as well. Although the symptoms often resolve without medication, antihistamines, cimetidine, or oral corticosteroids may be prescribed.

Food

About 70 percent of people with food allergies are under 30, and most are children under the age of 6. Nine out of 10 food allergies are caused by the proteins found in one of these five substances: cow's milk, egg whites, peanuts, wheat, and soybeans. Other common allergens include berries, shellfish (iodine), corn, beans, and yellow food dye No.5.

Symptoms of food allergies are stomach cramps, diarrhea and nausea, and in severe cases, vomiting, swelling of the tongue, and respiratory congestion. For severe reactions, an injection of epinephrine is administered to dilate the bronchial passages. Other than in such emergencies, the treatment for food allergies is simply to avoid the offending substance.

Insects

Insect sting allergies are caused by female membrane-winged insects—the only kind that sting. The sting may be from a honey bee, wasp, hornet, yellow jacket or ant, which uses the stinger—a modified egg depositor—to inject the venom and allergens. The venom contains histamine, a substance similar to that released by the body during an allergic reaction, typically causing pain, redness, swelling, itching, and warmth at the site. Toxic reactions, usually associated with multiple stings, may cause muscle cramping, headache, fever, and drowsiness as well.

Severe systemic reactions can also cause difficulty swallowing, labored breathing, hoarseness and thickened speech, as well as weakness and confusion. In the most severe cases, the sting may lead to anaphylactic shock. Treatment with antihistamines and corticosteroids is sufficient in most cases, but people known to be hypersensitive to insect bites often carry epinephrine in an easy-to-use self-injectable syringe.

About the Authors of This Section

Marilyn Dix Smith is director of Health Decision Strategies, Princeton, NJ. William McGhan is professor, Philadelphia College of Pharmacy and Science. They are, respectively, executive director and founding president of the Association for Pharmacoeconomics and Outcomes Research.

Section 3.2

The Hidden Costs of Sniffles and Sneezes

By Leighton Collis, in *HR Magazine*, July 1997. Copyright © 1997 Society for Human Resource Management. Reprinted with permission.

The weather is beautiful, the flowers and trees are in bloom. What could possibly go wrong today?

Try asking your watery-eyed workers. You know, the ones with the boxes of tissues and bottles of over-the-counter (OTC) antihistamines on their desks.

Allergies affect 40 million U.S. citizens and cost employers billions of dollars. Much of that cost goes unnoticed because it is driven by absenteeism and lost productivity, not direct treatment costs. But once noticed, the expenses associated with allergies stick out like a sore thumb—or a red nose.

Data from a number of studies suggest that, each year, allergies are responsible for:

- More than $5.7 billion in aggregate costs to employers.

- A loss of 3.4 million workdays due to absenteeism.

- The equivalent of 22.4 million workdays lost from reduced productivity.

- A 50 percent increase in the likelihood of work-related accidents or workers' compensation claims involving those who treat their symptoms with OTC medications that have sedating side effects.

To determine how much allergies cost their organizations, employers must look at the expenses incurred by all their benefit programs. Workers with allergies usually incur modest expenses for initial doctor visits, but the accumulated costs for sick pay, salary continuation, short- and long-term disability and workers' compensation—as well as for overtime, rework and training—can be quite high.

"If you look at costs as they are identified within individual benefit programs you're going to miss the collective impact," states Linda Culliton, head of managed time loss practice, William M. Mercer, Inc. "Imagine filling a row of water glasses from a pitcher of water, each glass getting a small splash. When you look into each glass individually, the amount of water is small. But pour all those glasses into one and you get a very different picture."

Of the costs associated with allergies, absenteeism is one of the easiest to track. Employees take 3.4 million days of sick leave every year because of allergies, estimates the National Center for Health Statistics.

Lost productivity—another result of allergies—is more difficult to measure, but may represent an even greater cost to employers than absenteeism. For example, one study suggests that the equivalent of 22.4 million workdays are lost because of reduced productivity caused by taking OTC antihistamines. That would mean employers may lose 6½ times more from this reduced productivity than they do from absenteeism.

Can that figure be accurate? It can, and the secret to understanding that statistic lies in understanding allergic reactions and their treatment.

Symptoms and Treatment

One in 10 U.S. workers has allergies, according to the National Center for Health Statistics. Allergy sufferers usually feel as if they have the flu or a severe cold. Symptoms may persist for two or more weeks and range from simple drowsiness to general fatigue, watering eyes, sneezing and nasal congestion. During an allergy attack, people take longer to make decisions, have reduced fine motor skills, and experience diminished peripheral vision.

For 75 percent of those with allergies, this ongoing "cold" will be something they experience every year as pollen counts rise.

People with allergies have three treatment options:

- Remove the allergens and irritants from their environment.

- Treat the condition with pharmaceuticals, such as antihistamines and nasal inhalant steroids.

- Receive immunotherapy allergy shots with increasing doses of the offending allergen to raise resistance.

All three options are relatively inexpensive.

By far, pharmaceuticals are the treatment of choice. Drugs are ordered in 92 percent of all doctor visits for hay fever. The most effective medication is available only by prescription. However, 70 percent of people with allergy symptoms treat themselves with OTC sedating antihistamine and do not consult a physician.

"The idea that over-the-counter drugs are enough is a fallacy," says Andrew Green, M.D., director of Allergy at Mercy Hospital in Buffalo, N.Y. Green says that OTC medications "aren't adequate because of significant side effects."

The principal side effects of OTC sedating antihistamines are cognitive impairment, drowsiness, and loss of attention, which compound the natural symptoms of allergies. On the job, symptoms and antihistamine side effects can have significant consequences for employees and employers.

Employers in manufacturing and transportation are especially at risk. Workers who operate machinery, fly planes, or drive trucks or cars may endanger themselves and those around them. People using OTC sedating antihistamines are 50 percent more likely to have a work-related accident, according to a clinical study conducted by the Group Health Cooperative of Puget Sound, in Seattle.

The degree of impairment following even a single dose of a sedating antihistamine is comparable to that of a blood alcohol level of 0.05 percent—half the legal intoxication limit in many states. In fact, 36 states prohibit driving while under the influence of OTC and prescription antihistamines.

Replacing Lost Labor

Workers are 25 percent less productive for two weeks each year when they use sedating drugs to manage allergy symptoms, reports *The American Journal of Managed Care*. That fact translates into a $700 cost each year—twice the direct cost of medical claims for allergies alone.

Federal Motor Carrier regulations recognize the danger associated with sedating antihistamines and restrict the operation of trains, trucks, and heavy equipment by workers taking those medications. Police and firefighters are similarly restricted. The Federal Aviation Administration grounds pilots for 24 hours after they have taken sedating antihistamines.

For employers whose workers are governed by such regulations, the cost of allergies can be especially high. That's because they will need to find someone to fill in for the employees who are experiencing allergy symptoms.

"The cost of replacement labor can be more than 100 percent of the cost of the worker," says Culliton. "In some industries, it can be as much as 150 percent. Just imagine the cost of an airline pilot," she says.

Businesses in the manufacturing, transportation, and education industries are most directly affected. However, location is also an important factor in determining how much allergy costs will affect an organization. Businesses in areas with high pollen counts or pollution, such as southern California, Texas, and heavily industrialized areas, will have a higher number of allergy sufferers.

Direct Medical Costs

Employees and their dependents with medically diagnosed allergies incur average annual health care expenses of $3,181, according to William M. Mercer Inc. Of that amount, $311 is attributable to allergy treatment, a figure that rises to $700 for allergies and related conditions such as asthma and sinusitis. So allergies can drive up to 22 percent of an allergy patient's total health care costs.

The figures cited above reflect costs for inpatient and outpatient medical care, as well as for prescription drugs, but not OTC medication. Prescription drug costs for allergies total $2 billion, with a direct effect on an employer's bottom line.

Effect on Families

Half of all allergy patients are children. And hay fever is the most frequently reported chronic condition among people under age 18 (64.6

out of every 1,000 children have hay fever). Researchers estimate that 2 million school days are lost each year because of allergies. Inevitably, a parent or guardian must stay home with a sick child, but data on work time lost as a result of children's illnesses are elusive.

Because employers' policies vary widely on using company sick time for a sick child, it is not unusual for a parent to call in "sick."

"There are two important questions for employers," states Culliton. "First, is there something that can be done to manage the illness—education or early intervention? Second, how can employers support parents with sick kids so they don't have to cheat the system?"

Getting on the Radar Screen

Employers and health care organizations must recognize the complete costs of allergies and their complications, in terms of direct health care, absenteeism, and lost productivity. Otherwise, employers may miss an opportunity to improve both their profits and the safety of their workforces. More effective treatment of the condition should result in lower overall costs to employers through reduced absenteeism, fewer job-related accidents, improved productivity, and improved employee well-being.

Solutions begin with relatively simple measures. The first is a better understanding of treatment. For chronic sufferers, allergies should be managed by a physician, rather than treated with OTC medication. Physicians and pharmacists can recommend nonsedating antihistamines and address the side effects of treatment, thereby reducing the loss in productivity and accident risks.

More comprehensive solutions range from implementing wellness programs to disease management education focusing on functional health outcomes in addition to clinical outcomes. In addition, employers may want to review their air quality for allergens and irritants. OSHA regulations set minimum standards for clean air, but employers may want to exceed those standards for removing or reducing allergens in the workplace.

Furthermore, paid-time-off plans that group sick time, vacation time, holidays, and personal time under a single umbrella can help employers better manage "cheating" and support parents at the same time. Employers can also integrate their medical benefits with a paid-time-off program.

Employers evaluating an asthma disease-management program should consider adding an allergy component because of the prevalence of asthmatics with allergies. (More than 56 percent of asthma patients also have allergies, and the two upper respiratory disorders may share similar triggers.) Implementing a joint program will return dividends in lower long-range health care costs and higher workforce productivity. Ultimately, employees and their families will be healthier, with an all-around better quality of life.

About the Author of this Section

Leighton Collis is an associate in the communications practice for William M. Mercer, Inc., a management consulting firm based in Boston, Mass.

Section 3.3

Antihistamines in the Workplace

By Iain M. Cockburn, Howard Bailit, Ernst Berndt, and Stan Finkelstein, in *Business and Health*, March 1999, p. 49(2). © 1999 Medical Economics Publishing Company. Reprinted with permission from *Business & Health*, vol. 17, no. 3, Medical Economics Co., Montvale, N.J.

Picture two coworkers, both claims processors at a major homeowners insurance company and both among their department's highest performers. But outstanding job performance is not the only characteristic they share. Like some 13 million employees and up to 30 percent of Americans, both suffer from allergic rhinitis.

And, like their counterparts in companies across the U.S., the coworkers—we'll call them Phyllis and Mary—take antihistamines to alleviate symptoms, and show up for work. But that's where the similarities end.

Different Drugs

There are several different types of antihistamines on the market. The primary distinction is between the older-generation sedating drugs and the newer-generation medications, known as H_1 antagonists but more commonly described simply as non-sedating antihistamines. What's more, both sedating and non-sedating antihistamines are available with a stimulant—typically, a decongestant such as pseudoephedrine—or without it.

Mary takes a non-sedating drug; her medication, like all antihistamines in this category, is available only by prescription. Phyllis takes one of the older-generation drugs, which alleviate allergy symptoms but cause significant sedation. Her medication is sold by prescription, but sedating antihistamines are sold over the counter as well. Drug prices vary considerably. So does the employee payout, depending on the design of the employer-based health benefit.

The kind of drug Phyllis has chosen is relatively inexpensive ($1–$1.50 per day), and she is responsible for only a small copayment. Mary, on the other hand, pays out of pocket for the full price of the more costly nonsedating drug ($2.50–$3 per day) she takes, since this type of antihistamine is not covered under her firm's pharmacy benefit. Anyone at their company who opts for an OTC antihistamine (typically cheaper but available only in smaller doses) picks up the tab for that, too.

At first glance, it seems as though the company policy of reimbursing for the medication with the lowest unit cost makes sense. But take a second look and you'll find the considerations—and final costs—are far more complex.

What to Measure

Few would argue against the medical benefits of treatments that minimize side effects, for example, or fail to realize that the medication an employee takes can have a significant effect on her productivity.

But how do you measure such things? That's what our recently completed research project—a study of the workplace productivity of clerical workers with allergies based on treatment with sedating or non-sedating drugs—aimed to find out. Our goal was twofold: to uncover the economic implications of drug choice and to determine whether a solid cost-benefit argument can be made for using the more expensive non-sedating antihistamines. The research, conducted at the MIT Sloan School of Management's Program on the Pharmaceutical Industry, was presented at the 55th annual meeting of the American Academy of Allergy, Asthma and Immunology in Orlando, Florida.

In deciding whether to encourage use of a higher-cost medication with fewer side effects, a company might compare the dollar value of the avoided productivity loss (the incremental benefit) with the greater expenditure for the drug (the incremental cost). Previous research turned up large, statistically significant effects of antihistamine use on individual performance based on psychological tests that gauge psychomotor function. Our cost/benefit comparisons suggest that the use of more costly non-sedating antihistamines makes sense for many companies as well.

It's important to note that we measured productivity objectively, not based on employee self-reporting but on employer-generated productivity data: the number of claims processed daily by some 680 claims processors at a large insurance company. The data was gathered by a third party and blinded to avoid any possibility of breaching the workers' privacy.

The job of an insurance claims processor consists largely of checking and entering data from claims forms into a computer. This made it easy to track the number of claims processed each day by each full-time employee.

It was also relatively straightforward to estimate the productivity impact of the antihistamine choice. First we identified the date an employee filled a prescription for an antihistamine—we were unable to track the use of OTC drugs—then we averaged the difference between the employee's actual daily output over the following week and the expected output based on the number of claims that employee otherwise processed each day. (We looked only at work completed, without using follow-up data to determine accuracy or error rates.)

Table 3.1. Allergies, Antihistamines and Productivity: Baseline figures for the workers studied revealed an average output of approximately 186 claims per person per day. In the week after filling a prescription, average per person productivity rose by 4 to 6 percent for those taking non-sedating antihistamines—and fell by about 8 percent among those taking sedating antihistamines.

Drug type	Effect on output	Approx. # of claims	Estimated cost
Non-sedating antihistamine	+ 4-6%	+8-11 per person per day	$3.50 per person per day gained
Sedating antihistamine	-8% per day	-15 per person per day lost	$5.50 per person

What We Found

Overall, the productivity of workers taking sedating antihistamines was about 12 percent below that of workers taking non-sedating antihistamines. Ironically, our study revealed a boost in productivity of around 5 percent among employees on the nonsedating drugs—not a huge difference but still statistically significant.

Which leads us back to the original question: Does the extra cost of the non-sedating antihistamine make sense from a business perspective?

To answer it, we first considered the size of the impact on productivity: in this case, the lost output in numbers of claims that would otherwise have been processed each day. Second, we looked at the dollar value to the company of each unit of output, easily calculated in our study by dividing daily pay (claims processors earned, on average, $11.50 per hour) by daily output during periods when the employee was not on antihistamines. Finally, we calculated the daily value of the lost output. We found this to range from under $7 to close to $11, with an average of about $9 per day. That's a significant economic burden associated with the workplace consequences of antihistamine choice, and well above the additional $1-$1.50 required to pay for a non-sedating antihistamine. Unless an employee's pay varies according to his or her daily or weekly performance—not the case at the company we studied—that burden falls squarely on the employer.

About the Authors of this Section

Iain M. Cockburn, PhD, is a professor at the University of British Columbia, Faculty of Commerce and Business Administration; Howard L. Bailit, DMD, PhD, is a professor at the University of Connecticut Health Center; Ernst R. Berndt, PhD, is a professor at the Massachusetts Institute of Technology, Sloan School of Management; and Stan Finkelstein, MD, is a senior research scientist at the MIT Sloan School and co-director of the Program on the Pharmaceutical Industry. The research was supported by Hoechst Marion Roussel, Schering Plough, the Alfred P. Sloan Foundation and Jannsen Pharmaceutica.

Chapter 4

The Allergic Response

The allergic response is a defensive reaction of the immune system against certain innocuous substances—called allergens—that the body mistakes for harmful parasites. An estimated 20% to 25% of Americans suffer from this misguided reaction against inoffensive substances that include pollens, animal danders, foods, insects and their venoms, and medications. The economic cost alone to our society is billions of dollars for medical care.

Symptoms of allergy are highly varied, because different allergens stimulate the immune system at different sites in the body. The respiratory system is the most common site of allergic reactions, with allergens in the upper airways causing sneezing and nasal congestion (allergic rhinitis, including hay fever), while allergens in the lower airways cause bronchoconstriction and wheezing (asthma). Food allergens cause immune activation in the gastrointestinal (GI) tract, leading to nausea, vomiting, abdominal cramps, and diarrhea. Local immune activation in the skin results in contact dermatitis. The most serious form of allergic reaction—anaphylaxis—occurs when an allergen enters the circulation and causes allergic manifestations at sites distant from the site of entry. In severe anaphylaxis, normal bodily functions are so disrupted that the patient may die.

From "Focus on ... The Etiology of Allergy," by Lynn Wilson, in *Medical Sciences Bulletin,* September 1995 © 1995 by Pharmaceutical Information Associates, Ltd., 2761 Trenton Rd., Levittown, PA 19056. Available online at: http://pharminfo.com/pubs/msb/allergy_et.html. Reprinted with permission. Reviewed and revised by David A. Cooke, M.D., January 24, 2001.

Physiologically, the allergic response occurs in three stages: sensitization, mast cell activation, and prolonged immune activation. During Stage 1, when the allergen first meets the immune system, no allergic reaction is produced; instead, the system is primed for subsequent encounters with that particular allergen. Macrophages degrade the allergen and display the fragments to T lymphocytes (T cells); T cells secrete interleukin-4, which promotes maturation of B lymphocytes into plasma cells; plasma cells secrete immunoglobulin E (IgE) antibodies specific for that allergen. These antibodies attach to receptors on circulating basophils and on mast cells (immune cells derived from the bone marrow that reside close to blood vessels and the epithelium).

Stage 2 represents a later encounter between the allergen and the immune system. The allergen binds to IgE antibodies on mast cells. When it connects with two IgE molecules, the result is the activation of various enzymes that induce mast cell granules to release their contents—substances such as histamine, platelet-activating factor, prostaglandins, and leukotrienes—and these substances trigger the allergy attack. Individuals prone to allergies are known to have abnormally high levels of IgE antibodies.

Stage 3 is characterized by prolonged immune activation. Tissue mast cells and neighboring cells synthesize chemotactic [involving movement of cells in relation to chemical agents] and adhesion molecules that induce circulating basophils, eosinophils, and other cells to migrate into that tissue, generating a new wave of symptoms. These recruited cells secrete chemicals of their own that sustain inflammation, cause tissue damage, and recruit other immune cells.

Anaphylaxis occurs when an acute, explosive release of mediators from mast cells causes severe allergic symptoms within minutes of allergen exposure. Anaphylaxis is a medical emergency; without prompt medical attention, death can occur soon after the onset of symptoms. Shock is the major cause of death, although swelling of the vocal cords can kill by closing off the trachea. Other common reactions include pruritus (itching), urticaria (hives), and bronchoconstriction. GI manifestations can also occur, although they are less common. Symptoms may be preceded by an aura, and patients who suffer from recurrent anaphylactic episodes report that the particular symptoms experienced are almost always the same with each attack. Treatment is usually with an injection of epinephrine to inhibit mediator release, open airways, and block vasodilation.

For decades, allergies have been treated with antihistamines, but today researchers at pharmaceutical and biotechnology companies are looking well beyond histamine. They are investigating drugs to block the activity of a wide variety of mediators of the allergic response, including leukotrienes, prostaglandins, cytokines (interleukins, platelet-activating factor, and granulocyte-macrophage colony stimulating factor), adhesion molecules (integrins, selectins, and immunoglobulin adhesion molecules), and the enzymes involved in their production. Enzymes targeted for inhibition include 5-lipoxygenase (involved in the synthesis of leukotrienes), phospholipase A2 (involved in the secretion of both leukotrienes and prostaglandins), protein kinase C (involved in mast cell degranulation), serine protease tryptase (involved in the kinin cascade), and tyrosine kinase (involved in IgE activity). These efforts have shown some fruit; three new medications are now available that block allergic reactions via the leukotriene pathways. Ultimately, it should be possible to tailor allergy therapy to the individual patient, selecting drugs to alleviate a symptom complex or combat a particular allergen.

References

Frankland, AW. *Clin Exp Allerg.* 1995; 25: 580-581.
Lichtenstein, LM. *Sci Am.* 1993; 269: 116-124.
Danheiser, SL. *Genet Eng News.* 1995; 15: 42-43.

Chapter 5

The Allergy Receptor

Introduction

For many people, the rites of spring have historically involved stocking up on plenty of antihistamines and tissue, but that may not be the case in the future. Researchers at Northwestern University in Chicago and Harvard Medical School in Boston have determined the precise shape of the receptor protein for immunoglobin E (IgE), the antibody that is responsible for the springtime sniffles and other allergic symptoms that afflict some 20% of the U.S. population. This may be the first step toward developing an allergy medication that stops the allergic response before it happens, rather than merely treating the symptoms.

The study was reported in the December 23, 1998 issue of *Cell*. Theodore S. Jardetzky, an assistant professor in the Department of Biochemistry, Molecular Biology, and Cell Biology at Northwestern, was the principal investigator for the team. His collaborators were Jean-Pierre Kinet, a professor of pathology at Harvard Medical School who first cloned the gene for the IgE receptor in 1986, and Scott Garman, a postdoctoral fellow in the Northwestern Department of Biochemistry, Molecular Biology, and Cell Biology.

Excerpted from "Forum," *Environmental Health Perspectives*, Vol. 107, No. 6, June 1999; published by the National Institute of Environmental Health Sciences (NIEHS), a subagency of the National Institutes of Health.

Allergy Prevalence

About 50 million people in the United States have some form of allergy. Many allergies, such as hay fever and eczema, are more inconvenient than life-threatening, but some allergic responses, such as anaphylaxis, can result in death. Allergies are also strongly suspected of playing a role in asthma. According to the National Institute of Allergy and Infectious Diseases, 90% of asthmatic children and 50% of asthmatic adults also have allergies. According to the Centers for Disease Control and Prevention, asthma accounts for almost 500,000 hospitalizations each year and is the foremost reason that children miss school. And the problem is growing—asthma prevalence in the United States is expected to rise by 5% each year.

Allergic Responses

Allergic responses are mediated by IgE, which is one of five classes of antibodies. As IgE circulates through the blood and the lymph, it binds to receptors found on the surface of mast cells (a type of white blood cell). There, IgE acts as an antenna, patrolling its airspace for allergens. When an antibody picks up the signal of a nearby allergen, the mast cell responds by releasing histamine and other powerful chemicals that cause an inflammatory response in surrounding tissues.

Mast cells are found throughout the body but are most highly concentrated in tissues that are exposed to the outside world, such as the skin and nasal and lung linings. So when an allergic response occurs, those tissues are most likely to be affected, resulting in the rashes, welts, runny noses, and watery eyes traditionally associated with allergies.

Imaging the IgE Receptor

The IgE receptor had previously defied imaging because it has a heterogenous sugar coating that solubilizes the receptor and prevents it from crystallizing into a structure that can be examined through x-ray diffraction. To counteract this problem, the scientists expressed the human IgE receptor gene in cultured insect cells from the cabbage looper and the fall armyworm, which attach fewer sugars to the molecule. Next, they applied a technique called multiple isomorphous replacement, in which IgE receptor crystals were soaked in one of two solutions containing either gold or platinum. The large, heavy atoms of the metals were absorbed into the crystals, adding mass in the form of electrons to the receptor at key points and making it possible to calculate its image. According to Jardetzky, by comparing data that correspond to the receptor by itself to another set of data that reflects the changes effected by the binding of one of these heavy metals to the receptor, the researchers can calculate the structure of the receptor.

The researchers then used the very high intensity x-rays of the Advanced Photon Source at Argonne National Laboratory in Illinois to scrutinize the IgE crystals. The Advanced Photon Source is a synchrotron, which uses magnetic fields to maintain charged particles in an orbit. The orbiting particles give off energy in the form of x-rays. Special detectors measure the x-rays as they bounce off the crystal being analyzed, and computers convert the data into an image of the crystal.

The researchers found that the receptor has an inverted "V" shape. At one end of the V is a spike that attaches the receptor to the cell membrane. The IgE antibody binds at the upward-pointing elbow of the V shape. Jardetzky and colleagues are currently investigating several potential inhibitors and are working on capturing an image of IgE bound to its receptor. "It may be more fruitful for drug development if we can get a picture of this 'lock and key' mechanism," says Jardetzky. "From that, it may emerge that it is better to design an inhibitor for the antibody than for the receptor."

Implications for Treating Allergies

Because allergic responses result only from IgE binding to the IgE receptor, therapeutic strategies aimed at inhibiting IgE-receptor interactions could provide a single treatment to fight multiple conditions such as asthma and sinusitis. The researchers believe that blocking the IgE receptor from binding the IgE antibody will short-circuit the allergy cycle.

Because the IgE-receptor interaction controls only the allergy branch of the body's immune response, it could be inhibited without compromising the entire immune response, says Kinet. The IgE receptor is thought to play some as-yet undefined role in immunity to parasitic infections. Jardetzky allows that inhibition of the IgE-receptor interaction may result in susceptibility to parasitic infections, particularly in developing nations, where such diseases are endemic. However, notes Kinet, IgE is not the only natural defense the body has against parasites. The advantages offered by such an inhibitor, he says, would far outweigh the disadvantages.

Chapter 6

Genetic Mutation and Allergic Susceptibility

Genetic Mutation Identified

Allergic diseases are among the major causes of illness and disability in the United States, affecting as many as 40 to 50 million Americans. Researchers have known for some time that allergies have a genetic link, but information about which genes are responsible has been limited.

Now, scientists at Washington University School of Medicine in St. Louis, Missouri, have identified a genetic mutation that appears to make people more susceptible to allergies.

This is one of the strongest associations so far between any one particular gene and allergies," said Talal Chatila, M.D., associate professor of pediatrics and senior author of the study, which appears in *The New England Journal of Medicine* (December 1997). "We have found that if you have this mutation, you are 10 times more likely to be allergic."

In the short term, this finding will help advance studies to identify highly susceptible individuals, Chatila said. The discovery also could lead to more targeted medications for allergies.

"Scientists Identify Genetic Mutation That Makes People Allergic," *Doctors Guide to the Internet*, December 11, 1997; © 1999 P\S\L Consulting Group Inc. Reprinted by permission. *Doctor's Guide to the Internet* is at http://www.docguide.com.

The Immune System and Allergy

The immune system normally defends the body against invading agents such as bacteria and viruses, but it sometimes confuses other foreign substances such as dust mites and certain foods with harmful intruders. When allergic people first come into contact with such allergens, their immune systems mobilize to respond.

First they generate large amounts of a type of antibody—a disease-fighting protein—called immunoglobin E (IgE). The IgE molecules then attach themselves to mast cells in tissues and basophils in blood. When an allergen encounters the IgE, it attaches to the antibody like a key fitting into a lock. This signal tells the mast cell or basophil to release, and in some cases to produce, powerful inflammatory chemicals like histamine, prostaglandins and leukotrienes.

The production of these chemicals in various parts of the body, such as the respiratory system, initiates an allergic reaction such as seen in asthma. IgE is key to this process because it triggers the chain of events that leads to symptoms.

Another key protein is interleukin-4, which induced immune cells to make IgE. Chatila and his colleagues studied the receptor for interleukin-4. Using techniques called single-strand polymorphism analysis and DNA sequencing, they searched for variations in the gene for one of the subunits of the interleukin-4 receptor. Then they determined how common the variant was in patients with severe allergic inflammatory disorders and healthy adults.

Genetic Discovery

One variant occurred at high frequency in patients with allergic inflammatory disease and in adults with various allergies but at a low frequency in adults with no allergies. This genetic alteration occurred at the tail end of the interleukin-4 receptor, Chatila and his colleagues discovered. The consequence, they showed, was that the receptor becomes hyperresponsive when stimulated with interleukin-4.

"This mutation makes the receptor function better, so it signals the cells to make IgE antibodies more effectively than it would have done otherwise," Chatila said. "Therefore, people with this altered receptor gene are more likely to develop allergies."

Environmental factors also play a role in whether an individual develops allergies. Previous studies have established that avoiding particular allergens in childhood substantially decreases the risk. Breastfeeding also helps guard a child against allergies.

Additional Research Needed

Identifying the altered receptor gene could greatly aid studies of allergic reactions. "This finding will help us identify individuals at high risk of developing allergies and evaluate intervention strategies aimed at protecting these individuals from developing allergic disorders," Chatila said.

The genetic finding also could help researchers develop better medications to treat allergies. Because the identified target is unique, Chatila said, drugs could be developed that are more specific and have fewer side effects.

In future studies, Chatila and colleagues will study other mutations along the pathway between the activation of the interleukin-4 receptor and the production of IgE to find out what happens if a person has more than one mutation. They hope to determine if different combinations of mutations predispose individuals to specific allergies.

This discovery is an important first step. "We know that the process by which some people develop allergies is not random but is genetically determined," Chatila said. "This study helps clarify the basis for this genetic predisposition."

Part Two

Allergic Disorders and Related Symptoms

Chapter 7

What Are Allergies?

Rarely is a medical term used as frequently and casually as "allergy." It pops up in everyday conversation to describe what we don't like—school, work, or just about anything else. But medically speaking, *allergy* has a very specific meaning: a reaction to something that your *body* doesn't like.

Allergies are an abnormal sensitivity to a substance called an allergen that is eaten, inhaled, or touched, that most other people can tolerate without trouble. Usually, the immune system does a good job of distinguishing between the many nontoxic substances in our environment and the viruses, bacteria, and other trouble-makers that threaten health. For example, when harmful bacteria enter the respiratory system, the immune system mounts a defense in which protective proteins called *antibodies* attach themselves to the outer surface of the bacteria and target them for destruction. Yet it usually leaves alone those substances that don't harm us.

But in people with allergies, the immune system sometimes makes a mistake and launches attacks against a perfectly harmless substance, such as ragweed pollen, animal dander, or certain foods or drugs. Hence the word allergy comes from the Greek *allos,* meaning *other*. It was first used in 1906 to refer to an "altered reaction" in the body's immune system. Since then, allergies have been called a lot of things . . . sometimes in language that would make a sailor blush.

From "What Are Allergies?" Johns Hopkins Health, October 1, 1998. Available at http://www.intelihealth.com. ©1996-2000 by InteliHealth Inc. Reprinted with permission of InteliHealth.

While many mild allergies are more of a nuisance than anything else, they can be disruptive enough to require ongoing vigilance and medical treatment. Occasionally, they can be life-threatening.

The Action of a Reaction

Most people know their allergies by the reaction they cause—the sneezing, wheezing, and other effects that are none too pleasing. What they may not know is that what happens to their body is a result of what's happening inside it.

Basically, an allergic reaction is what happens when your immune system tries to do its job: mount a defense against what it believes is a hostile invader. During a period of *sensitization,* the time when you are exposed to a specific allergen, the immune system produces antibodies—chemicals that are produced by a type of white blood cell whose job is to fight infection and other invaders of the body. Unfortunately, in those with allergies, these cells may produce antibodies against a certain food or pollen.

The body produces five different classes of antibodies, or *immunoglobulins*—IgA, IgM, IgG, IgD, and IgE—and each class serves a different function. Those formed in response to allergens belong to the IgE class, which normally function to attack parasitic worms. The IgE antibodies bind to the allergen, such as pollen molecules, as well as two types of defensive cells: *mast cells* (found in the nose, skin, lungs, and gastrointestinal tract) and *basophils* (found mostly in the blood).

These cells then release a series of chemicals called *mediators,* which cause the sneezing, runny nose, itching, and other symptoms of an allergic reaction. Probably the best known of these mediators is *histamine.*

Because some mediators work very quickly, reactions occur almost instantly after exposure to an allergen; and most reactions occur where the allergens enter the body. So if you inhale an allergen, you'll experience symptoms along the respiratory tract. If you're allergic to a food, you'll likely feel it in your gut, while touching an allergen tends to result in a skin rash.

Some other substances are called in for reinforcement. A type of white blood cell called [an] *eosinophil* is attracted to the site of the reaction. The result is a more intense reaction—such as swelling or inflammation, which can be more difficult to treat. (Once an allergen enters the bloodstream, though, its effects can be more far-reaching. So a food allergen may not only cause gastrointestinal problems, but can also cause hives or a skin rash.)

Who's at Risk

If you have allergies, you're in good company. The National Institute of Allergy and Infectious Diseases estimates that 50 million Americans—one in five of us—has some form of regular allergy:

- Nearly half of people with allergies—at least 10 percent of the entire U.S. population—have hay fever, medically known as *allergic rhinitis*. This reaction to outdoor airborne allergens like pollens occurs on a seasonal basis. A second type of airborne allergy called *perennial allergic rhinitis,* occurs year-round and is more of a response to indoor allergens such as pet dander or dust mites.

- Roughly 5 to 10 percent of the U.S. population—at least 15 million Americans—have asthma. Up to 90 percent of children with asthma also have allergies.

- About half of us get a reaction to poison ivy, with about 50 million affected yearly.

- Approximately 6 to 10 million Americans are allergic to cats or other pets.

- About 2 million have had allergic reactions to insect stings.

- Approximately 1 in 12 children under age 6 have symptoms of food allergies, but only about one in 25 has confirmed food allergies. Between 1 and 2 percent of adults have food allergies.

Costs

All told, allergies rank sixth in cost on the list of chronic diseases in the United States. Each year, Americans lose 3½ million work days because of allergies at a cost of $639 million. Children lose about 2 million school days. Allergies cost about $2 billion a year in treatment, tests, medications, and allergy shots, and require nearly 8½ million physician visits.

How Allergies Develop

How people become allergic is still something of a mystery. Experts know it begins with what is called *sensitization*—a period that ranges from a few weeks to several decades, in which repeated exposure to a particular allergen activates the immune system to attempt to fight what is usually a perfectly innocuous substance. Because this period of sensitization varies so much, one person can develop a contact allergy during infancy while another may not be sensitized until adulthood. Still, most allergies become apparent in childhood—especially inhalant reactions like hay fever. Some children can outgrow one allergy only to develop another later in life. Adults seldom develop new allergies after age 40, but rarely "outgrow" those they have, although sometimes reactions become less severe with age.

Risk Factors

Regardless of when they begin or what symptoms they cause, most allergies seem to be caused by the same risk factors.

Heredity. If you have allergies, chances are you're carrying on a family tradition. A child with one allergic parent has a 30 to 50 percent chance of developing allergies, although he may get a different type of allergy than his folks. His chances of developing allergies rise as high as 60 to 80 percent if both parents have them.

Still, children from the same family may not get the same allergies. Studies show that only 25 to 50 percent of identical twins share the same type of allergy. In many cases, one twin will have allergies and the other won't. This means environment is an important factor, too.

Environment. While your genes make you more vulnerable to an allergy, it's your environment that sets it all in motion. Specifically, it's being in a place where you are exposed to high levels of a particular allergen—especially early in life. Infants and young children exposed to a lot of pollen, for instance, are more likely to get hay fever than those less exposed . . . even when heredity is taken into account. So if you have allergies and one of your children is exposed to dust mites during infancy, chances are he'll be more likely to develop dust mite allergies than another child of yours who wasn't around mites— or an exposed child of someone not allergic. It's always a combination of *both* factors that paves the way for allergies to develop.

Are emotions to blame? One of the frustrating aspects of dealing with allergies is the pervasive myth that the disorder is psychosomatic, an "all in your head" phenomenon instead of a "real" medical problem.

Although an allergy is a physical disorder, sometimes reactions can be set off by an emotional or psychological response. For example, studies indicate that people with allergies can develop reactions if they merely revisit a place where they once had a bad allergy attack. This phenomenon, known as a "conditioned response," is not unique to allergies. Patients receiving chemotherapy for cancer may become nauseated just walking into the hospital even if they're not going to see the doctor. As far as allergy is concerned, a conditioned response is as "real" as it would be if the allergen actually were present. Your immune system is simply responding to a signal from your brain triggered by the remembered danger.

Certain drugs—especially those taken for asthma—can cause severe systemic effects as well as emotional or mood changes. Many antihistamines used to control allergy symptoms cause drowsiness (although newer, non-sedating types control allergy symptoms without causing drowsiness). Others can make you restless, nervous, or anxious. And the oral corticosteroids used to treat asthma can lead to depression or agitation in some patients.

What's more, managing an allergy can place certain limitations on your lifestyle. Teenagers and young people, in particular, may chafe at restrictions that embarrass them, make them feel different from their friends, or less free to enjoy themselves. But even adults can feel uncomfortable if they have to limit activities in order to avoid allergens or irritants (such as cigarette smoke) that can trigger reactions. These restrictions are likely to be more of a burden for people with asthma.

Chapter 8

You and Your Stuffy Nose

Nasal congestion, stuffiness, or obstruction to nasal breathing is one of man's oldest and most common complaints. While it may be a mere nuisance to some persons, to others it is a source of considerable discomfort, and it detracts from the quality of their lives.

Medical writers have classified the causes of nasal obstruction into four categories, recognizing that overlap exists between these categories and that it is not unusual for a patient to have more than one factor involved in his particular case.

Infection

An average adult suffers a common "cold" two to three times per year, more often in childhood and less often the older he gets as he develops more immunity. The common "cold" is caused by any number of different viruses, some of which are transmitted through the air, but most are transmitted from hand-to-nose contact. Once the virus gets established in the nose, it causes release of the body chemical histamine, which dramatically increases the blood flow to the nose—causing swelling and congestion of nasal tissues—and which stimulates the nasal membranes to produce excessive amounts of mucus. Antihistamines and decongestants help relieve the symptoms of a "cold," but time alone cures it.

During a virus infection, the nose has poor resistance against bacterial infections, which explains why bacterial infections of the nose and sinuses so often follow a "cold." When the nasal mucus turns from clear to yellow or green, it usually means that a bacterial infection has taken over and a physician should be consulted.

Acute sinus infections produce nasal congestion, thick discharge, and pain and tenderness in the cheeks and upper teeth, between and behind the eyes, or above the eyes and in the forehead, depending on which sinuses are involved.

Chronic sinus infections may or may not cause pain, but nasal obstruction and offensive nasal or postnasal discharge is often present. Some persons develop polyps (fleshy growths in the nose) from sinus infections, and the infection can spread down into the lower airways leading to chronic cough, bronchitis, and asthma. Acute sinus infection generally responds to antibiotic treatment; chronic sinusitis usually requires surgery.

Structural Causes

Included in this category are deformities of the nose and the nasal septum, which is the thin, flat cartilage and bone that separates the nostrils and nose into its two sides. These deformities are usually due to an injury at some time in one's life. The injury may have been many years earlier and may even have been in childhood and long since forgotten. It is a fact that 7 percent of newborn babies suffer significant nasal injury just from the birth process; and, of course, it is almost impossible to go through life without getting hit on the nose at least once. Therefore, deformities of the nose and the deviated septum should be fairly common problems—and they are. If they create obstruction to breathing, they can be corrected with surgery.

One of the most common causes for nasal obstruction in children is enlargement of the adenoids: tonsil-like tissues that fill the back of the nose up behind the palate. Children with this problem breath noisily at night and even snore. They also are chronic mouth breathers, and they develop a "sad" long face and sometimes dental deformities. Surgery to remove the adenoids and sometimes the tonsils may be advisable.

Other causes in this category include nasal tumors and foreign bodies. Children are prone to inserting various objects such as peas, beans, cherry pits, beads, buttons, safety pins, and bits of plastic toys into their noses. Beware of one-sided foul smelling discharge, which can be caused by a foreign body. A physician should be consulted.

Allergy

Hay fever, rose fever, grass fever, and "summertime colds" are various names for allergic rhinitis. Allergy is an exaggerated inflammatory response to a foreign substance which, in the case of a stuffy nose, is usually a pollen, mold, animal dander, or some element in house dust. Foods sometime play a role. Pollens cause problems in spring (trees) and summer (grasses) or fall (weeds) whereas house dust allergies and mold may be a year-around problem. Ideally the best treatment is avoidance of these substances, but that is impractical in most cases.

In the allergic patient, the release of histamine and similar substances results in congestion and excess production of watery nasal mucus. Antihistamines help relieve the sneezing and runny nose of allergy. Many antihistamines are now available without a prescription. The most familiar brands include Chlor-Trimeton®, Benadryl®, or Dimetane® (although most are also available in generic forms). Newer, nonsedating antihistamines, which require a prescription include Claritin®, Zyrtec®, and Allegra®.

Decongestants shrink congested nasal tissues. Examples include Sudafed®, Guaifed®, and Entex® that are available without a prescription in several generic forms. Combinations of antihistamines with decongestants are also available. All these preparations have potential side effects, and patients must heed the warnings of the package or prescription insert. This is especially important if the patient suffers from high blood pressure, glaucoma, irregular heart beats, difficulty in urination, or is pregnant.

Allergy shots are the most specific treatment available, and they are highly successful in allergic patients. Skin tests or at times blood tests are used to make up treatment vials of substances to which the patient is allergic. The physician determines the best concentration for initiating the treatment. These treatments are given by injection. They work by forming blocking antibodies in the patient's blood stream, which then interfere with the allergic reaction. Many patients prefer allergy shots over drugs because of the side effects of the drugs.

Patients with allergies have an increased tendency to develop sinus infections and require treatment as discussed in the previous section.

Vasomotor Rhinitis

"Rhinitis" means inflammation of the nose and nasal membranes. "Vasomotor" means blood vessel forces. The membranes of the nose have an abundant supply of arteries, veins, and capillaries, which have a great capacity for both expansion and constriction. Normally these blood vessels are in a half-constricted, half-open state. But when a person exercises vigorously, his/her hormones of stimulation (i.e., adrenaline) increase. The adrenaline causes constriction or squeezing of the nasal membranes so that the air passages open up and the person breathes more freely.

The opposite takes place when an allergic attack or a "cold" develops: The blood vessels expand, the membranes become congested (full of excess blood), and the nose becomes stuffy, or blocked.

In addition to allergies and infections, other events can also cause nasal blood vessels to expand, leading to vasomotor rhinitis. These include psychological stress, inadequate thyroid function, pregnancy, certain anti-high blood pressure drugs, and overuse or prolonged use of decongesting nasal sprays and irritants such as perfumes and tobacco smoke.

In the early stages of each of these disorders, the nasal stuffiness is temporary and reversible. That is, it will improve if the primary cause is corrected. However, if the condition persists for a long enough period, the blood vessels lose their capacity to constrict. They become somewhat like varicose veins. They fill up when the patient lies down and when he/she lies on one side, the lower side becomes congested. The congestion often interferes with sleep. So it is helpful for stuffy patients to sleep with the head of the bed elevated two to four inches accomplish this by placing a brick or two under each castor of the bedposts at the head of the bed. Surgery my offer dramatic and long time relief.

Summary

Stuffy nose is one symptom caused by a remarkable array of different disorders, and the physician with special interest in nasal disorders will offer treatments based on the specific causes. Additional information and suggestions can be found in the American Academy of Otolaryngology–Head and Neck Surgery (AAO-HNS) pamphlets "Hayfever, Summer Colds and Allergies" and "Antihistamines."

Order the print version of this information (sold in packs of 100) through our online catalog [www.entnet.org].

Chapter 9

Rhinitis

Chapter Contents

Section 9.1

Allergic and Non-Allergic Rhinitis

Text prepared by the National Jewish Medical and Research Center, 1-800-222-LUNG; © 1995 National Jewish Medical and Research Center. Reprinted with permission from National Jewish Medical and Research Center. Reviewed by David A. Cooke, M.D. January 24, 2001.

Do you suffer from a runny or stuffy nose much of the time? You may not have given it much thought because it typically is not a serious condition. It can, however, be quite annoying. This condition is known as rhinitis. Approximately 40 million people in the U.S. suffer to one degree or another from rhinitis. Although hay fever, or seasonal allergic rhinitis, is the condition that most people are familiar with, there are different types of rhinitis. This text reviews these conditions and current treatments.

Classifications

Atopic Rhinitis

There are three types of atopic (associated with allergic-like symptoms) rhinitis.

1. **Seasonal Allergic Rhinitis** (also known as hay fever): This is triggered by allergy to pollens, including trees in spring, grasses in summer, and weeds in fall. Symptoms include sneezing, itching, tickling in the nose, runny or stuffy nose, and watery or itchy eyes. Seasonal rhinitis is diagnosed primarily by your medical history. Skin testing is not always indicated, especially if your symptoms are mild.

2. **Perennial Rhinitis (year-round) with Allergic Triggers:** These triggers include indoor allergens such as mold, house dust mite, cockroach, and animal dander. Symptoms are the same as seasonal allergic rhinitis but are experienced throughout the year. The health care provider makes the diagnosis for perennial rhinitis by your medical history and positive skin tests to relevant allergens.

3. **Perennial Rhinitis with Non-Allergic Triggers:** This type of rhinitis is not well understood. Although not triggered by allergy, it's an allergic-like condition with increased eosinophils (a special type of white blood cell associated with allergy) in the lining and secretions of the nose. Symptoms are the same as perennial rhinitis with allergic triggers. Diagnosis is determined from negative skin tests and a nasal smear test positive for eosinophils. Nasal polyps can be a complication of this condition.

Idiopathic Non-Allergic Rhinitis

This is also known as vasomotor rhinitis. A person with this type reacts to temperature and humidity changes, smoke, odors, and emotional upsets. Symptoms are primarily nasal congestion and postnasal drip. Diagnosis comes after negative skin tests and nasal smear negative for eosinophils.

Infectious Rhinitis

This can occur as an acute viral respiratory infection (cold) which may clear rapidly or continue with symptoms up to six weeks. Some people develop the complication of an acute or chronic bacterial sinus infection, usually associated with blocked sinus drainage. Symptoms of infectious rhinitis are an increased amount of colored (yellow-green) and thickened nasal discharge and nasal congestion. The diagnosis of an acute or chronic sinus infection is confirmed by an abnormal sinus x-ray or CT scan.

Other types

1. **Rhinitis Medicamentosa:** This type is associated with long-term use of decongestant nasal sprays or recreational use of cocaine. Symptoms typically are nasal congestion and postnasal drip. A person who has taken a decongestant nasal spray for months or years is using this treatment inappropriately. These medications are intended for short-term use only. Overuse can cause rebound congestion, which leads to increased nasal obstruction. It is very important for a person with rebound congestion to work closely with a physician to gradually withdraw the nasal spray.

2. **Mechanical Obstruction:** This is most often associated with a deviated septum or enlarged adenoids. If you have chronic

nasal obstruction that is one-sided, a medical evaluation is recommended.

3. **Hormonal.** This is generally associated with pregnancy or untreated hypothyroidism.

Diagnosis

Often a person may have more than one type of rhinitis. In making the diagnosis, an evaluation by your doctor may include:

- **History:** Specific symptoms and when they occur, family history, and work history.

- **Physical exam**

- **Nasal smears:** Microscopic exam of nasal secretions, especially eosinophils.

- **Allergy testing:** Skin testing by a board-certified allergist is generally indicated for someone with recurrent symptoms. A positive skin test indicates the presence of IgE antibody, which can react with specific substances to produce an allergic reaction. In most cases, an allergic person will react to more than one substance.

- **Sinus x-ray:** About 40 percent of persons with perennial rhinitis will have changes on the sinus x-ray. This can indicate the presence of sinusitis (inflammation of the sinuses) with or without infection or nasal polyps.

Complications

Complications of seasonal allergic rhinitis are rare. The condition may be associated with bronchial asthma, but evidence that rhinitis specifically predisposes you to asthma is not convincing. Two epidemiologic studies in the United States found that asthma followed allergic rhinitis in 1 to 10 percent of the cases, which suggests that the subsequent development of asthma in rhinitis sufferers may be only slightly more common than in the overall population. In childhood, bronchial asthma may precede the onset of allergic rhinitis. Persons with rhinitis are prone to recurrent respiratory, sinus, and ear infections.

Treatment and Environmental Control

Avoidance of triggers is clearly the most important treatment for allergic rhinitis. Although total avoidance is usually not possible (except for family pets), you can take a few steps to significantly reduce your exposure to allergens.

Pollens

Keep your doors and windows closed during your allergy season. The use of central air conditioning dramatically reduces the level of indoor pollen and can also lessen indoor humidity. Lower humidity reduces both mold and dust mite allergen concentrations. Pollen and mold counts can vary throughout the day. Peak times are:

- **Grass:** Afternoon and early evening

- **Ragweed:** Early midday

- **Mold spores:** Some types peak during warm, dry, windy afternoons; other types occur at high levels during periods of dampness and rain and peak in the early morning hours

It may help to limit your outdoor activities during the times of highest pollen and mold counts.

Molds

Mold can grow in damp areas of your home, such as the kitchen, bathroom, or basement. If you are allergic to mold, take measures to lessen mold growth. These include:

- Ventilate these areas well.

- Clean damp areas frequently, using a weak, chlorine bleach solution as needed.

- Use a humidifier with caution because frequent use increases growth of mold and dust mites within your home. Clean your humidifier routinely as it can become a source for mold and bacteria growth.

- Consider a dehumidifier if your basement is damp, or if you live in a very humid climate.

Dust Mites

If you are allergic to house dust mites and live in a humid area:

- Cover your mattress and box spring in zippered, dust proof encasings.

- Wash your pillows, sheets, and blankets weekly in hot water. Mites will survive lukewarm water.

Pets

Dander from pets, particularly cats and dogs, is a major year-round allergen. If you are allergic to your pet, the obvious recommendation is removal of the pet from your home. If you choose to keep it, completely exclude the animal from your bedroom and keep the doors and heating ducts closed. Keep in mind that the more restricted the area in which the pet is allowed, the less allergic exposure you will have.

Irritants

Many irritants (non-allergenic substances) can also trigger rhinitis symptoms. Reducing exposure to irritants is recommended for persons with allergic or non-allergic rhinitis. Cigarette smoke is a strong respiratory irritant and it is important that no one smoke in your home. You may need to avoid aerosol sprays, perfumes, dusty or polluted environments, strong cleaning products, and other sources of strong odors.

Commonly Used Medication for Rhinitis

The goal of medical treatment is to reduce symptoms and use medications with few or no side effects.

Commonly available preparations include:

- Beconase AQ®, Vancenase DS AQ® (beclomethasone)

- Nasacort® (triamcinolone)

- Nasarel® (flunisolide)

- Flonase® (fluticasone)

- Rhinocort® (budesonide)

- Nasonex® (mometasone)

- Nasalcrom® (cromolyn sodium): This nonprescription nasal spray reduces milder symptoms of nasal discharge and sneezing. This is also a preventive medication and does not relieve symptoms immediately.

- Atrovent® (ipratropium bromide): This prescription medication occasionally benefits those with non-allergic rhinitis.

- Oral Corticosteroids: These prescription tablet/syrup preparations are very effective in treating and preventing symptoms of rhinitis. However, the side effects of oral steroids, especially with long-term use, limit their use. Your doctor may prescribe a short course (three to seven days) for more severe symptoms. It is important to note that the corticosteroids used in respiratory treatment are not the same as the anabolic steroids used by athletes.

- Nasal Wash: A salt water nasal wash is helpful in removing mucus from the nose. The salt water nasal wash is often done before using nasal medications. It temporarily reduces symptoms of nasal congestion and postnasal drainage.

Immunotherapy

Immunotherapy ("allergy shots") consists of a series of injections containing the allergens believed to be triggering allergy symptoms. The objective is to reduce your sensitivity to these allergens so that you experience fewer symptoms. Treatment usually begins with injections of a weak solution given once or twice a week, with the strength gradually increasing. When the strongest dosage is reached, the injection is then usually given once a month.

Immunotherapy has proven effective against the following allergens:

- Grass pollen

- Ragweed pollen

- Birch pollen

- Mountain cedar pollen

- House dust mite

- Cat and dog dander

- Alternaria mold spores

Skin testing, or RAST testing, can identify your specific allergens. Immunotherapy is specific against only the allergens used in the treatment. For example, if someone with allergy to both ragweed pollen and grass pollen is treated for ragweed only, this person will continue to experience rhinitis triggered by grass pollen. Physicians generally recommend immunotherapy for allergic rhinitis in someone with clear-cut allergy to very specific allergens who responds poorly to treatment or whose symptoms persist over several seasons or throughout the year. Doctors at the National Jewish Medical and Research Center recommend that allergy testing and immunotherapy be done by a board-certified allergist.

Note

This information in this section is provided to you as an educational service of LUNG LINE®, a service of the National Jewish Medical and Research Center. It is not meant to be a substitute for consulting your own physician.

National Jewish Medical and Research Center is the nation's leading treatment center for respiratory diseases and immune disorders. LUNG LINE® 1-800-222-LUNG (5864) is available Monday-Friday from 8:00 AM–5:00 PM, Mountain Time. Registered nurses can answer questions and provide educational literature on respiratory and immunologic diseases. LUNG LINE® also provides information on the treatment options available at National Jewish.

Section 9.2

Rhinitis Update: A Guide to Treatment

Excerpted from "Rhinitis Update: A Guide to Treatment," by Mark S. Dykewicz, in *Consultant,* Vol. 39, No. 5, May 1999, pp. 1446-9. © 1999 by Cliggott Publishing Co., 134 W. 29th St., New York, NY 10001. Reprinted with permission.

Fundamental to the management of rhinitis is the identification and avoidance of provoking factors, which include a wide range of allergic, nonallergic, and infectious triggers. Effective treatment is also greatly facilitated by appropriate use of pharmacologic agents [medications].

Environmental Control Measures

Effective treatment of rhinitis includes identification of triggers — such as allergens, irritants, and medications — and the implementation of effective avoidance measures. Whenever possible, enlist family cooperation.

The major classes of allergic rhinitis triggers include the following:

- **Pollens.** Tolerance of unavoidable triggers (such as airborne pollen) may be improved by avoidance of other allergens. Tell patients to keep doors and windows closed and to keep air-conditioning vents closed when air-conditioning is used. Remind them that indoor pollen levels are increased by window or attic fans, and that a shower or bath after outdoor activity removes pollen from the hair and skin.

- **Molds.** Make sure patients understand that exposure to outdoor molds is increased by walking in uncut fields and that activities such as mowing and threshing may result in very high levels of exposure. Indoor molds proliferate in damp homes, basements, cold outside walls, sinks, shower stalls, carpeting, bedding, and upholstered furniture. Mold-sensitive patients should avoid console humidifiers and cool-mist vaporizers, which are reservoirs for mold unless kept scrupulously clean.

Chemical and physical measures to control indoor mold usually fail unless relative humidity and condensation are reduced.

- **House dust mites.** Encourage patients to avoid having carpets and upholstered furniture in their homes, to wash bedclothes in hot water (above 54.4° C [130° F]), and to decrease indoor humidity to reduce levels of dust mite allergen. They should cover mattresses, box springs, and pillows in zippered, allergen-proof casings.

- **Animal allergens.** The key to preventing exposure to cat or dog allergen is to remove the animal from the home. A trial removal is usually deceptive because it takes 20 weeks or longer for the allergen to dissipate. If the patient or patient's family is not willing to part with the animal, the next option is to confine the animal to an uncarpeted room—but not the patient's bedroom.

- **Insect allergens.** Cockroaches are a significant cause of respiratory allergy. When ordinary sanitation methods and "roach traps" fail, recommend extermination. Changing homes may be a necessary last resort.

Pharmacologic Therapy

It is important to establish the correct diagnosis before beginning therapy. Initial treatment of mild rhinitis may include avoidance measures and single-agent or combination pharmacologic therapy. Compliance with treatment is enhanced when:

- The patient has written instructions.
- Fewer daily doses are required.
- The patient schedules when doses are to be taken.
- There is a good physician-patient relationship.

When the onset of symptoms can be anticipated (as in the case of seasonal rhinitis), consider prophylactic use of medications to lessen the impact of exposure.

Antihistamines. Second-generation antihistamines are now preferred to first-generation antihistamines in most cases. Sedation and performance impairment—side effects associated with first-generation antihistamines—have been shown to cause problems ranging from learning difficulties to occupational and traffic accidents. Even when administered at bedtime, these agents can cause significant daytime sedation; decrease alertness; and impair performance in reaction time, visual-motor coordination, memory, learning, and driving. Alcohol, sedatives, hypnotics, and antidepressants may potentiate these effects.

However, there are some circumstances in which the use of first-generation antihistamines may be appropriate. When small children are agitated from the discomfort of rhinitis, mild sedation may be beneficial. The anticholinergic side effects of first-generation antihistamines are sometimes desirable because they may help reduce nasal secretions, but dry mouth and urinary retention may result.

The second-generation antihistamines—astemizole, cetirizine, fexofenadine, and loratadine—decrease sneezing, itching, nasal discharge, and the ocular symptoms of allergic conjunctivitis (Table 9.1.). Although they are probably no more effective than the first-generation agents, they do not have the same sedating effects.

Astemizole (and terfenadine, which was withdrawn from the U.S. market in 1998) may produce undesirable side effects at higher than

Table 9.1. Guidelines for the Use of Second-Generation Oral Antihistamines

Agent	Usual adult dosage	Available with decongestant?	Reduce dosage with liver disease?	Reduce dosage with renal impairment?
Astemizole	10 mg/d	No	Avoid	No
Cetirizine	5 or 10 mg/d	No	5 mg/d	5 mg/d
Fexofenadine	60 mg twice daily	Yes	No	60 mg/d
Loratadine	10 mg/d	Yes	Start at 10 mg every other day	Start at 10 mg every other day

Adapted from Dykewicz MS et al. *Ann Allergy Asthma Immunol.* 1998.[1]

recommended doses or if taken concurrently with azole antifungals (such as fluconazole, itraconazole, and miconazole), some macrolides (such as erythromycin and clarithromycin), or ciprofloxacin. Instruct patients to take antihistamines 2 to 5 hours before allergen exposure. Although effective on an "as-needed" basis, they work best when taken regularly. Nasal congestion is not relieved by oral antihistamines.

Intranasal antihistamines are appropriate first-line treatment for the symptoms of allergic rhinitis or in combination with intranasal corticosteroids or oral antihistamines. Unlike oral antihistamines, they may help reduce nasal congestion. However, patients may find their taste bitter, and they may cause sedation.

Azelastine is the first intranasal antihistamine preparation approved for use in the United States. Recommended dosing is 2 sprays in each nostril twice daily for patients 12 years or older.

Oral and intranasal decongestants. An oral decongestant, such as pseudoephedrine or phenylephrine may be needed to manage nasal congestion. Prescribe these agents with caution for patients with arrhythmias, coronary heart disease, hypertension, hyperthyroidism, glaucoma, diabetes, or urinary dysfunction. Side effects may include elevated blood pressure, palpitations, loss of appetite, tremor, and sleep disturbance. The disadvantage of antihistamine-decongestant formulations is that the dose of each ingredient cannot be adjusted.

Intranasal decongestants can be useful for short-term (2 to 3 days) control of nasal congestion associated with rhinitis. These agents are not usually associated with systemic sympathomimetic reactions.

Intranasal corticosteroids. These agents most effectively control the symptoms of allergic rhinitis (Table 9.2.). Intranasal corticosteroids are particularly useful for treating more severe allergic rhinitis and—except for intranasal dexamethasone—generally are not associated with significant systemic side effects in adults. Compared with first- and second-generation antihistamines, intranasal corticosteroids provide less relief of ocular symptoms but more effectively improve allergic rhinitis symptoms.

Although local side effects are minimal if the patient is instructed in the proper use of these agents, nasal irritation and bleeding may occur. Tell patients to direct the spray away from the nasal septum to prevent repetitive direct application. Examine the nasal septum periodically to ensure that mucosal erosions do not develop; in rare instances, these may lead to nasal septal perforation.

Oral and parenteral corticosteroids. Although systemic corticosteroids are not appropriate for treating chronic rhinitis, short oral courses (3 to 7 days) may help manage very severe or intractable nasal symptoms or significant nasal polyposis. Adrenal suppression in adults is avoided with short courses at dosages equivalent to 40 mg/d of prednisone. The use of parenteral corticosteroids (particularly if administered recurrently) is discouraged because of greater potential for long-term corticosteroid side effects. Before initiating treatment with systemic corticosteroids, consider the use of intranasal corticosteroids.

Intranasal cromolyn. Pretreatment with this agent before an anticipated allergen exposure will result in considerable diminution or ablation of the nasal allergic response. If the patient has a seasonal allergy, be sure to use cromolyn as early in the allergy season as possible. Cromolyn is also effective when used regularly during the period of exposure normally associated with allergic symptoms. The

Table 9.2. Recommended Dosages of Intranasal Corticosteroids

Agent	Dose per inhalation (μg)	Initial adult dosage
Beclomethasone	42	1 or 2 sprays per nostril twice daily
Budesonide	32	2 sprays per nostril twice daily or 4 sprays per nostril daily
Flunisolide	25	2 sprays per nostril twice daily
Fluticasone	50	2 sprays per nostril daily or 1 spray per nostril twice daily
Mometasone	50	2 sprays per nostril daily
Triamcinolone acetonide	55	2 sprays per nostril daily
Dexamethasone sodium phosphate	84	2 sprays per nostril 2 or 3 times daily

Adapted from Dykewicz MS et al. *Ann Allergy Asthma Immunol.* 1998.[1]

starting dosage is 1 spray in each nostril every 4 hours (during waking hours), until relief is evident. Usually, benefit is noted within 4 to 7 days, but severe cases may require several weeks of treatment for maximum effect. Maintenance treatment usually requires dosing three or four times daily.

Cromolyn is generally less effective than intranasal corticosteroids,[2] but because of its good safety profile, it is appropriate for very young children and for pregnant women. Intranasal cromolyn and intranasal antihistamines provide comparable control of allergic rhinitis.

Intranasal anticholinergics. These agents may effectively reduce rhinorrhea, but they have no effect on other nasal symptoms. Although side effects are minimal, dryness of the nasal membranes may occur. Ipratropium is the most extensively studied intranasal anticholinergic. The recommended regimen is 2 sprays in each nostril two or three times a day.

Oral antileukotriene agents. The role of these agents in the treatment of allergic rhinitis remains to be determined.

Allergen Immunotherapy

Immunotherapy may be appropriate for persons with yearly recurrent seasonal symptoms, perennial symptoms due to allergic factors, and/or significant progression of symptoms. It is generally unnecessary for persons with sensitivity to only one seasonal allergen when seasonal exposure is short.

With rare exceptions, immunotherapy is inappropriate for preschool children and elderly persons. Severe pulmonary and cardiovascular disease and the concurrent use of beta blockers are also contraindications.

Immunotherapy is best administered only by professionals familiar with the procedure who are prepared to manage anaphylaxis. Treatment should not be indefinite; generally, a 3- to 5-year period is appropriate.

Concomitant Asthma

Clinical evidence has shown that treatment of rhinitis can improve the status of coexisting asthma. For example, an intranasal corticosteroid can prevent a seasonal increase in bronchial hyperresponsiveness in patients with allergic rhinitis and asthma. In placebo-controlled trials, conventional dosages of cetirizine, fexofenadine, loratadine, and oral decongestants improved asthma symptoms and pulmonary function in patients with concomitant allergic rhinitis.

Persons with concomitant asthma may be candidates for immunotherapy, but their asthma should be well controlled when this therapy is administered. Referral to an allergist-immunologist is appropriate for these patients.

Special Groups of Patients

Special diagnostic and therapeutic considerations are warranted for children, the elderly, pregnant women, athletes, and those with rhinitis medicamentosa.

Children. When treating a child with allergic rhinitis, initiate preventive nonpharmacologic measures whenever possible. Oral antihistamines and intranasal cromolyn remain the first-line choices for childhood allergic rhinitis. As in adults, second-generation antihistamines provide a greater benefit-to-risk ratio, but not all of these agents have been approved for use in young children.

Intranasal corticosteroids are the most effective agents for rhinitis in children as well as in adults. However, because some intranasal corticosteroids may have a temporary adverse effect on growth in children, use these agents at the lowest possible effective dosage, monitor height routinely, and combine therapeutic approaches to minimize the dosage.

The elderly. Allergic rhinitis is an uncommon cause of perennial rhinitis in persons older than 65 years. More commonly, rhinitis in the elderly is attributable to cholinergic hyperreactivity (which may be worse after eating), congestion associated with antihypertensive drug therapy, or sinusitis. Discontinuation of an antihypertensive medication responsible for nasal congestion should be considered but may not always be feasible.

Second-generation antihistamines, such as fexofenadine and loratadine, which are not associated with significant anticholinergic effects, sedation, performance impairment, or adverse cardiac effects, are better choices than sedating antihistamines.

Pregnant women. The most common causes of nasal symptoms during pregnancy are allergic rhinitis, sinusitis, rhinitis medicamentosa, and vasomotor rhinitis. Chlorpheniramine and tripelennamine

63

have been the preferred antihistamines for use during pregnancy, and pseudoephedrine is the preferred decongestant. However, advise patients that it is probably best to avoid oral decongestants in the first trimester; studies have linked first-trimester use with infant gastroschisis.

Nasal cromolyn is useful for allergic rhinitis and may merit first consideration because it is topically applied and has an excellent safety profile. Vasomotor rhinitis is often adequately controlled by intranasal saline instillation, appropriate exercise, and pseudoephedrine.

Athletes. Athletes and their physicians should be aware that all oral decongestants and oral or parenteral corticosteroids are banned by the U.S. Olympic Committee (USOC). Oral antihistamines are allowed by the USOC but may be banned by the international federations of certain sports. If intranasal corticosteroids are administered to Olympic-class athletes, physicians must send written notification of the indication for use to the USOC.

Rhinitis medicamentosa. Use intranasal corticosteroids for patients with this syndrome, and advise them to discontinue topical decongestants as soon as symptoms abate. Occasionally, a short course of oral corticosteroids may be necessary in adults to allow for discontinuation of the topical decongestants.

When to Refer to an Allergist-Immunologist

- Medications are ineffective or produce adverse reactions.

- There is a co-morbid condition (such as asthma or chronic sinusitis).

- Symptoms interfere with the patient's ability to function or decrease quality of life.

- Symptoms have persisted for more than 3 months.

- There are complications of rhinitis (such as otitis media, sinusitis, or nasal polyposis).

- Further definition of allergic/environmental triggers of the patient's rhinitis symptoms is indicated, or patient requires more intense education.

- Allergen immunotherapy is a consideration.

References

1. Dykewicz MS, Fineman S, Skoner DP, et al. Diagnosis and management of rhinitis: parameter documents of the Joint Task Force on Practice Parameters in Allergy, Asthma, and Immunology, *Ann Allergy Asthma Immunol,* 1998;81:463-518.

2. Welsh PW, Stricker WE, Chu-Pin C, et al. Efficacy of beclomethasone nasal solution of ragweed allergy, *Mayo Clin Proc,* 1989;62:125-134.

—by Mark S. Dykewicz

Dr. Dykewicz is associate professor of internal medicine and director of the training program in allergy and immunology at Saint Louis University School of Medicine, St. Louis. He was an editor of the rhinitis parameter documents of the Joint Task Force on Practice Parameters in Allergy, Asthma, and Immunology.

Chapter 10

Sinusitis

Chapter Contents

Section 10.1

Understanding Sinusitis

"Sinusitis," a fact sheet produced by the national Institute of Allergy and Infectious Diseases (NIAID), April 2001. Press releases, fact sheets and other NIAID-related materials are available on the NIAID Web site at http:// www.niaid.nih.gov.

What is sinusitis?

You're coughing and sneezing and tired and achy. You think that you might be getting a cold. Later, when the medicines you've been taking to relieve the symptoms of the common cold are not working and you've now got a terrible headache, you finally drag yourself to the doctor. After listening to your history of symptoms, examining your face and forehead, and perhaps doing a sinus X-ray, the doctor says you have sinusitis.

Sinusitis simply means your sinuses are infected or inflamed, but this gives little indication of the misery and pain this condition can cause. Health care experts usually divide sinusitis cases into:

- Acute, which lasts for 3 weeks or less

- Chronic, which usually lasts for 3 to 8 weeks but can continue for months or even years

- Recurrent, which is several acute attacks within a year

Health care experts estimate that 37 million Americans are affected by sinusitis every year. Health care workers report 33 million cases of chronic sinusitis to the U.S. Centers for Disease Control and Prevention annually. Americans spend millions of dollars each year for medications that promise relief from their sinus symptoms.

What are sinuses?

Sinuses are hollow air spaces in the human body. When people say, "I'm having a sinus attack," they usually are referring to symptoms in one or more of four pairs of cavities, or sinuses, known as paranasal sinuses. These cavities, located within the skull or bones of the head surrounding the nose, include the:

- Frontal sinuses over the eyes in the brow area
- Maxillary sinuses inside each cheekbone
- Ethmoid sinuses just behind the bridge of the nose and between the eyes
- Sphenoid sinuses behind the ethmoids in the upper region of the nose and behind the eyes

Each sinus has an opening into the nose for the free exchange of air and mucus, and each is joined with the nasal passages by a continuous mucous membrane lining. Therefore, anything that causes a swelling in the nose—an infection, an allergic reaction, or an immune reaction—also can affect the sinuses. Air trapped within a blocked sinus, along with pus or other secretions, may cause pressure on the sinus wall. The result is the sometimes intense pain of a sinus attack. Similarly, when air is prevented from entering a paranasal sinus by a swollen membrane at the opening, a vacuum can be created that also causes pain.

What are the symptoms of sinusitis?

The location of your sinus pain depends on which sinus is affected.

- Headache when you wake up in the morning is typical of a sinus problem.

- Pain when your forehead over the frontal sinuses is touched may indicate that your frontal sinuses are inflamed.

- Infection in the maxillary sinuses can cause your upper jaw and teeth to ache and your cheeks to become tender to the touch.

- Since the ethmoid sinuses are near the tear ducts in the corner of the eyes, inflammation of these cavities often causes swelling of the eyelids and tissues around your eyes, and pain between your eyes. Ethmoid inflammation also can cause tenderness when the sides of your nose are touched, a loss of smell, and a stuffy nose.

- Although the sphenoid sinuses are less frequently affected, infection in this area can cause earaches, neck pain, and deep aching at the top of your head.

Most people with sinusitis, however, have pain or tenderness in several locations, and their symptoms usually do not clearly indicate which sinuses are inflamed.

Other symptoms of sinusitis can include:

- Fever

- Weakness

- Tiredness

- A cough that may be more severe at night

- Runny nose (rhinitis) or nasal congestion

In addition, the drainage of mucus from the sphenoids or other sinuses down the back of your throat (postnasal drip) can cause you to have a sore throat. Mucus drainage also can irritate the membranes lining your larynx (upper windpipe). Not everyone with these symptoms, however, has sinusitis.

On rare occasions, acute sinusitis can result in brain infection and other serious complications.

What are some causes of acute sinusitis?

Most cases of acute sinusitis start with a common cold, which is caused by a virus. These viral colds do not cause symptoms of sinusitis, but they do inflame the sinuses. Both the cold and the sinus inflammation usually go away without treatment in 2 weeks. The inflammation, however, might explain why having a cold increases your likelihood of developing acute sinusitis. For example, your nose reacts to an invasion by viruses that cause infections such as the common cold or flu by producing mucus and sending white blood cells to the lining of the nose, which congest and swell the nasal passages.

When this swelling involves the adjacent mucous membranes of your sinuses, air and mucus are trapped behind the narrowed openings of the sinuses. When your sinus openings become too narrow, mucus cannot drain properly. This increase in mucus sets up prime conditions for bacteria to multiply.

Most healthy people harbor bacteria, such as *Streptococcus pneumoniae* and *Haemophilus influenzae*, in their upper respiratory tracts with no problems until the body's defenses are weakened or drainage from the sinuses is blocked by a cold or other viral infection. Thus, bacteria that may have been living harmlessly in your nose or throat can multiply and invade your sinuses, causing an acute sinus infection.

Sometimes, fungal infections can cause acute sinusitis. Although fungi are abundant in the environment, they usually are harmless to healthy people, indicating that the human body has a natural resistance to them. Fungi, such as *Aspergillus*, can cause serious illness in people whose immune systems are not functioning properly. Some people with fungal sinusitis have an allergic-type reaction to the fungi.

Chronic inflammation of the nasal passages also can lead to sinusitis. If you have allergic rhinitis or hay fever, you can develop episodes of acute sinusitis. Vasomotor rhinitis, caused by humidity, cold air, alcohol, perfumes, and other environmental conditions, also may be complicated by sinus infections.

Acute sinusitis is much more common in some people than in the general population. For example, sinusitis occurs more often in people who have reduced immune function (such as those with immune deficiency diseases or HIV infection) and with abnormality of mucus secretion or mucus movement (such as those with cystic fibrosis).

What causes chronic sinusitis?

If you have asthma, an allergic disease, you may have frequent episodes of chronic sinusitis.

If you are allergic to airborne allergens, such as dust, mold, and pollen, which trigger allergic rhinitis, you may develop chronic sinusitis. In addition, people who are allergic to fungi can develop a condition called "allergic fungal sinusitis."

If you are subject to getting chronic sinusitis, damp weather, especially in northern temperate climates, or pollutants in the air and in buildings also can affect you.

Like acute sinusitis, you might develop chronic sinusitis if you have an immune deficiency disease or an abnormality in the way mucus moves through and from your respiratory system (for example, immune deficiency, HIV infection, and cystic fibrosis). In addition, if you have severe asthma, nasal polyps (small growths in the nose), or a severe asthmatic response to aspirin and aspirin-like medicines such as ibuprofen, you might have chronic sinusitis often.

How is sinusitis diagnosed?

Because your nose can get stuffy when you have a condition like the common cold, you may confuse simple nasal congestion with sinusitis. A cold, however, usually lasts about 7 to 14 days and disappears without treatment. Acute sinusitis often lasts longer and typically causes more symptoms than just a cold.

Your doctor can diagnose sinusitis by listening to your symptoms, doing a physical examination, and taking X-rays, and if necessary, an MRI or CT scan (magnetic resonance imaging and computed tomography).

How is sinusitis treated?

After diagnosing sinusitis and identifying a possible cause, a doctor can suggest treatments that will reduce your inflammation and relieve your symptoms.

Acute Sinusitis

If you have acute sinusitis, your doctor may recommend:

- Decongestants to reduce congestion
- Antibiotics to control a bacterial infection, if present
- Pain relievers to reduce any pain

You should, however, use over-the-counter or prescription decongestant nose drops and sprays for only few days. If you use these medicines for longer periods, they can lead to even more congestion and swelling of your nasal passages.

If bacteria cause your sinusitis, antibiotics used along with a nasal or oral decongestant will usually help. Your doctor can prescribe an antibiotic that fights the type of bacteria most commonly associated with sinusitis.

Many cases of acute sinusitis will end without antibiotics. If you have allergic disease along with infectious sinusitis, however, you may need medicine to relieve your allergy symptoms. If you already have asthma then get sinusitis, you may experience worsening of your asthma and should be in close touch with your doctor.

In addition, your doctor may prescribe a steroid nasal spray, along with other treatments, to reduce your sinus congestion, swelling, and inflammation.

Chronic Sinusitis

Doctors often find it difficult to treat chronic sinusitis successfully, realizing that symptoms persist even after taking antibiotics for a long period. In general, however, treating chronic sinusitis, such as with antibiotics and decongestants, is similar to treating acute sinusitis.

Some people with severe asthma have dramatic improvement of their symptoms when their chronic sinusitis is treated with antibiotics.

Doctors commonly prescribe steroid nasal sprays to reduce inflammation in chronic sinusitis. Although doctors occasionally prescribe them to treat people with chronic sinusitis over a long period, they don't fully understand the long-term safety of these medications, especially in children. Therefore, doctors will consider whether the benefits outweigh any risks of using steroid nasal sprays.

If you have severe chronic sinusitis, your doctor may prescribe oral steroids, such as prednisone. Because oral steroids are powerful medicines and can have significant side effects, you should take them only when other medicines have not worked.

Although home remedies cannot cure sinus infection, they might give you some comfort.

- Inhaling steam from a vaporizer or a hot cup of water can soothe inflamed sinus cavities.

- Saline nasal spray, which you can buy in a drug store, can give relief.

- Gentle heat applied over the inflamed area is comforting.

When medical treatment fails, surgery may be the only alternative for treating chronic sinusitis. Research studies suggest that the vast majority of people who undergo surgery have fewer symptoms and better quality of life.

In children, problems often are eliminated by removal of adenoids obstructing nasal-sinus passages.

Adults who have had allergic and infectious conditions over the years sometimes develop nasal polyps that interfere with proper drainage. Removal of these polyps and/or repair of a deviated septum to ensure an open airway often provides considerable relief from sinus symptoms.

The most common surgery done today is functional endoscopic sinus surgery, in which the natural openings from the sinuses are enlarged to allow drainage. This type of surgery is less invasive than conventional sinus surgery, and serious complications are rare.

How can I prevent sinusitis?

Although you cannot prevent all sinus disorders—any more than you can avoid all colds or bacterial infections—you can do certain things to reduce the number and severity of the attacks and possibly prevent acute sinusitis from becoming chronic.

- You may get some relief from your symptoms with a humidifier, particularly if room air in your home is heated by a dry forced-air system.

- Air conditioners help to provide an even temperature.

- Electrostatic filters attached to heating and air conditioning equipment are helpful in removing allergens from the air.

If you are prone to getting sinus disorders, especially if you have allergies, you should avoid cigarette smoke and other air pollutants. If your allergies inflame your nasal passages, you are more likely to have a strong reaction to all irritants.

If you suspect that your sinus inflammation may be related to dust, mold, pollen, or food—or any of the hundreds of allergens that can trigger an upper respiratory reaction—you should consult your doctor. Your doctor can use various tests to determine whether you have an allergy and its cause. This will help you and your doctor take appropriate steps to reduce or limit your allergy symptoms.

Drinking alcohol also causes nasal and sinus membranes to swell.

If you are prone to sinusitis, it may be uncomfortable for you to swim in pools treated with chlorine, since it irritates the lining of the nose and sinuses.

Divers often get sinus congestion and infection when water is forced into the sinuses from the nasal passages.

You may find that air travel poses a problem if you are suffering from acute or chronic sinusitis. As air pressure in a plane is reduced, pressure can build up in your head blocking your sinuses or Eustachian tubes in your ears. Therefore, you might feel discomfort in your sinus or middle ear during the plane's ascent or descent. Some doctors recommend using decongestant nose drops or inhalers before your flight to avoid this problem.

What research is going on?

Scientific studies have shown a close relationship between having allergic rhinitis and chronic sinusitis. In fact, some studies state that up to 80 percent of adults with chronic sinusitis also had allergic rhinitis. There is also an association between asthma and sinusitis. Some researchers think that as many as 75 percent of people with asthma also get sinusitis. The National Institute of Allergy and Infectious Diseases (NIAID) conducts and supports research on allergic diseases as well as bacteria and fungus that can cause sinusitis. This research is focused on developing better treatments and ways to prevent these diseases.

Scientists supported by NIAID and other institutions are investigating whether chronic sinusitis has genetic causes. They have found that the alterations in genes which cause cystic fibrosis may also contribute to chronic sinusitis. This research focus will give scientists new insights into the cause of the disease in some people and points to new strategies for diagnosis and treatment.

Another NIAID-supported research study is trying to determine whether fungi may play a role in causing many cases of chronic sinusitis. This research also will help scientists develop better medicines to treat chronic sinusitis.

Section 10.2

Colds and Allergies May Mask More Serious Sinus Infection

From *Doctor's Guide to the Internet*, © 1999 P\S\L Consulting Group, Inc. Reprinted with permission. *Doctor's Guide to the Internet* is at http://www.docguide.com.

Millions of Americans who think they have colds or allergies may actually be suffering from sinusitis, a more serious condition that requires medical therapy, according to a survey released today by the American Academy of Otolaryngology—Head and Neck Surgery (AAO-HNS). Consequently, many people do not see a doctor for treatment that can prevent future complications.

The survey of more than 1,000 cold and allergy sufferers, conducted by Yankelovich Partners, found that almost one-third (29%) had three or more of the common symptoms of sinusitis, which if bacterial can only be treated effectively with prescription antibiotics. Sinusitis affects 06 million Americans annually.

"Symptoms of sinusitis can mimic those of colds and allergies, so it takes an educated patient to tell the difference," said Jack Anon, MD, clinical assistant professor, Department of Otolaryngology, University of Pittsburgh College of Medicine, and chairman of the AAO-HNS Rhinology and Paranasal Sinus Disease Committee. Sinusitis symptoms include facial pressure or pain, headache, thick yellow-green nasal discharge, bad breath, sore teeth, or cold symptoms lasting more than 10 days. Anyone experiencing three or more of these symptoms should see a doctor."

The survey findings indicate a large number of people do not know what sinusitis is, nor that it can be easily and quickly treated with a visit to the doctor. Nearly half of those surveyed (41%) had never even heard of sinusitis. Among those who claim to have had the infection, 78 percent were treating themselves with over-the-counter medications and more than a third (39%) said they never saw a physician.

A companion survey of 200 primary care physicians, also released today by the AAO-HNS, found that more than half of doctors are concerned about self-treatment of sinusitis. "Self-treatment and failure to see a doctor will only prolong the infection and increase the chances of repeated infection which can lead to serious damage requiring surgery," said Dr. Anon.

Successful sinusitis treatment requires a full course of antibiotic therapy; however, physicians believe that nearly 40 percent of patients fail to finish their prescriptions. Conversely, only 13 percent of patients surveyed admitted to not finishing their prescriptions.

Some physicians believe the antibiotic itself may be causing problems. "Older antibiotics and those that treat only one of the bacteria that cause sinusitis can be less effective in curing the infection," said Dr. Anon. "As antibiotic resistance to *Streptococcus pneumoniae*, the primary pathogen causing sinusitis, continues to increase, we will need better antibiotics to treat this infection." More than half of physicians surveyed echoed his call for improved antibiotics to treat the infection. Sufferers report trying more than 11 different medications over the years of treatment.

Acute bacterial sinusitis occurs when sinus cavities become irritated and inflamed, often during a cold or allergy attack. The inflamed tissues prevent the sinuses from draining properly, causing congestion. Bacteria multiply in the blocked sinus, leading to infection.

The survey found that sinusitis takes a heavy toll on sufferers' quality of life. The average sinusitis sufferer had three to four infections per year; more than one-third estimate they have had 20 or more infections in their lifetime. The average sufferer missed almost two days of work per infection.

Chapter 11

Asthma

Breathing is something that most people take for granted. Without giving it a thought, we pull an invisible stream of gases, aerosols, particles, microbes, pollen, and dust into our lungs with every breath. But not everyone breathes easily. For the more than 14 million Americans with asthma, breathing becomes difficult when sensitive airways are inflamed and constricted. The number of people with asthma increased by 42% in the last decade, according to a recent report by the Centers for Disease Control and Prevention (CDC). Not only is asthma becoming more prevalent, but it is also more severe. According to the National Heart, Lung, and Blood Institute (NHLBI), the number of people who die of asthma jumped 58% between 1979 and 1992. Emergency room visits and hospital admissions for asthma are increasing. Children, ethnic minorities, and the urban poor are at the greatest risk. Researchers suspect that a variety of factors such as air contaminants and heightened exposure to aeroallergens in airtight homes trigger bouts of asthma or cause chronic airway inflammation that may lead to permanent lung dysfunction.

What could be making a respiratory disease, triggered by an allergic response and aggravated by a multitude of factors, more common, more acute, and potentially more fatal?

From "The Attack of Asthma," by Elaine Friebele, in *Environmental Health Perspectives,* Vol. 104, No. 1, January 1996. Available online at http://ehpnet1.niehs.nih.gov/docs/1996/104-1/focusasthma.html. Produced by the National Institute of Environmental Health Sciences (NIEHS), a subagency of the National Institutes of Health.

The rising number of asthmatics might be attributed to increased awareness among physicians, said Gale Weinman of the NHLBI. "Physicians may now be recognizing ailments previously diagnosed as a cold or bronchitis as the long-term, chronic illness of asthma. However, increased diagnosis of asthma cannot [totally] explain the rise in its prevalence," she said.

"We're looking at a disproportionate rise in the incidence and mortality of asthma in ethnic minorities and those living in poverty," said Darryl Zeldin, a clinical investigator of asthma in the National Institute of Environmental Health Sciences (NIEHS) Laboratory of Pulmonary Pathobiology. "Most researchers believe that there must be some environmental component to that. In the lower socioeconomic groups, individuals are being exposed very early in life to allergens. Once sensitized, repeated exposure to these allergens leads to chronic airway inflammation and asthma. But most likely there are multiple factors."

More Common, More Deadly

When people with asthma encounter allergens, environmental irritants, cold air, or viral infections, a complex cascade of events leads to airway inflammation and constriction. As air is forced past smaller and constricted openings, asthmatics develop an audible wheeze, shortness of breath, chest pain, and often coughing. Long-term exposure to irritants without medical intervention can lead to permanent reductions in lung function, damage to lung tissue, severe breathing discomfort, and lower resistance to infection, according to the American Lung Association (ALA).

For the 70-75% of asthmatics who have allergic asthma, their respiratory systems have developed a very specific response to specific allergens. Nonallergic asthmatics, on the other hand, may wheeze after exercising or taking aspirin, and show little sensitivity to allergens. Asthma and allergies appear to be inherited separately, but they are mysteriously associated. Most asthmatics can name at least one person in their family who has asthma or allergies. At least half of the people with asthma have allergic rhinitis, or inflammation of the nasal membranes, and 35% have atopic dermatitis, known as eczema.

Asthma is a more manageable disease than it was three decades ago. "The philosophy of asthma management has changed," said Peter Gergen, director of the Office of Epidemiology and Clinical Trials at the National Institute of Allergy and Infectious Diseases. "The role of inflammation in asthma became more accepted. The use of anti-inflammatory drugs and the monitoring of peak flow [a measure of the ability to exhale air from the lungs] has been increasing through the 1980s." Rather than focusing on asthma attacks already in progress, physicians emphasize prevention of wheezing and maintenance of optimal lung function, said Gergen. The National Asthma Education Program, sponsored by the NHLBI, has provided physicians and patients with guidelines for treating asthma and helped change their understanding and management of the disease.

Still, during the last three decades, asthma prevalence and morbidity in the United States has been rising. "The paradox of asthma is that we've had good treatment and quite adequate medications, and yet we're still having this problem," said Gergen. From 1982 to 1992, the number of people 5-34 years old who were afflicted with asthma increased by 52%, according to a recent CDC report. This seems to follow an earlier trend found by Gergen and associates in the 1970s, when asthma prevalence among 6-11 year olds increased by 58%.

The increase in asthma is not unique to the United States. Asthma appears to be growing worse in other economically developed countries as well. In Great Britain, deaths and hospital admissions due to asthma doubled between 1979 and 1985. In Finland, the proportion of military recruits with asthma increased 20-fold between 1961 and 1989. Sweden and Denmark also saw increasing death rates from asthma through the 1970s.

Health statistics are only one measure of asthma's high cost. Health care expenses for asthma reach $6.2 billion per year, or nearly 1% of all U.S. health care expenses in 1985, according to a 1992 study by Kevin Weiss, director of research at the Rush Presbyterian St. Luke's Medical Center in Chicago, published in the *New England Journal of Medicine*. Of that amount, $1.6 billion was spent for inpatient hospital costs.

Asthma exacts an equally significant personal cost. Asthma is the number one cause of absenteeism for school children and a common reason for adult absenteeism from work. In 1985, adults with asthma lost nearly 3 million work days, at a cost of $285 million, according to an analysis by Weiss.

Though death from asthma is relatively rare, it is becoming more frequent. Asthma mortality in the United States declined by nearly 8% per year during the 1970s, but by 1977, the trend reversed, and the number of deaths due to asthma began to climb steadily, increasing about 6% per year. Asthma killed 1,674 Americans in 1977, but by 1991 the death rate had risen to 5,106 (from 0.8 to 2.0 per 100,000 people). Although most asthmatics who die of the disease are over 50 years old, rates of asthma death have increased in almost all age groups, according to Michael Sly, chairman of Allergy and Immunology at the Children's National Medical Center in Washington, DC.

Most asthma deaths occur in urban areas. In 1905, 21% of asthma deaths among 5-34 year olds occurred in New York City and Cook County, Illinois (which includes Chicago), where only 6.8% of the U.S. population in this age group resided, according to Weiss. David Lang and Marcia Polansky of the Hahnemann University Hospital reported in a 1994 study in the *New England Journal of Medicine* that a disproportionate number of the asthma deaths in Pennsylvania occurred in Philadelphia, where mortality was clustered in poorer neighborhoods.

Although some evidence suggests that asthma's death toll could be leveling off, the rising rate of hospital admissions and emergency room and doctor's office visits for asthma suggests that the disease is becoming more severe. Between 1965 and 1983, hospitalization rates for asthma increased by 50% in adults and over 200% in children. Approximately 4.5% more children were hospitalized for asthma each year from 1979 to 1987, Gergen and Weiss found.

Disproportionate Risk

Blacks, Hispanics, and people living in urban environments seem to be at the greatest risk for asthma. Using data on the U.S. population from the National Health and Nutrition Examination Survey, Gergen and coworkers found that asthma occurs more frequently in black children than in white, and more often in urban areas than rural ones. The prevalence of asthma in these groups was not associated with gross family income, education level of the head of household, poverty index ratio, or crowding, the researchers found. In the 1980s, three times as many black children as white children under four were hospitalized because of asthma. Blacks 5-34 years of age are five times more likely to die of asthma than whites.

As depicted in a recent *New York Times* article about inhaler use in the South Bronx, Puerto Ricans in the United States suffer from asthma far more frequently than other ethnic groups. One in every five (20.1%) Puerto Rican children (6 months to 11 years) in the United States had asthma in 1982-1984, compared to 4.5% of Mexican-American, 8.8% of Cuban, 9.1% of black, and 6.5% of white children. Researchers have proposed that the high prevalence of asthma among Puerto Ricans could result from a possible genetic predisposition, or from the high rate of smoking among Puerto Rican women of childbearing age.

Blacks and Hispanics in Philadelphia had higher rates of death from asthma, but only in areas with higher poverty rates, according to Lang and Polansky. A study by Lawrence Wissow and colleagues at the Johns Hopkins University Hospital suggests that black children in Maryland are more likely to be hospitalized for asthma, but this tendency may be more strongly related to poverty than to race. The hospitalization rate for asthma in Maryland increased three times faster for blacks than for whites during the 1979-1982 period, but when poverty was considered as a factor, many of the racial differences in hospitalization rates disappeared. A higher proportion of children on Medicaid, or with no health insurance, were hospitalized for asthma than children with private health insurance.

These findings raise important questions about why the economically disadvantaged are at greatest risk of dying from asthma. "Poverty is associated with all sorts of diseases," said Gergen. "Poor people in the United States die more than the rich of all causes, and the gap is widening. General health is poorer, as well as access to medical care. Exposure, environmental quality of life, stress, and social factors all play a role," said Gergen.

Environmental Culprits

Spurred by the alarming statistics, researchers are focusing on direct exposures to allergens indoors where people are spending more of their time. Allergen levels are thought to be higher in less well-ventilated homes, where moisture accumulates, allowing mildew and molds to grow. Research shows that cumulative exposure to dust mites, which live in bedding, upholstery, and carpets, causes some people to develop allergic sensitivity, including asthma and airway hyperresponsiveness. The levels of cockroach antigen generally found in suburban homes are too low to sensitize individuals, but the 10-fold higher levels found in inner-city dwellings are enough to cause sensitization and appear to be associated with asthma.

"We're also concerned about second-hand tobacco smoke," said Alfred Munzer, pulmonary specialist at Washington Adventist Hospital and former president of the ALA. "There is increasing evidence that childhood exposure to environmental smoke can be a predisposing factor to developing asthma." The Harvard Six Cities Air Pollution Health Study demonstrated that in families where parents smoke, the frequency of coughing and wheezing in their children is increased by up to 30%. A 1986 study reported in the *American Review of Respiratory Diseases* that was conducted in Tecumseh, Michigan, showed parental smoking was associated with increased prevalence and risk of asthma in children.

Infants of women who smoke have higher levels of the antibody immunoglobulin E (IgE) in umbilical cord blood compared to infants of nonsmokers, indicating an immune reaction. Whether children born to smoking mothers develop asthma pre- or postnatally is an unanswered question. The increase in asthma prevalence in western countries is correlated with more women of childbearing age smoking, according to a 1990 British study in the *British Medical Journal*.

Increasing asthma incidence cannot totally be explained by smoking in the United States, however. Between 1965 and 1990, cigarette smoking in the United States declined by 40%. Though the greatest number of smokers are 25-44 years of age, poorly educated, and live below the poverty level, according to statistics from the CDC's Office on Smoking and Health, the proportion of smokers in this group is also following a downward trend.

The National Inner City Asthma Study (NICAS), underway in seven U.S. cities, sponsored by the National Institute of Allergy and Infectious Diseases (NIAID), may soon add to our understanding of the disease. During the first phase of NICAS, begun in 1991, health researchers surveyed people with asthma in selected cities to identify factors in their lives most strongly associated with asthma. These included access to medical care, the patient's understanding of the disease and its potential severity, and factors in the home that exacerbate asthma. Results are still being analyzed, but initial conclusions indicate that cockroach antigen is a more prevalent allergen in inner-city households than dust mite antigen.

In the second phase of NICAS, co-sponsored by the NIEHS, researchers will intervene to reduce allergen exposure inside inner-city residences. George Malindzak of the NIEHS is an administrator for the second phase. "We know that some components of indoor air have a definite provocative effect on asthma," Malindzak said. "We're now looking into things that people with asthma can do for themselves to alleviate asthma episodes."

The NIEHS is involved in recommending ways to reduce dust mites and cockroaches and evaluating allergy symptoms and lung function in children who are susceptible to recurrent wheezing. NICAS data should provide some insight into the soaring asthma rates among the poor and minorities in inner cities.

Other studies are exploring the influence of a child's surroundings during the vulnerable first weeks and months of life. It is precisely during this period, scientists believe, that the environment of a child with a genetic predisposition can tip the scales toward developing a full-fledged allergy.

"Sensitization is the critical point," said Harvard School of Public Health researcher Douglas Dockery, who is working on another study funded by NIAID. "You have to have a combination of genetic factors which puts you at risk but also a challenge via environmental exposure that sensitizes you," said Dockery. Indeed, evidence suggests that increased exposure to dust mites in early life is associated with increased allergic responses and asthma.

Using a sample of newborn children whose parents have a history of asthma and allergies, Dockery and coworkers will follow the infants' health while monitoring their home exposure to dust mites, cockroaches, and other antigens. "Asthma is clearly a multifactorial process," said Dockery. "A lot of things could be contributing. I believe nutritional factors are important. There is also the whole maintenance issue and the need for empowerment of these people who have asthma and need appropriate clinical support."

In some urban areas, more than half of the children with asthma may receive all their medical care at the emergency room, and many are never diagnosed. "The fact that many inner-city asthmatics end up in the hospital shows that something is wrong with the treatment," said Gergen. The uninsured have poor access to long-range care programs that would provide help in managing the disease and preventing acute episodes.

Increasing awareness of asthma and improving treatment are the aims of the National Asthma Education Program, a major effort of the NHLBI since 1989. In addition to training professionals about asthma management, the program is working with communities and organizations to educate people about asthma, including school staff, teachers, and coaches.

Breathing Bad Air

"The consensus seems to be that the environment is playing a tremendous role in the increasing prevalence of asthma," said Munzer. In addition to the provocation of asthma by allergens, he says, "air pollution is a big factor."

The nation's air has improved dramatically in the past 25 years. Emissions of soot and smog-forming volatile organic compounds have decreased significantly in the United States since 1970 despite crowded highways where more vehicles are driven twice as many miles. Release of sulfur oxide has decreased by 30% since 1970. Between 1988 and 1993, overall industrial emissions of toxic compounds decreased by 22%.

The distribution of asthma in other countries also fails to implicate pollution as an aggravating factor. Some of the highest asthma mortality rates occur in Australia and New Zealand, which have excellent air quality. Asthma is more prevalent in rural areas of the Scottish highlands, which have some of the lowest ozone concentrations in the world, than in more urban and polluted parts of the United Kingdom, according to a recent report.

Several U.S. studies of air quality and respiratory disease have also come up empty-handed in linking asthma to air pollution. In a comparison of school children in the Six Cities Study, measurements of lung function and asthma prevalence did not differ significantly between cities in relation to air quality. Philadelphia's soaring numbers of asthma deaths from 1978 to 1991 were starkly contrasted with the city's declining average annual air pollutant levels in the study by Lang and Polansky.

In spite of overall improvements in air quality, many Americans are not breathing risk-free air, according to EPA Administrator Carol Browner. Almost 100 million people live in areas where the air does not meet national air quality standards. Eighty percent of Hispanics and 65% of blacks live in "nonattainment areas" for air standards. For more sensitive populations, like those with asthma, polluted air presents a daily challenge.

"It is clear that for people with asthma, episodes of air pollution will aggravate that preexisting condition, resulting in more symptoms, more use of medications, and more hospital visits," said Dockery. "We can show that it is related to day-to-day variations in air quality."

In the Six Cities Study, scientists found that the odds of having bronchitis increased with greater concentrations of fine particulates (particles less than 15 micrometers in diameter). Moreover, the 10% of children with asthma or persistent wheeze accounted for 42% of the bronchitis episodes.

Another study by Dockery and Harvard researcher C.A. Pope substantiated these findings. When fine particle concentrations reached the current air quality standard of 150 micrograms per cubic meter ($\mu g/m^3$), school children experienced increased respiratory symptoms, and those with asthma doubled their use of asthma medications.

The question remains whether small particles in the atmosphere provoke asthma episodes. In Seattle, Washington, a study by Joel

Schwartz of the Harvard School of Public Health and coworkers showed that the PM_{10} level (number of particles less than 10 micrometers in diameter) on the previous day was a significant predictor of the number of emergency room visits for asthma. At 30 $\mu g/m^3$—the mean concentration of PM_{10} in Seattle during the study period—PM_{10} exposure appeared to be responsible for approximately 12% of the emergency visits for asthma, according to Schwartz.

Higher PM_{10} levels in other communities also present a serious concern. In 1992, nearly one-fifth of Americans with asthma lived in areas where PM_{10} levels exceeded the national standard of 150 $\mu g/m^3$, and nearly one-half were exposed to levels exceeding 55 $\mu g/m^3$, according to the ALA.

No one understands why small particles may provoke asthma. "Larger particles get trapped by our defense mechanisms, but these fine particles behave almost like a gas, going very deep into the lungs," said Munzer.

"It is puzzling that we observed the same effects—mortality, hospital admissions, aggravation of asthma, and reduced pulmonary function—associated with particles in Los Angeles, Philadelphia, and Steubenville, Ohio," said Dockery. "Clearly, the particles in these cities have a different chemical makeup, but all of the particles in the different communities come from combustion—whether from automobile engines, as in Los Angeles, from industry and power plants in Philadelphia, or from steel mills in Steubenville," he said.

In 1993, the ALA sued the EPA for failing to follow the Clean Air Act requirement to review the PM_{10} standard five years after its establishment in 1987. "If EPA tightens the current particulate standards, as recent scientific evidence suggests it should, potentially tens of thousands of hospitalizations, respiratory problems, and premature deaths can be avoided each year," said Ronald H. White, ALA director of environmental health.

Mark Utell, of the University of Rochester Medical Center and a member of the EPA's Clean Air Scientific Advisory Committee, which reviews EPA staff recommendations and PM_{10} criteria documents, believes that the toxicity of particulates should be more completely understood before standards are lowered. "There is no real toxicological basis for understanding how PM_{10} is linked with the epidemiological results. We need a stronger framework for understanding associations that occur with PM_{10}, at concentrations as low as 30 micrograms per cubic meter," said Utell.

The ALA also sued the EPA for failing to review the federal ozone standard. The ALA estimates that the health of 2 million children under age 18 who have asthma is potentially at risk because they live in high-smog areas (ozone is the main component of smog). EPA staff scientists conclude that a more stringent standard is needed to protect public health. In the second staff paper of the review, the agency has recommended that the old standard of 0.12 ppm be lowered to an average concentration of 0.07-0.09 ppm over an 8-hour time period, with 1-5 exceedances allowed per year.

Ozone is a powerful oxidant and respiratory irritant. Studies in recent years have linked ozone levels well below current U.S. health standards to a decline in lung function, respiratory symptoms, and increased hospital admissions and emergency room visits for respiratory problems. Other pollutants, such as sulfur dioxide, the main component of acid aerosols, and nitrogen dioxide, an indoor pollutant from gas stoves, clearly exacerbate asthma. Results of the Six Cities Study associated acid aerosols with respiratory symptoms, changed pulmonary function, and mortality.

"An important question is whether pollutant gases can enhance a person's susceptibility to being sensitized [to allergens]," said Paul Nettesheim, chief of the Laboratory of Pulmonary Pathobiology at the NIEHS. Animal studies have shown that ozone, sulfur dioxide, and components of diesel exhaust fumes irritate cells lining the airways and increase an animal's sensitivity to inhaled allergens. Irritation of the bronchi by pollutants like ozone could make it easier for antigens to penetrate the airway lining and reach lymphocytes and other cells involved in the allergic response, Nettesheim said.

David Peden, an investigator at the Center for Environmental Medicine and Lung Biology of the University of North Carolina at Chapel Hill School of Medicine, has examined how ozone exposure might exacerbate the response of people who are allergic to dust mites when they are in contact with the allergen. His results suggest that ozone would worsen the asthmatic response. But whether ozone exposure increases the likelihood of developing allergies in general is still open to question.

One study showed people with asthma to be more sensitive to ragweed pollen when they were exposed to substantial amounts of ozone. "One could say . . . if not for ozone, these people with asthma could make it all the way through the ragweed season without trouble," said Jane Koenig of the University of Washington School of Public Health, a coauthor of the paper with Schwartz. "Then you have to ask, how does one decide what your main stimulus is to control? Ragweed would be hard to control. Ozone might be a little easier."

Summary

While many factors that provoke asthma, such as air pollution and cigarette smoking, are decreasing, the disease is becoming more prevalent. Its increasing severity is concentrated in urban pockets where children live under poor conditions, are frequently exposed to allergens and air pollution episodes, and have sporadic medical care. Research suggests that education, controlling exposure to antigens in the indoor environment, and improving urban air quality could improve the quality of life for these children.

—by Elaine Friebele

Chapter 12

Dermatitis

Chapter Contents

Section 12.1

Contaot Dcrmatitio

From "Contact Dermatitis Is a Costly Skin Disease," by Laura E. Skellchock, M.D., in *Skin Care Today for the Health Professional*, Vol. 1. No. 1. Copyright © 1995 Healthline Publishing, Inc.; reprinted with permission. Reviewed and revised by David A. Cooke, M.D., January 23, 2001.

Contact dermatitis causes more than 90 percent of all occupational skin disease in this country. This potentially disabling rash most often affects workers in industry, construction, hairdressing, food preparation, floristry, housekeeping, and health care. Rubber, epoxy, soaps, solvents, adhesives, and metals are chief culprits on the job. Nonoccupational offenders include glue in shoes, fragrances in personal hygiene products, and dyes in clothing.

A typical dermatologist spends up to 10 percent of each day treating contact dermatitis patients, who make an estimated 11 million visits to physicians every year. The uncomfortable, often chronic skin rash can cause patients to lose considerable time from work, or to perform below par when they are at work. Some patients must retrain for new positions. Others lose their jobs altogether. Still others stay in jobs that make them sick, enduring continued exposures and suffering increased disability.

Costs of Contact Dermatitis

All told, contact dermatitis costs the nation an estimated $300 million a year. That includes $238 million for professional treatment and $74.3 million for nonprescription corticosteroid preparations. Adding to society's costs are governmental monitoring and regulation of occupational chemicals.

Clearly, diagnosing the underlying cause of dermatitis is best not only for the patient, but for society. Early, accurate diagnosis can avoid unnecessary physician visits and wasteful, inappropriate treatments.

Two Types of Contact Dermatitis

There are two major types of contact dermatitis: irritant and allergic. Even the most experienced dermatologist can have difficulty distinguishing the two, as the signs, symptoms, and even histopathology overlap. A detailed history is essential and should include the patient's occupation, domestic activities, hobbies, and use of personal care products and clothing. Often, activities of other family members can add diagnostic clues.

Irritant Contact Dermatitis

An irritant is any substance that damages and causes an inflammatory reaction in the skin by direct action through a nonimmune mechanism. Several factors help determine the severity of the skin reaction. They include properties of the irritant, such as pH, solubility, physical state (gas, liquid, or solid), and host factors. Host factors include the area of affected skin, oil gland, and sweat gland activity, and the presence of or tendency toward other skin disease.

Environmental factors such as temperature and humidity also play a role, but irritant dermatitis can occur in anyone if the concentration of an irritant is high enough and the exposure is long enough. The hands and forearms are affected most often.

Clinical findings in irritant contact dermatitis vary from mild erythema (redness), itching, and chapping to severe blistering and ulceration. The worst cases can be categorized as chemical burns, but most cases are mild. Mild cases may be insidious in onset. The dermatologist should be alert to the fact that chronic irritant dermatitis may be indistinguishable from allergic contact dermatitis. Even when a patient clearly has an irritant dermatitis, definitive diagnosis frequently can pick up an additional allergic etiology.

Allergic Contact Dermatitis

Statistics suggest that allergic contact dermatitis (ACD) occurs less frequently in the workplace than irritant contact dermatitis. But the statistics may be misleading. Many cases of ACD go undiagnosed and therefore unreported.

Allergic response requires repeated exposures to an allergen. It usually takes at least four to five days of exposure for allergic sensitization to occur in a nonsensitized individual, but it can take weeks or months. The number of potential allergens is vast; in a 1983 National

Research Council report, 65,725 chemicals were identified, including 3,350 pesticides, 3,410 cosmetics, 1,815 drugs, 8,627 food additives, and 10,000 commercial chemicals. However, about 30 allergens cause up to 80 percent of all cases of ACD. In particular, about 10 percent of all women who are allergy tested are allergic to nickel, a common ingredient of inexpensive jewelry. Rubber additives, preservatives, and fragrances are other common allergens.

Factors affecting clinical presentation of ACD include the allergen, the patient's immune status, the exposure route, and the therapy. Although ACD is usually not life-threatening, very acute and serious reactions may develop. For example, latex gloves and condoms can cause contact urticaria. This potentially life-threatening reaction has become more common with the increasing use of gloves and condoms to prevent the transmission of the HIV virus.

By history alone, experienced dermatologists can predict 80 percent of nickel allergies and 50 percent of colophony and fragrance sensitivities. But dermatologists can predict only 10 to 20 percent of reactions to other allergens. The only sure way to differentiate between allergic and irritant dermatitis is to identify the allergen through skin patch testing. While allergy testing is sometimes offered using a blood test known as RAST, it is generally not considered to be as accurate as skin patch testing. Once the allergen has been identified, the patient can try to avoid the substance altogether.

A new patch test is available for patient use. The "T.R.U.E. TEST" is a convenient and comprehensive diagnostic tool that should help physicians simplify the diagnosis and management of contact dermatitis. Compared to the patch test already available, this new test is easier to use and permits more standardized allergen placement.

Despite its immense psychosocial and economic costs, contact dermatitis can be controlled and often prevented with the help of a dermatologist. Patients, employers, and society all benefit when this potentially disabling rash is diagnosed promptly and accurately.

About the Author of This Section

Dr. Skellchock is Clinical Associate Professor of Dermatology at the University of California, San Francisco, and a dermatologist at Kaiser Permanente in Oakland, California.

Section 12.2

Recognizing Atypical Presentations of Allergic Contact Dermatitis

From "Recognizing Allergic Contact Dermatitis," by Marti Jill Rothe and Jane M. Grant-Kels in *Consultant*, December 1997, vol. 37, no. 12, p. 3028(5). ©1997 Cliggott Publishing Company; reprinted with permission.

Case Studies

Contact dermatitis is often uncomplicated and easy to recognize. However, it may sometimes have a florid, alarming, or atypical presentation, as the following three cases illustrate.

Case 1. A 70-year-old man presented with a swollen, itchy right eye. He denied having fever, eye pain, visual disturbances, and discharge; he did not recall any trauma to the site. He also denied exposure to contactants, such as eye drops, and the use of new medications.

Examination showed prominent edema and erythema affecting the right upper and lower eyelids. There were several erythematous papules affecting the right side of the nose and linear papules and vesicles affecting the left forearm. The patient's ophthalmologist did not identify evidence of ocular inflammation or infection.

The patient later recalled gardening several days before the rash developed. A diagnosis of poison ivy was made. The patient responded to prednisone, 60 mg every morning for 4 days, followed by gradual taper over 2 weeks.

Case 2. A 48-year-old man complained of an itchy eruption on his hands that began after he changed a flat tire and then wiped his hands on some leaves. He had been applying a triple antibiotic containing neomycin, bacitracin, and polymyxin B to his hands for abrasions sustained while he was changing the tire. Examination showed purpuric blisters and erosions as well as confluent purpura and edema of the thumb. Linear erythema was present on the forearms and legs.

The patient was presumed to have poison ivy complicated by contact allergy to neomycin and possibly bacitracin. A hand surgeon who
was consulted failed to identify infection or vascular compromise and
supported the diagnosis of contact dermatitis and the initiation of
systemic corticosteroid therapy. The patient's purpura, blistering, and
erythema resolved with prednisone, initiated at 80 mg/d and tapered
by 20 mg every 4 days. Patch testing was positive for neomycin and
negative for bacitracin.

Case 3. A 35-year-old machinist presented to his physician with
several weeks of a progressively worsening eruption on the feet that
was causing him to have difficulty in walking. He noted that he had
been wearing leather work boots for 12-hour shifts at the machine
shop and that hot and humid conditions were causing his feet to perspire excessively.

Examination showed weeping, crusted erosions over the dorsal
surface of the feet with maceration of the toe webs; hyperkeratosis
and edema of the soles; and psoriasiform plaques affecting the scalp,
elbows, knees, and legs. A few small blisters were noted on the me-
dial and lateral aspects of the fingers. Bacterial culture from the feet
showed large numbers of *Staphylococcus aureus* organisms sensitive
to erythromycin and cephalosporins.

The patient was treated with a regimen of cephalexin, 500 mg PO
bid [by mouth, twice a day]; aluminum acetate wet dressings for 15
minutes three times daily, followed by clobetasol gel to the dorsal feet
and topical antifungal and antibacterial gels to the toe webs; and bed
rest with leg elevation. He showed marked improvement within 10
days. A patch test was positive for potassium dichromate—a leather-
tanning agent.

Discussion

Diagnostic Considerations

The value of a thorough cutaneous examination is apparent in
these dramatic cases of allergic contact dermatitis. If the focus of the
examination had been limited to the patients' presenting complaints,
signs critical to diagnosis and treatment would not have been recognized.

In Case 1, the differential diagnosis of periorbital erythema and
edema included herpes zoster, erysipelas, and angioedema. In Case
2, the differential diagnosis of acral purpura included vasculitis, emboli,

and infection. The observation of linear vesicles and papules affecting other sites was essential in establishing the diagnosis of poison ivy. Identification of concomitant psoriasis in Case 3 was significant because examination limited to the feet may have prompted the initiation of systemic corticosteroid therapy; a severe flare of psoriasis may have been precipitated on corticosteroid withdrawal.

Secondary Allergies

Case 2 is a striking example of a primary contact dermatitis complicated by secondary contact allergy to medicaments. Common secondary sensitizers include diphenhydramine, benzocaine, and neomycin. Patients who become sensitized to topical medicaments are at risk for a widespread cutaneous hypersensitivity reaction when these or structurally related agents are administered orally or parenterally. Patients with contact dermatitis not uncommonly apply topical diphenhydramine; they may also take over-the-counter oral ethanolamine antihistamines, such as diphenhydramine, dimenhydrinate, and clemastine fumarate.

Benzocaine, a strong sensitizer, is an ester-type local anesthetic. Sensitization can result from the use of benzocaine-containing remedies for poison ivy, hemorrhoids, toothaches, vaginitis, burns, and warts. Patients allergic to benzocaine may also be allergic to other ester anesthetics, including tetracaine; paraphenylenediamine (a hair and fur dye); sunscreens that contain para-aminobenzoic acid; and sulfonamides. Benzocaine does not cross-react with lidocaine, mepivacaine, or other amide anesthetics, which are rare topical sensitizers.

Sensitization to neomycin is most likely when it is used for prolonged periods for stasis or venous ulcers, external otitis, or dermatitis. Concomitant sensitization to bacitracin may also occur when patients use triple antibiotic preparations. Neomycin may cross-react with other aminoglycosides, such as gentamicin and tobramycin, whether administered topically or systemically.

Identifying Causative Substances

Identification of a causative allergen or irritant may be facilitated by familiarity with the most common causes of contact dermatitis affecting specific sites of the body. For example, eyelid dermatitis (ectopic contact dermatitis) is more often associated with cosmetics such as nail polish, which are brought by the hand to the lid, than with cosmetics such as eye shadow, which are applied directly to the lid. Contact dermatitis resulting from allergy to paraphenylenediamine hair dyes, ammonium persulfate bleaches, and poison ivy may manifest as pronounced eyelid edema without facial dermatitis.

The allergens most frequently implicated in shoe dermatitis are adhesives (e.g., colophony, paratertiary butylphenol formaldehyde resin), leather-tanning agents (e.g., potassium dichromate), and rubber accelerators (e.g., mercaptobenzothiazole, thiurams). Initially, shoe dermatitis affects the aspect of the foot in direct contact with the allergen, but it may spread with chronicity. A vesicular reaction of the hands is common in patients with shoe dermatitis.

Table 12.1. Culprit contactants and affected body sites.

Site	Contactants
Eyelids	Eye and hair cosmetics; nail polish; ophthalmic preparations; poison ivy; matches
Scalp	Hair dye; permanent-wave products
Forehead	Rubber in bathing caps and hat bands
Ear	Neomycin for otitis; nickel in earrings and eyeglasses; nail polish; plastic hearing aids; fragrance
Neck	Nickel in necklaces and zippers; nail polish; fragrance
Waist and umbilicus	Nickel in buttons or snaps; rubber in elastic
Axillae	Deodorants; antiperspirants; fragrance
Vulva	Deodorants; chemical contraceptives; rubber in condoms; dyes and textile finishes; medicaments
Penis	Fragrance; chemical contraceptives; poison ivy
Anus	Medicaments; methylcholoroisothiazolinone/ methylisothiazolinone in moist toilet paper; fragrance

Adapted from Rietschel, RL and Fowler, JF Jr. Fisher's Contact Dermatitis, *4th ed. Baltimore: Williams & Wilkins; 1995: chap 6.*

Hyperhidrosis, which predisposes to shoe dermatitis, may be treated to try to prevent flares once acute dermatitis is controlled. Allergen avoidance (e.g., patients who are allergic to rubber may wear all-leather shoes; leather-allergic patients may wear all-plastic or all-fabric shoes) is critical for long-term management.

Awareness of other unusual presentations of contact dermatitis is helpful in identifying the culprit allergen. For example, erythema multiforme may result from allergy to tropical woods; purpuric dermatitis may result from allergy to rubber antioxidants in elastic and paraphenylenediamine in hair and fur dye.

Patch Testing

This is a useful tool for identifying causative allergens. Patch tests—strips of hypoallergenic tape impregnated with allergens or to which allergens have been applied—are placed on the patient's back and removed after 48 hours. The test sites are evaluated at the time of removal and then 4 to 7 days after the patches were applied. Patients are generally tested for any suspected allergens and for reaction to a panel of 20 to 24 standardized allergens. Those who have positive reactions are given lists identifying potential exposures to the allergen and, when appropriate, potential substitutes for the allergen.

Treatment

Successful treatment of severe contact dermatitis with prednisone usually requires an initial dosage of about 1 mg/kg/d, depending on the patient's weight and the extent of the dermatitis, with gradual taper over 2 to 3 weeks. Lower initial dosages and more rapid taper can lead to a profound rebound of dermatitis.

About the Authors of This Section

Dr. Rothe is associate professor of dermatology and director of phototherapy and clinical services in the department of dermatology at the University of Connecticut Health Center in Farmington. Dr. Grant-Kels is professor and chair, department of dermatology, and director of dermatopathology at the same institution.

Chapter 13

Allergic Conjunctivitis

What is allergic conjunctivitis and what causes it?

Allergic conjunctivitis is an allergy in your eyes. Conjunctivitis is swelling and redness of the clear membrane (covering) of the eyelid and eye. If you have allergic conjunctivitis, your eyes may become red and swollen. They may itch or even hurt, and may "water," or make tears. You may have a runny nose and you may sneeze a lot.

These symptoms are started by an allergen, which is a substance that irritates your body. Your body reacts to the allergen by releasing chemicals, such as histamine, which cause many of your allergic symptoms. Some common allergens and irritants include pollen from trees, grass and ragweed; animal skin and hair; skin medicines; air pollution and smoke.

Will allergic conjunctivitis damage my eyesight?

Allergic conjunctivitis is irritating and uncomfortable, but it will not damage your eyesight. It's not a good idea to wear contacts while you have allergic conjunctivitis, because you might get worse or get an eye infection. Instead, wear your glasses until you get relief from your symptoms.

What can I do to avoid getting these symptoms?

Try your best to avoid the allergens that start your symptoms. Stay indoors when pollen levels are high. You can sometimes find out when pollen and other allergen levels are high from the weather report on TV or the radio, or in the newspaper. Keep your doors and windows closed during the summer months and use an air conditioner.

Can I do anything to help the symptoms?

You can treat mild symptoms yourself with medicines you buy over-the-counter at the grocery store or drug store (no prescriptions are needed). Lubricating eye drops (sometimes called artificial tears) can wash out your eyes and make the swelling go down. Antihistamines in tablet form (such as Benadryl, Chlor-Trimeton, etc.) can reduce the itching, redness, swelling, and discomfort. You can also put a cold compress over your eyes for relief (use a washcloth or small towel soaked in cold water or wrapped around ice cubes).

What other treatments are available?

If cold compresses and over-the-counter medicines don't help, your doctor may prescribe medicine for you. Your doctor might suggest eye drops that contain an antihistamine-decongestant combination. This medicine relieves your symptoms and stops them from coming back. Drops are available in over-the-counter forms (some brand names: Clear Eyes ACR, Naphcon-A, Visine Allergy) and in prescription forms (brand name: Vasocon-A). These medicines should only be used for less than 2 weeks.

Another new medicine, ketorolac tromethamine (brand name: Acular), can be used even while you are taking other eye medicines, such as those used for glaucoma. However, ketorolac may not be a good choice for you if you are allergic to aspirin or ibuprofen, or if you have a bleeding disorder. Levocabastine (brand name: Livostin) and olopatadine (brand name: Patanol) are other medicines. They help itchy, watery eyes and may keep symptoms from returning.

If these medicines don't give you enough relief, your doctor may suggest desensitization therapy: your allergic reaction is reduced or stopped when you take small doses of the allergen. The small doses are slowly increased. This is one way to control long-term (chronic) allergic conjunctivitis. Another medicine that can be used is steroid eye drops but, because these can have serious side effects, they are used only in people with severe allergic conjunctivitis.

Do these medicines have side effects?

All of the eye drops listed above can cause burning and stinging at first when you put them in, but this goes away in a few minutes. Each medicine has side effects that don't happen often, so talk with your doctor before you decide which medicine to use. Don't wear contact lenses while using any of the eye drops.

Chapter 14

Anaphylaxis

Chapter Contents

Section 14.1

Anaphylaxis—Severe Allergic Reaction

From "Med Facts: Anaphylaxis," produced by the National Jewish Medical and Research Center, 1-800-222-LUNG; © 1995 National Jewish Medical and Research Center. Reprinted with permission from National Jewish Medical and Research Center. Available online at http://www.njc.org/MFhtml/ANA_MF.html. Reviewed and revised by David A. Cooke, M.D. February 6, 2001.

Many people experience allergy symptoms which are only a minor annoyance. However, a small number of highly allergic individuals are susceptible to a life-threatening allergic reaction known as anaphylaxis. Anaphylaxis, the most serious type of allergic reaction, is extremely rare. Symptoms usually appear rapidly—within seconds or minutes—after exposure to an allergen (a substance which causes an allergic reaction). In a few cases, however, reactions have been delayed as much as 12 hours.

Symptoms of Anaphylaxis

In anaphylaxis, cells of the immune system release massive amounts of chemicals—particularly histamine. As a result, blood vessels dilate and begin to leak fluid into surrounding tissues, producing swelling. Several organs can be affected:

- The skin frequently shows symptoms first. Hives, itching, swelling, redness, or a stinging or burning sensation may develop.

- The loss of fluid from blood vessels causes a drop in blood pressure and the individual may feel light-headed or even lose consciousness.

- Anaphylaxis can cause obstruction of the nose, mouth, and throat. Individuals may first notice hoarseness or a lump in the throat. If the swelling is very severe, it shuts off the air supply and the individual experiences severe respiratory distress.

- The airways in the lungs can constrict, causing chest tightness, shortness of breath, and wheezing—the classic symptoms of asthma.

- The gastrointestinal tract often reacts, especially if the allergen is something that was swallowed. The person may experience nausea, vomiting, cramping, and diarrhea.

- Women may experience pelvic cramps due to contractions of the uterus.

It's worth repeating that anaphylaxis is rare. The vast majority of people with allergies will never have an anaphylactic reaction.

Triggers of Anaphylaxis

An anaphylactic reaction is usually triggered by a limited number of allergic exposures. These include injection, swallowing, inhaling, or skin contact with an allergen by a severely allergic individual.

Examples of injected allergens are bee, hornet, wasp, and yellow jacket stings; certain vaccines which have been prepared on an egg medium; and allergen extracts used for diagnosis and treatment of allergic conditions. Antibiotics such as penicillin can trigger a reaction by injection or ingestion (swallowing).

Typically, a severe reaction caused by a food allergy occurs after eating that particular food, even a small bite. Skin contact with the food rarely causes anaphylaxis. Foods most commonly associated with anaphylaxis are peanuts, seafood, nuts, and, in children particularly, eggs and cow's milk.

An anaphylactic reaction from an inhaled allergen is rare. An increasingly recognizable example is when an allergic individual inhales particles from rubber gloves or other latex products.

For some people, two or more factors may be needed to cause anaphylaxis. Recently, it has been recognized that some persons have experienced an anaphylactic reaction if they eat a certain food and then exercise. Neither the food alone nor exercise alone causes any problem for these individuals.

When exposed to a foreign substance, some people suffer reactions identical to anaphylaxis, but in which no allergy is involved. These reactions are called anaphylactoid (meaning anaphylaxis-like) reactions. While the immune system must be "primed" by previous exposure to cause anaphylaxis, anaphylactoid reactions can occur with no previous exposure at all. An example of something that can bring on this kind of reaction is radiographic contrast material (the dye injected into arteries and veins to make them show up on an x-ray).

Fortunately, health care providers don't need to distinguish be tween anaphylactic and anaphylactoid reactions during an emergency because the treatment is the same.

Prevention of Anaphylaxis

To prevent anaphylaxis, it is important to avoid the allergen that causes the reaction. That may not be easy since stinging insects can find their way indoors and allergenic foods can be concealed in a wide variety of preparations.

Precautions can lower the risk of anaphylaxis and minimize the severity of reactions. For many people, immunotherapy ("allergy shots") can help. For example, immunotherapy for bee, wasp, hornet, and yellow jacket stings gives effective protection 98% of the time. There is some risk when an individual with past episodes of anaphylaxis is injected with an allergen, but experienced health care professionals working in a controlled setting can make that risk negligible.

If immunotherapy is not practical or available for a particular allergen, the physician has other options. For example, if someone has experienced an anaphylactic reaction to penicillin, the physician might order skin tests before giving certain other types of antibiotics. In most cases, different classes of antibiotics are available. Individuals who have a history of severe reactions to medications should take a new medication orally (by mouth) whenever possible, because the risk of anaphylaxis is higher with an injection.

Rarely, someone may get an infection that requires treatment with an antibiotic known to cause anaphylaxis in that individual. In this case, rapidly increasing oral (by mouth) doses of the antibiotic under carefully controlled conditions can often desensitize the person.

Physicians sometimes suggest that individuals who have had an anaphylactic reaction carry an epinephrine syringe designed for self-administration. This is particularly important if the allergen that causes the reaction is difficult to avoid. This type of medication, available by prescription only, is sold under the name Ana-Kit®, EpiPen®, or EpiPen Jr.® (for children). We recommend that the patient, and any person who might be in a position to administer the injection, receive training in the use of these syringes. We also recommend that anyone at risk for anaphylaxis wear a Medic-Alert® bracelet.

Some medicines given for high blood pressure (called beta blockers) can partially counteract the effects of epinephrine, making the treatment of anaphylaxis more difficult. Allergic individuals with high blood pressure may need to ask their physician about switching to a different type of high blood pressure medication.

Treatment of Anaphylaxis

If you suspect that an anaphylactic reaction is occurring, immediately seek medical help. Treatment must begin before blood pressure and breathing problems become life-threatening.

Epinephrine is the most important medication for the treatment of anaphylaxis. It is injected under the skin or into a muscle. Epinephrine works rapidly to make blood vessels contract, preventing them from leaking more fluid. It also relaxes airways, helping the individual breathe easier, relieves cramping in the gastrointestinal tract, and stops itching and hives.

Even if the individual responds to the epinephrine, it is vitally important to go to an emergency room immediately! Other treatments may be given such as oxygen and medications to improve breathing. Intravenous fluids may be necessary to restore adequate blood pressure. Additional medications may be given to counteract the effects of histamine and to help prevent a delayed allergic reaction.

About National Jewish Medical and Research Center

Allergists at National Jewish have been evaluating, treating, and researching anaphylaxis and other allergic reactions for many years. A comprehensive allergy evaluation at National Jewish generally can identify the cause or causes of the reaction. National Jewish physicians may perform specific skin testing for antibiotics, foods, or other allergens to determine the cause. In addition, they are able to perform double-blind food challenges, if indicated. Based on each individual's evaluation, the physician develops a management plan which includes specific things to avoid, alternative recommendations, treatment, and intensive education.

One of the allergic reactions currently being evaluated at National Jewish is latex sensitivity. Latex allergy may be severe, leading to anaphylaxis. Some individuals may develop allergic eye, nose, skin, or chest symptoms, as well as anaphylaxis, when exposed to airborne particles of latex. Due to the widespread use of rubber gloves by health care workers, allergic reactions to latex are on the increase. Occupational pulmonary physicians and allergists at National Jewish evaluate patients and develop specific treatment plans for individuals with latex allergy. In some cases, specific inhalation challenges may be done. Our experienced specialists also recommend administrative and environmental controls to prevent exposure to latex both in the workplace and the home.

If you would like additional information on allergies or an evaluation at National Jewish, please call LUNG LINE® (1-800-222-LUNG) to speak with one of our nurses.

Section 14.2

Preventing and Controlling Anaphylaxis

From "Office Emergencies: Strategies to Prevent—and Control—Anaphylaxis," by Len Scarpinato, in *Consultant,* Vol. 38, No. 11, November 1998, pp. 2639-45. © 1998 by Cliggott Publishing Co., SCP Communications, Inc., 134 W. 29th St., New York, NY 10001. Reprinted with permission.

Note: This section describes how anaphylaxis is prevented and controlled in a doctor's office. Although it is written for physicians, people concerned about the management of anaphylaxis will be introduced to issues they may wish to discuss with their doctors.

Few office emergencies are as dramatic—and frightening—as anaphylaxis, the multi-organ system response to an exogenous antigen exposure in a previously sensitized person. The immediate systemic hypersensitivity reaction produced when mast cells and basophils release their powerful mediator substances into the circulation can result in respiratory distress, circulatory collapse, or shock within minutes of exposure to an offending antigen. Cutaneous manifestations of intense allergy, such as urticaria, pruritus, and angioedema, often help make the diagnosis obvious (Table 14.1).

However, gastrointestinal discomfort, such as nausea, vomiting, cramping abdominal pain, and explosive diarrhea, may confuse the clinical picture. This is unfortunate, because the patient experiencing anaphylaxis is more likely to have gastrointestinal symptoms than rhinitis, headache, substernal pain, or pruritus without rash. Similarly, absence of a clear history of exposure to an allergen may mean that anaphylaxis is not considered among the first diagnostic possibilities (Table 14.2). Knowledge of exposure to a known allergen, however, is not essential for diagnosis.

Here I will outline the steps that I have found effective in preventing anaphylaxis and anaphylactoid reactions. I then describe an aggressive management approach that can be used when this potential catastrophe strikes in an office setting. But first, it is worthwhile to review the risk factors and high-risk settings that increase the likelihood of this archetypal office emergency.

Table 14.1. Signs and Symptoms of Anaphylaxis

Abdominal cramps	Headache	Substernal pain
Angioedema	Hypotension	Syncope
Diarrhea	Itch (rashless)	Upper airway edema
Dizziness	Nausea	Urticaria
Dyspnea	Rhinitis	Vomiting
Flushing	Seizure	Wheezing

Table 14.2. Differential Diagnosis of Anaphylaxis

Flush syndromes	Panic attack
Food allergy	Pheochromocytoma 'Red man' syndrome (from vancomycin)
Globus hystericus	
Hereditary angioedema	Shock from other causes
Medication reactions	
Medullary thyroid carcinoma	Syndromes of excess histamine production
Munchausen's stridor	Urticaria syndrome
Neurologic urgency (seizure, stroke)	Vocal cord dysfunction syndrome

High-Risk Settings and Prevention

Some 700 people—almost two per day—die in this country every year because of anaphylaxis or anaphylactoid reactions. The incidence is probably increasing because many new drugs are introduced every year and because polypharmacy is becoming increasingly commonplace.

The pathophysiologic hallmarks of anaphylaxis are increased vascular permeability, vasodilation, laryngeal and mucosal edema, and bronchial constriction. From a practical point of view, there is little difference between anaphylaxis, which is an IgE-mediated event, and an anaphylactoid reaction, which is not mediated by IgE and is not necessarily an immune phenomenon. When the possibility of either exists, steps may be taken to reduce risk, and therapy is generally the same for both.

Risk Factors

The most important causes of anaphylaxis in primary care are insect bites and stings, penicillin injections, allergen immunotherapy, allergenic foods, and contact with latex (Table 14.3). Agents frequently responsible for anaphylactoid reactions include aspirin and other NSAIDs; injected diagnostic agents, such as radiocontrast media (especially iodinated forms); intravenous muscle relaxants; and plasma expanders (Table 14.4). Anaphylactoid reactions also can follow exercise and exposure to cold. The two terms—"anaphylaxis" and "anaphylactoid reaction"—are often used interchangeably, and anaphylaxis is used to mean both for the remainder of this article.

Three caveats need to be kept in mind:

- As many as one third of patients have biphasic anaphylaxis, in which a second or late phase occurs hours or days after the initial episode.

- Anaphylaxis is more likely when exposure to an antigen is stopped and then continued later (an example of this is the intermittent use of insulin for a woman with gestational diabetes).

- Injection is usually associated with more frequent and serious anaphylaxis than is ingestion, although anaphylaxis can occur regardless of how an antigen is administered. This is why a penicillin shot or an insect sting usually—but not always—results in a more rapid evolution of symptoms than oral penicillin or a food allergy.

Prevention

Patients who have had anaphylactic episodes should wear a Medic-Alert bracelet or necklace and carry in their wallets or purses an identification card that lists drug allergies. (Medic-Alert items are available from Medic-Alert, 2323 Colorado Avenue, Turlock, CA 95382.) The most important general measure to reduce the likelihood of anaphylaxis is a thorough allergy history. Such a history needs to include drug allergies and other exposures, including incidents related to latex and other chemicals.

Because cross-reactivity occurs, however, it is not enough to simply take the history at face value. For example, a patient who has had an anaphylactic episode from aspirin is almost certainly going to be sensitive to any other drug that inhibits prostaglandin synthetase—including all NSAIDs. Similarly, patients sensitive to penicillin are at increased risk for similar sensitivity to cephalosporins and other beta-lactam antibiotics, and patients who have reactions to sulfa-containing antibiotics need to be careful about taking chlorthiazide diuretics, sulfonylureas, furosemide, and dapsone.

Oral administration of medication is less likely to result in anaphylaxis than is parenteral administration, so oral forms should be selected when possible. A wise practice is to have patients remain in the office for 20 to 30 minutes after any injection—just in case anaphylaxis develops.

Certain medications that reduce blood pressure can potentiate anaphylaxis, making it more likely and more severe. In addition to

Table 14.3. Key Causes of Anaphylaxis

- Foods
- Insect bites and stings
- Latex
- Medications (especially injectables)

Table 14.4. Causes of Anaphylactoid Reactions

- Medications
- Dialysis
- Physical stimuli (cold, exercise)
- Plasma expanders
- Protamine reactions
- Radiocontrast media
- Transfusion reactions

Table 14.5. Office Anaphylaxis Treatment Kit. Be sure to have these medications and materials on hand:

Medications

- Aerosol β_2-adrenergic bronchodilator and compressor nebulizer
- Aminophylline
- Cimetidine or ranitidine (injectable)
- Diphenhydramine (injectable)
- Dopamine
- Epinephrine, aqueous solution, 1:1,000 dilution (1-mL ampules and multidose vials)
- Epinephrine, aqueous solution, 1:10,000 dilution (preloaded in syringes for IV use)
- Fluids (2,000 mL of crystalloid or 1,000 mL of hydroxyethyl starch)
- Glucagon
- Hydrocortisone or methylprednisolone (injectable)
- Oxygen tank with mask or nasal prongs
- Saline, normal (10-mL vial for epinephrine infusion)
- Sodium bicarbonate

Materials

- Ambu bag
- Defibrillator
- Disposable syringes (1 mL, 5 mL)
- Electrocardiography machine
- Endotracheal tube
- Gloves (non-latex)
- Intravenous access kit with large-bore catheter
- Laryngoscope
- Needle (#12)
- Oral airway
- Suction apparatus
- Tourniquet

Adapted from Lieberman PL. *Medscape Respiratory Care.* 1997.[1]

beta-adrenergic blocking agents, these include angiotensin-converting enzyme inhibitors and angiotensin blockers. Medications that complicate the treatment of anaphylaxis by interfering with epinephrine activity include monoamine oxidase inhibitors and tricyclic antidepressants. If possible, all of these drugs should be discontinued or modified for a day or two when a treatment or procedure that increases the risk of anaphylaxis (for example, those that require injectable medications or antibiotic prophylaxis) is necessary.

For patients known to be susceptible to anaphylaxis, pretreatment is possible. The protocol is to give 50 mg of prednisone orally 13, 7, and 1 hour before the study or treatment; 300 mg of cimetidine or ranitidine orally 2 to 3 hours beforehand; and 50 mg of diphenhydramine intramuscularly and 25 mg ephedrine orally 1 hour beforehand. The need for the study should be documented and informed consent obtained. Note, however, that while this regime has been found effective in many settings, it has not proved useful in preventing latex anaphylaxis. Other preventive techniques, such as provocation challenge regimens and desensitization, are generally best left to allergy/immunology specialists.

Another option might be any of the "patient injectable" anaphylaxis treatments, such as Epipen and AnaKit. A prescription is necessary, and patients, their family members, and their friends need to be taught how to use these devices.

Managing Anaphylaxis

Therapy for anaphylaxis consists of early and aggressive use of epinephrine, plus cardiopulmonary resuscitation. Oxygen, glucagon, antihistamines (both H_1-receptor and H_2-receptor blocking agents), corticosteroids, colloid and other volume expanders, glucagon, and inhaled ß$_2$-adrenergic bronchodilators also have roles in anaphylaxis management. Every primary care office should be equipped with a basic therapeutic armamentarium intended for this emergency (Table 14.5).

Overall Approach

As in any emergency situation, the priorities are the "ABCs" — airway, breathing, and circulation. The immediate imperatives are to assess the patient's status—particularly the airway, vital signs, and level of consciousness—and give epinephrine (Table 14.6). Epinephrine is usually injected subcutaneously into the patient's upper arm, and the site is gently massaged to help disperse the medication.

The airway needs to be secured if there is danger of compromise. Unless the patient is already wheezing, he or she should be placed in the supine position. If there is wheezing, an upright position may be better. The blood pressure and pulse as well as pulse oximetry, which are monitored continuously, guide positioning. Give the patient supplemental oxygen. If anaphylaxis followed an injection, a tourniquet may be placed on the extremity proximal to the injection site to limit antigen absorption. During treatment, the tourniquet may be released for 3 minutes every 5 minutes but not applied for more than 30 minutes.

Respiratory, vascular, or cardiac complications warrant sampling of arterial blood for blood gas measurements and placement of an intravenous line for fluid replacement. Consider a central line if it is apparent that the periphery is "clamped down" from the anaphylaxis. If the patient is in respiratory distress, consider aerosol bronchodilator therapy and intravenous aminophylline. Antihistamines may reduce pruritus, urticaria, and angioedema when given at the onset of symptoms, and diphenhydramine may be given intravenously. An H_2-receptor blocker, in addition to epinephrine and dopamine, may help manage hypotension. Corticosteroids do not influence the immediate anaphylactic response but may have a role in controlling the late effects.

When massive regional swelling but no systemic evidence of anaphylaxis develops in a person who has been stung by an insect, the major differential diagnosis is cellulitis. Anaphylaxis is unlikely in this setting. This type of reaction occurs because the venom (especially of hymenoptera) contains hyaluronidase, a proteolytic enzyme that dissects through tissue planes. Therapy for such a patient consists of local ice, elevation of the involved site above the level of the heart, and sometimes use of diphenhydramine or another H_1-receptor blocking antihistamine to control pruritus.

Table 14.6. Imperatives in Anaphylaxis

- Assess "ABCs" —airway, breathing, circulation
- Assess vital signs
- Assess level of consciousness
- Give epinephrine
- Consider other therapeutic modalities as appropriate

Specific Modalities

The only therapy to give immediately with the onset of anaphylaxis is epinephrine (Table 14.7). Other therapeutic modalities are given depending on the evaluation of the patient and the evolution of the condition (Table 14.8). Massive fluid resuscitation with crystalloids or colloids is indicated when hypotension persists despite initial therapy with epinephrine and antihistamines.

Epinephrine is the mainstay of treatment. Give it subcutaneously or intramuscularly, two or three times at intervals of 10 to 15 minutes. The dosage for adults is 0.3 to 0.5 mL of a 1:1,000 aqueous solution, which corresponds to 0.3 to 0.5 mg of drug. The dosage for children is 0.01 mL/kg of a 1:1,000 aqueous solution every 15 to 20 minutes.

Intravenous epinephrine can be dangerous, but if there is no response to other therapy and the patient is markedly hypotensive, it may be considered. Repeated small boluses are preferable to continuous infusion. The dosage is 0.3 to 0.5 mg of a 1:10,000 aqueous solution (note the different concentration) in a bolus every 3 to 5 minutes.

Table 14.7. Epinephrine Dosing in Anaphylaxis

Age group	Dosage
Adults	Subcutaneously or intramuscularly: 0.3 - 0.5 mL of a 1:1,000 aqueous solution
	Intravenously*: 0.3 - 0.5 mg of a 1:10,000 aqueous solution in a bolus every 3-5 min
Children	Subcutaneously or intramuscularly: 0.01 mL/kg of a 1:1,000 aqueous solution every 15-20 min
	Intravenously*: 1 mL of a 1:10,000 solution; maximum concentration, 100 mg/mL

*Contraindicated in patients with malignant cardiac dysrhythmias (for example, in Wolff-Parkinson-White syndrome) or who are known to be severely hypertensive at baseline.

Table 14.8. Other Medications for Anaphylaxis Control

Medication	Dosage
Corticosteroids	
Hydrocortisone	
Adults	100-1,000 mg IV
Children	10-100 mg IV
Methylprednisolone	
Adults	80-125 mg IV
Children	40 mg IV
Prednisone	
Adults	60 mg PO
Children	30 mg PO
Antihistamine	
Diphenhydramine	
Adults	50-100 mg IM, IV, PO
Children	2 mg/kg/d IM, IV
Fluids	
Hydroxyethyl starch	
Adults	500 mL rapidly, more by slow infusion if necessary
Children	Not used
Lactated Ringer's or normal saline	
Adults	1-2 L at rate of 5-10 mL/kg
Children	Up to 30 mL/kg within 1 h
Glucagon	1-5 mg as IV bolus, then 5-15 mg/min
H_2-receptor blocker	
Cimetidine	1 mg/kg IV or 100 mg q3h PO
Ranitidine	4 mg/kg IV or 100-200 mg q3-4h PO

A premixed intravenous preparation of epinephrine in a preloaded syringe is available. To mix the intravenous solution yourself, dilute 1 mL of 1:1,000 in 10 mL of saline. Intravenous administration is contraindicated in the patient with malignant cardiac dysrhythmias (as seen in Wolff-Parkinson-White syndrome, for example) or who is known to be severely hypertensive at baseline.

When intravenous administration is desired but access is impossible, sublingual injection is a possibility. Inject 0.3 to 0.5 mL of a 1:1,000 aqueous solution into a site in the posterior third of the tongue. When injection of a drug caused anaphylaxis, absorption may be slowed by injecting 0.1 to 0.3 mL of a 1:1,000 aqueous solution directly into the site.

Diphenhydramine is the H_1-receptor blocking antihistamine of choice. It is useful for controlling cutaneous symptoms and hypotension. It may be given intramuscularly or intravenously; for adults, oral dosing can be used in the late stages of treatment. The adult dose is 50 to 100 mg; the pediatric dose is 2 mg/kg/d.

Diphenhydramine can also be used for local wound care in a patient allergic to lidocaine. The dosage is 50 mg of diphenhydramine diluted in 3 mL of saline, which is injected subcutaneously as needed.

It is also important for patients to have diphenhydramine on hand when they leave your office after being treated for anaphylaxis. Oral diphenhydramine is adequate in most instances and does not require a prescription. However, the dose needs to be 50 to 100 mg, not 25 mg (the amount in a single capsule), and patients need to understand this. Those patients whose symptoms rebound or who are hospitalized with hemodynamic collapse may require oral diphenhydramine therapy for up to 3 days after.

H_2-receptor antagonist antihistamines are advantageous in the management of urticaria and other manifestations of anaphylaxis and should be given in addition to—not in place of diphenhydramine.

Intravenous administration of cimetidine or ranitidine is recommended. The dosage is 1 mg/kg of cimetidine or 4 mg/kg of ranitidine, given slowly to avoid worsening hypotension. In less emergent situations, H_2-receptor antagonists may be given orally. The oral dosage for cimetidine is 100 mg every 3 hours and for ranitidine is 100 to 200 mg every 3 to 4 hours.

Glucagon may be indicated for hypotension in patients who have been taking beta-blockers. It has both chronotropic and inotropic effects on the heart and acts independently of catecholamine receptors. It is given intravenously in a bolus followed by a slow infusion. The bolus dose is 1 to 5 mg; the infusion dosage is 5 to 15 μg[microgram]/min;

the duration is determined by the clinical response (i.e., reversal of the blood pressure back to normal levels).

Fluid resuscitation is guided largely by response to medication. When epinephrine and antihistamines fail to control hypotension, the cause of the fluid shift is probably increased vasopermeability rather than vasodilation. Adults need 1 to 2 L of lactated Ringer's or normal saline at a rate of 5 to 10 mL/kg; children should receive up to 30 mL/kg within the first hour of treatment. Hydroxyethyl starch may be given, but the amount is usually less; for an adult, give 500 mL rapidly and more by slow infusion as necessary.

The need for fluid replacement may be greater when the patient has been treated with a beta-blocker. Some patients may require as much as 5 to 7 L of fluid before their condition becomes stable.

Other agents may be used in special circumstances. For example, beta-adrenergic agents may be indicated when wheezing cannot be controlled by epinephrine. Similarly, dopamine may be necessary for hypotension; the dosage is 2 to 20 μg/kg/min.

Corticosteroids may reduce the risk of late reactions and prolonged inflammation. For adults, 100 to 1,000 mg of hydrocortisone may be given intravenously; for children, the dose is 10 to 100 mg. An alternative is intravenous methylprednisolone; the adult dose is 80 to 125 mg, and the pediatric dose is 40 mg. Oral prednisone, which is appropriate for milder episodes, may be given instead at a dose of 60 mg for adults and 30 mg for children. Oral therapy generally lasts 3 to 7 days.

Reference

1.   Lieberman PL. Anaphylaxis. *Medscape Respiratory Care.* 1997;1(7):1-15.

For More Information

Austen KF. Diseases of immediate type hypersensitivity. In: Isselbacher KJ, Braunwald E, Wilson JD, et al, eds. *Harrison's Principles of Internal Medicine.* 13th ed. New York: McGraw-Hill Inc; 1994: 1631-1638.

Bochner BS, Lichtenstein LM. Anaphylaxis—current concepts. *N Engl J Med.* 1991;324:1785.

Chernow B. *Pocketbook of Critical Care Pharmacotherapy.* Baltimore: Williams & Wilkins; 1995.

Green MG (ed). *The Harriet Lane Handbook.* St Louis: Mosby Yearbook; 1991.

Kaplan AP. Anaphylaxis. In: Bennett JC, Plum F, eds. *Cecil Textbook of Medicine.* 20th ed. Philadelphia: WB Saunders Company; 1996:1417-1420.

Lieberman P. Specific and idiopathic anaphylaxis: pathophysiology and treatment. In: Bierman W, Pearlman D, Shapiro G, et al, eds. *Allergy, Asthma, and Immunology from Infancy to Adulthood.* 3rd ed. Philadelphia: WB Saunders Company; 1996:297-320.

Nelson HS, Lahr J, Rule R, et al. Treatment of anaphylactic sensitivity to peanuts by immunotherapy with injections of aqueous peanut extract. *J Allergy Clin Immunol.* 1997;99:744-751.

Patterson R, Harris KE. Distant referrals for idiopathic anaphylaxis. *Medscape Respiratory Care.* 1997;1(9):1-6.

Slater JE. Latex sensitivity. *Medscape Respiratory Care.* 1997;1(11):1-15.

—by Len Scarpinato

Dr. Scarpinato is associate professor of family and community medicine at the Medical College of Wisconsin in Milwaukee. He is also program director for the Racine Family Practice Residency Program.

Chapter 15

Multiple Chemical Sensitivity (MCS)

Chapter Contents

Section 15.1

MCS Is a Medical Mystery

From "Allergies—Multiple Chemical Sensitivity," in *Alphabetical Index of Health Topics*, National Institute of Environmental Health Sciences, March 1998, revised January 2000. Text available at http://www.niehs.nih.gov/external/faq/allergy.htm.

Question: Two years ago there was a chemical spill at my workplace, and many of my co-workers and I became ill immediately after the exposure. Since then, I haven't been the same. It feels like I can't think as clearly now, and I seem to be allergic to almost everything, including perfumes, cosmetics, detergents, and household cleaning products. I heard about multiple chemical sensitivity (MCS) on a radio talk show, and I think I am chemically sensitive. When I asked my doctor about MCS, he didn't have much to say about it. What can you tell me about multiple chemical sensitivity?

Answer: I can tell you that multiple chemical sensitivity (MCS) is something of a medical mystery. The medical community is divided over whether or not MCS actually exists.

Some physicians acknowledge MCS as a medical disorder that is triggered by exposures to chemicals in the environment, often beginning with a short term, severe chemical exposure (like a chemical spill) or with a longer term, small exposures (like a poorly ventilated office building). After the initial exposure, low levels of everyday chemicals such as those found in cosmetics, soaps, and newspaper inks can trigger physical reactions in MCS patients. These patients report a range of symptoms that often include headaches, rashes, asthma, depression, muscle and joint aches, fatigue, memory loss, and confusion.

Others in the medical community, however, do not accept MCS as a genuine medical disorder. The Centers for Disease Control, for example, do not recognize MCS as a clinical diagnosis. There is no official medical definition of MCS, partially because symptoms and chemical exposures are often unique and are widely varied between individuals. Some physicians are skeptical of concluding that low concentrations of the same chemicals that are tolerated by everyone else can cause dramatic symptoms in MCS patients. The American Medical Association denies that MCS is a clinical condition because conclusive scientific evidence is lacking.

Section 15.2

Symptoms and Health Status in Individuals with MCS

From "Symptoms and health status in individuals with multiple chemical sensitivities syndrome from four reported sensitizing exposures and a general population comparison group," by Ann L. Davidoff and Penelope M. Keyl, in *Archives of Environmental Health*, May-June 1996, vol. 51, no. 3, p. 201(13); © 1996 Helen Dwight Reid Educational Foundation.Reprinted with permission.

Ashford and Miller[1] postulated that three populations are at special risk for developing a persisting hypersusceptibility to very low levels of environmental chemicals:

1. People who experience nonspecific building-related illnesses,

2. Individuals who work in industry, and

3. Those who live in contaminated communities.

Such an altered response pattern has been called various names, including multiple chemical sensitivities (MCS) syndrome, environmental illness (EI), environmental or chemical hypersusceptibility, chemical hypersensitivity syndrome (CHS), environmentally induced illness, complex allergy, total allergy syndrome, and twentieth-century disease. We refer to the altered response pattern as MCS syndrome.

No case definition of MCS syndrome has gained wide acceptance. Several provisional case definitions have been proposed. In 1985, the Committee on Environmental Hypersensitivity Disorders, commissioned by the Ontario Ministry of Health, advanced the following working definition:[2] "Environmental hypersensitivity is a chronic (i.e., continuing for more than three months) multisystem disorder, usually involving symptoms of the central nervous system and at least one other system. Affected individuals are frequently intolerant to some foods and they react adversely to numerous chemicals and to environmental agents, singly or in combination, at levels generally tolerated by the majority. Affected persons have varying degrees of morbidity, from mild discomfort to total disability. Upon physical examination, the patient is normally free from any abnormal objective findings.

The research case definition by Mark Cullen[3] has been used widely in the United States. Cullen asserts that:

1. The disorder is acquired relative to some documentable environmental exposure(s), insult(s), or illness(es);

2. Symptoms involve more than one organ system;

3. Symptoms recur and abate in response to predictable stimuli;

4. Symptoms are elicited by exposures to chemicals of diverse structural classes and toxicologic modes of action;

5. Symptoms are elicited by exposures that are demonstrable (albeit of low level);

6. Exposures that elicit symptoms are very low—below those known to induce health effects; and

7. No single, widely available test of organ-system function can explain the symptoms.

A consensus case definition came from a survey by Nethercott et al.,[4] during which questionnaires were sent to 212 physicians and to other professionals knowledgeable about MCS syndrome by virtue of having contributed to the medical literature on the condition or by having served on a relevant task force, review board, editorial board, and so forth. Five criteria were considered major for diagnosing MCS syndrome by more than 50% of the respondents: (1) symptoms are reproducible with exposure, (2) the condition is chronic, (3) symptoms occur at low exposure levels, (4) symptoms resolve when incitants are removed, and (5) individuals respond to multiple unrelated substances.

Given the absence of a well-accepted case definition of MCS syndrome, it is not surprising that published data on prevalence do not exist. Mooser reported that clinician estimates of the prevalence of disruptive forms of MCS syndrome ran as high as 2-10% of the general population.[5] Among 114 individuals who were poisoned by organophosphates in industrial settings and who were diagnosed subsequently by physicians as having occupational disease attributable to organo-phosphates,[6] 19% of the individuals reported intolerance to low levels of environmental chemicals. With respect to 160 solvent-exposed workers admitted consecutively for clinical services, 13% reported such intolerances.[7]

Mild MCS-like conditions, which may not represent alterations from baseline, are widespread. It was suggested in a research survey, using a random national sample, that 7%-11% of the 600 office workers studied reported that they experienced significant building-related symptoms[8]—considered by some to constitute a less fully expressed pattern of the same syndrome. Sensitivity to chemicals has also been associated with upper and lower respiratory ailments (e.g., sinusitis, asthma, allergies); with metabolic conditions (hypothyroidism, hyperthyroidism, diabetes mellitus); and with drug use.[9,10] Finally, sensitivity to chemicals has been documented in the general population. In a study of male and female undergraduate students enrolled in an introductory class at the University of Arizona, 66% of 643 subjects reported feeling ill from one or more of five chemical odors, and 15% of the students reported being made ill by at least four of five odors.[11]

Although MCS syndrome is often associated with considerable disability,[1,12,13] the basis for the problem has not been elucidated, and controversy about its pathogenesis is widespread. Many observers have reported no evidence that the condition is based on a physiologically mediated response to environmental chemicals, and they have speculated that the symptomatology has a psychogenic etiology.[14-30] Diverse positions about underlying pathophysiology have been stated by other observers who view environmental stimuli as inducers of symptoms in affected persons.[31-49]

To date, the unique features of people who have reported MCS syndrome have been reported in four published and two unpublished studies.[2,23,24,50,52] The Committee on Environmental Hypersensitivity Disorders[2] placed newspaper advertisements in 16 Ontario newspapers, and they solicited testimonials from readers, affected individuals, and organizations and subsequently analyzed the letters received from 130 affected individuals. An unpublished review of 100 patients admitted consecutively to the largest environmental control unit in Carleton, Texas, has also been described.[50] Cone et al.[51] inspected the records of 400 patients who, during a period of approximately 3 years, consulted the Occupational Medicine Clinic at the University of California, San Francisco, after which the researchers published information derived from the case records of 13 clients. Cone and Sult[52] described a cohort of 250 casino workers, exposed to repeated pesticide applications to control a cockroach infestation, who consulted the ⟨illegible⟩ of 19 workers who were referred to the authors for interview and examination reported a new onset sensitivity or intolerance to perfumes, gasoline, and other solvent-containing materials. Terr[23,24] described the characteristics of patients who were referred for evaluation, primarily by employers or insurance carriers, because of claims of work-related environmental illness (of the 50 subjects in the 1986 study, 43 were included again in the 1989 study).

This article constitutes the first report of a systematic study of extensive self-reported information from standardized interviews with different samples of MCS syndrome subjects and a comparison group that comprised members of the general population. The MCS syndrome samples differed with respect to reported sensitizing exposures. The study enabled us to examine five descriptive questions:

1. Do diverse samples that report MCS syndrome from different sensitizing exposures resemble one another?

2. Do members of the general population report some degree of chemical sensitivity?

3. If so, is the chemical sensitivity in MCS syndrome similar to that observed in the general population?

4. Is MCS syndrome associated with a particular psychiatric history or status? and

5. Do MCS syndrome patients treated by clinical ecologists differ from other MCS syndrome patients?

Material and Method

Information about four sample groups of cases with MCS syndrome (i.e., organic solvent in industry origin, organophosphate pesticide origin, sick building syndrome origin, chlorine dioxide origin) and about one sample group from the general population was used for this study.

Multiple chemical sensitivities syndrome samples: Eligibility requirements for study cases in three of the MCS syndrome groups (i.e., organic solvent in industry origin, organophosphate pesticide origin, and sick building syndrome origin) included (a) having experienced a definite change in perceived sensitivity to chemicals following the exposure specified and (b) having to avoid three or more dissimilar situations involving environmental chemicals to feel good daily. In addition, subjects had to be between the ages of 30 and 60 years, had to have developed MCS syndrome during the previous 5 years, and had to be free of any medications that attenuated their responses to environmental chemicals.

Origin of Cases Identified

- **Organic solvents in industry:** Cases exposed in industrial settings to organic solvents were recruited by enlisting the aid of interested occupational physicians in Baltimore, upstate New York, California, Pennsylvania, and Louisiana. These physicians distributed letters that enlisted volunteers. Letters were also distributed to members of injured workers groups in New York, Massachusetts, and Rhode Island.

- **Organophosphate pesticide:** Cases were recruited by sending letters to persons who were listed on a registry of victims of pesticide poisonings. This registry was maintained by the National Coalition Against the Misuse of Pesticides, a District of Columbia-based organization. The same letters, also distributed to members of support groups, were formulated specifically for people who had identified themselves as being victims of pesticide poisonings.

- **Sick building syndrome:** Cases were recruited by distribution of letters to support groups for injured workers in a private research institute and in a government facility, both of which facilities were associated prominently with outbreaks of sick building syndrome. In some instances, physicians involved in the identification of cases with organic-solvent-in-industry onset referred MCS syndrome patients who had organophosphate pesticide or sick building syndrome onsets.

During the study period, consent forms were received from 201 possible MCS syndrome participants, from which cases were chosen randomly and screened. Subjects who qualified were classified with respect to exposure onset into one of three targeted onsets: (1) sick building syndrome, (2) organic solvent in industry, or (3) organophosphate pesticides. After 20 subjects from a targeted onset history were interviewed, we did not enroll any others with that onset history.

Chlorine dioxide: Ten workers in a potato processing plant in rural Wisconsin were studied. They developed conditions that resembled MCS syndrome after they were exposed chronically and acutely, by accident, to both chlorine dioxide gas and to chloroform, which was formed from the reaction between chlorine dioxide gas and organic material (in this case, potatoes). Pending litigation necessitated evaluation by one of the authors (ALD), who used instruments similar to those used for the other groups. All 10 subjects reported that following, but not before, exposure they were made more than "a little sick" by three or more chemicals.

General population sample: Sixty members from the general population were recruited. A random-number table was used to select 1,000 subjects from several Baltimore-area telephone directories. These subjects received letters that encouraged their participation in a telephone interview on health and common environmental chemical exposures. Subjects were offered an incentive of $25.00 for a completed interview. Respondents were informed that all members of a household who were between the ages of 30 and 60 years had to volunteer for the study, but that only one household member would be selected randomly. Matching was accomplished on the basis of three variables: (1) gender, (2) age, and (3) socioeconomic status (SES). In 55 cases, SES was defined by job status, using seven broad categories based on the 1980 Census Occupational Classification System; for 5 women, we defined SES by educational background (3 cases) or husband's occupational status (2 cases). Forty members of the general population were matched to the index subjects in the SBS onset MCS syndrome group, and 20 members of the general population were matched to the index subjects in the industrial-solvent-onset MCS syndrome group. This was done because these two groups represented the extremes with respect to gender distribution and SES. Members of the general population were not screened for sensitivity to chemicals.

We mailed 1,000 letters, 70 of which were undeliverable and were returned. Thirty-one individuals wrote to disqualify themselves because of their ages. Six individuals who volunteered either could not be reached (n=4) or declined to be interviewed, despite volunteering initially (n=2). One letter was returned by a residence that contained a physician's office. Twenty-three eligible households were discarded after the required number of subjects were obtained. The remaining households did not respond to our letter. The total number of respondents was 121. An exact response rate could not be determined because some households may have disqualified themselves on the basis of being "ineligible."

Survey instruments: Items were chosen initially for the questionnaire because pilot data suggested that they discriminated between individuals with MCS syndrome and the general population. Additional items were then chosen to reflect the five criteria of MCS syndrome endorsed by at least 50% of physician participants in the survey described previously. Questionnaires were adapted for a telephone interview used for the SBS-, organophosphate-pesticide-, and organic-solvent-in-industry-onset cases and in members of the general population. A self-administered questionnaire, derived from the same sources, but with some items deleted and some additional items included, was used for the chlorine-dioxide-onset cases who were studied several months following the study of the original participants.

Telephone interview: The duration of the telephone interview was between 20 and 75 minutes. Cases were asked 16 questions to ensure that they met the eligibility criteria. Otherwise, cases and controls answered the same questions about the following:

1. Demographic characteristics (e.g., age, gender, occupation, years of education, work setting).

2. Whether and to what degree they would feel sick in 12 situations that involved exposures to various environmental chemicals common in daily life. They were asked first about exposures of 4 hours, followed by exposures of 20 minutes. Outdoor exposures included being near someone who smoked cigarettes, being near a road being tarred, driving a new car, and driving in heavy traffic. Indoor exposures included shopping in an enclosed mall, being in a room newly sprayed with pesticides, being in a newly painted room, being near newly installed wall-to-wall carpet, and being around perfume. Six additional inquiries were made about chemical exposures that occurred for just seconds to several minutes (i.e., using a bathroom newly sprayed with a scented air freshener, reading a freshly printed newspaper, filling a gas tank with gasoline, walking down the detergent row at the grocery, trying on newly dry-cleaned clothing, and drinking a glass of chlorinated water).

3. Changes in tolerance to odors, alcohol, food, medications, and traditional allergens (e.g., pollen, dust, mold, cats).

4. The nature of responses to chemicals (e.g., frequency, consistency, latency, recovery period, time of earliest response).

5. Current symptomatology occurring at least once per week during the previous month and causes of these symptoms.

6. Life histories of medical conditions, including autoimmune, thyroid, and endocrine disorders.

7. Personal and familial mental health history.

At the conclusion of the interview, the interviewer administered the Positive Affect/Negative Affect Scale (PANAS), which consists of 20 adjectives. Ten of the adjectives are toned positively (e.g., interested, excited, strong, active), and 10 are toned negatively (e.g., hostile, scared, guilty). For each adjective, we asked subjects to indicate to what extent during the previous few weeks they had been feeling that way. The positive affect and negative affect scales have been shown to be very consistent internally, largely uncorrelated, and stable at appropriate levels during a 2 month period.[53] Normative data and factorial and external evidence of convergent and discriminant validity exist for the scales.

All questions were asked in a standardized manner and were closed ended.

Interviewers. Three paid interviewers conducted telephone interviews with members of the general population. One of the paid interviewers and one of the co-authors (ALD) conducted interviews with the MCS syndrome subjects. Given that the interviewers qualified the MCS syndrome subjects for the study, they were not blind to the subjects' group membership.

Statistical analyses. Using the SAS computer software package, we computed frequency distributions on categorical variables, and we computed means and standard deviations on continuous variables for each of the four MCS syndrome groups and for the general population. Pearson product-moment correlations were computed on psychiatric status, medical status, and PANAS data. We used likelihood ratio tests of heterogeneity for categorical data to assess (a) whether the four MCS syndrome samples originated from similar populations and

(b) whether the combined MCS syndrome samples and the general population sample came from similar populations. Likelihood ratio tests were used because they could be applied, even with small-cell frequencies.[54] Student t tests and likelihood ratio tests were used to assess the likelihood that ecologist-treated and ecologist-untreated subjects were different with respect to continuous and categorical variables, respectively.

Results

Demographic characteristics of the MCS syndrome and general population samples: Females predominated in the general population (75%) and in three of the four MCS syndrome groups (70-90%), whereas males predominated in the organic-solvent-in-industry MCS syndrome group (60%). The mean ages of the MCS syndrome subjects ranged from 42.6 to 51.7 years, and the mean age of the general population was 43.2 years. Professional managerial status predominated in two MCS groups (i.e., SBS onset, 95%; organophosphate-pesticide-onset, 60%) and in the general population (66.7%). Laborer status predominated in the industrial-solvent-onset group (85%) and in the chlorine-dioxide-onset group (100%). Correspondingly, education was highest in the MCS, SBS-onset group (mean=18.1 years); MCS, organophosphate-pesticide-onset group (mean=16.0 years); and general population group (mean: 15.8 years) group. Education was lowest in the MCS, industrial-solvent-onset group (mean=13.5 years) and in the chlorine-dioxide-onset group (mean=11.1 years). Exposure durations before onset of chemical sensitivities ranged from 2.0 to 4.3 years in the three MCS syndrome samples for which data were available. At the time of the evaluation, neither the general population nor chlorine-dioxide-onset MCS syndrome subjects had consulted a clinical ecologist, whereas 30% to 60% of the remaining MCS syndrome subjects had.

General health status: With respect to all health outcomes, negative reports were more characteristic of the MCS syndrome group subjects, compared with subjects in the general population. Whereas only 6.7% of the general population sample considered their health to be "fair" or "poor," 75%-100% of the MCS syndrome samples considered their health to be "fair" or "poor." MCS syndrome subjects did not consider fair to poor health to have always been characteristic of them. Between 80% and 100% of the MCS syndrome subjects felt that their health status had changed, compared with 18.3% of the general population. Consistent with the reports of fair to poor health, 65.0% to 75.0% of the MCS syndrome subjects reported being sick more than 22 hours during the preceding week (i.e., equivalent of being sick for all waking hours in any given 2-day period), compared with 8.3% of the general population subjects. On average, the MCS syndrome subjects reported being sick for 59.2-78.6 waking hours during the preceding week, compared with 9 hours for the general population subjects. Likewise, 85%-100% of MCS syndrome subjects reported more than 9 symptoms each week during the preceding 2 months, compared with 21.7% of the general population. On average, the MCS syndrome subjects reported 17.5-19.7 symptoms at least weekly; the general population reported, on average, 5.6 symptoms weekly. A higher percentage of MCS syndrome subjects (80%-90%) had ever been disabled for more than 3 months, compared with the general population (8.3%), and they experienced limitations on their social lives during much of the time of this study (i.e., MCS = 60%-80%, general population = 2.3%). With respect to all general health and illness status variables, the likelihood ratio tests suggested that the four MCS syndrome groups were not significantly different from one another, but collectively, they were significantly different from the general population sample.

Current health complaints were aggregated into the systems affected, and symptoms that belonged to every category were reported by larger percentages of MCS syndrome subjects than by general population subjects. Systemic, central nervous system (excluding headache), dermatologic, and lower respiratory symptoms were common in MCS syndrome subjects; these symptoms were relatively uncommon in the general population subjects. The symptom categories reported most often by the general population sample were reported much more frequently by the MCS syndrome samples: ear, nose, throat (MCS = 90%-100%, general population=63.3%); headache (MCS: 65-100%; general population: 41.7%); musculoskeletal (MCS = 80%-100%, general population = 31.7%); and gastrointestinal (MCS = 40%-95%, general population = 33.3%). Two symptom categories varied greatly in frequency among the MCS syndrome groups, but occurred rarely in the general population group: genitourinary (MCS = 20%-65%, general population = 1.7%); and circulatory (MCS = 25%-80%, general population = 5.0%). In addition, reports by the MCS and general population groups of physician-diagnosed thyroid conditions (20%-55% and 10%, respectively) and autoimmune conditions (20%-45% and 15%, respectively) were elevated in the three MCS syndrome samples. It should be noted that autoimmune conditions were not defined. Participants were simply asked to specify whether a doctor had ever stated that they had an autoimmune condition. Participants who reported affirmatively were asked to specify the conditions they had been told they had. Except for gastrointestinal disorders and diagnosed autoimmune disorders, likelihood ratio tests suggested that the four MCS syndrome groups were not significantly different from one another. Collectively, the MCS syndrome groups were significantly different from the general population sample on all symptom categories, but not with respect to diagnosed autoimmune disorders.

Changed tolerances: All subjects were asked about changes in tolerance for the following: chemical odors; alcoholic beverages; meals; medications; and after-contact with pollen, dust, molds, mildew, animals, grass, leaves, flowers, and other natural allergens. All four groups of MCS syndrome subjects were much more likely than the members of the general population group to say that two or more tolerances had changed (MCS = 90%-95%, general population = 28.8%). Change in odor tolerance was the most common tolerance change reported by MCS syndrome samples (MCS = 85%-100%, general population = 26.7%). Change in tolerance for allergens was also relatively common for all four MCS syndrome groups (70%-85%), but it was much less common (32.2%) in the general population group. The same trend was obtained for changed tolerances for food (MCS = 60%-90%, general population = 20%); alcohol (MCS = 40%-55%, general population = 8.3%); and medication (MCS = 30%-75%, general population = 13.3%). Without exception, likelihood ratio tests suggested that, in terms of changed tolerances, the four MCS syndrome groups were not significantly different from one another. Collectively, however, the MCS syndrome groups were significantly different from the general population sample.

Chemical sensitivity: Whereas both MCS syndrome and general population subjects were likely to report chemical sensitivities, the MCS syndrome subjects were more likely to attribute illness to chemical exposures on a daily basis (MCS = 70%-80%, general population = 1.7%) and to place recovery from the ill effects of chemical exposures at more than 12 hours from onset (MCS = 45%-60%, general population = 0%). These same trends were noted when we compared the MCS syndrome sample with a subset of the general population. This subset contained individuals who reported at least 6 20-minute-or-less exposures to environmental chemicals, which made them sick. Without exception, the likelihood ratio tests suggested that the four MCS syndrome groups were not significantly different from one another on these indices of illness after chemical exposure. Collectively, however, the MCS syndrome subjects were significantly different from the general population sample with respect to these indices.

Indices of illness following exposures that occurred greater than or equal to 20 minutes were considered relatively sensitive measures of chemical hypersensitivity. The average number of such brief exposures reported to sicken the MCS syndrome subjects ranged from 10.7 to 14.7. The general population subjects reported feeling sick after a mean of 3.8 such brief exposures, and the sensitive subset of the general population reported feeling sick after a mean of 8.9 brief exposures. Eighty to 100% of the MCS syndrome subjects reported that more than 6 chemical exposures of less than 21 minutes duration made them sick, whereas only 20% of the general population sample reported being made sick by more than 6 brief exposures. Between 90% and 100% of the MCS syndrome subjects reported more than four symptoms weekly that they attributed to chemical exposures (general population = 8.3%). On average, MCS syndrome subjects attributed 11.4 to 14.9 symptoms weekly, on average, to chemical exposures, whereas the general population subjects reported such attributions for 1.0 symptoms; the sensitive subset of the general population reported 1.7 such symptoms. The chemically attributed symptoms of 95% to 100% of the MCS syndrome subjects included symptoms in more than two systems, whereas the chemically attributed symptoms of only 8.3% of the general population sample included symptoms in more than two systems. With respect to the general population, an ear-nose-throat (ENT) symptom and headache were the most commonly reported responses to environmental chemicals; for the sensitive subset of the general population, the most commonly reported response to environmental chemicals was also upper respiratory. In addition to reporting multiple ENT symptoms and headache commonly, the MCS syndrome subjects reported experiencing symptoms in five categories frequently: (1) central nervous system, excluding headache; (2) systemic; (3) lower respiratory; (4) musculoskeletal; and (5) gastrointestinal. Without exception, the likelihood ratio tests suggested that the four MCS syndrome groups were not significantly different from one another on these indices of chemical sensitivity. Collectively, however, the MCS syndrome subjects were significantly different from the general population sample on these indices in every instance.

Psychiatric history and status: Evidence of longstanding somatic complaints or complaints of sickliness in childhood—operationalized in terms of frequency of subjects who reported experiencing three or more chronic health conditions before age 18 years—was seen relatively often (15%-55%) in all three MCS syndrome groups that were asked the questions, but was observed rarely (1.7%) in the general population sample. The difference between the collective MCS groups and the general population was significant. It is, nonetheless, noteworthy that one or no chronic health conditions in childhood were reported by the majority of subjects in both the general population sample (58%) and in two of the three MCS syndrome groups (50%-80%).

Periods of unusually intense or long-lasting stress before age 18 years were reported relatively frequently by two samples of MCS syndrome subjects: SBS-onset (50%) and organic-solvent-in-industry-onset (30%) groups. However, with respect to the reporting of intense early life stress, two MCS syndrome samples (i.e., organo-phosphate-pesticide-onset [20%] and chlorine-dioxide-onset [0%] groups) were comparable with, or lower than, the general population sample (18.3%). A similar pattern was seen for reporting of psychiatric problems among family members. In both cases, the likelihood ratio tests suggested that the four MCS syndrome groups were not significantly different from one another at the .05 level, and, collectively, the MCS syndrome groups were not significantly different from the general population sample.

The three samples of subjects interviewed by telephone were asked, "Has a doctor ever treated you for any kind of condition that she considered psychological or psychiatric?" Positive responders were then asked to specify the cause of the condition. A higher percentage of the general population sample (78.3%), compared with the MCS syndrome telephone samples (45-70%), reported never having received psychiatric treatment. However, 15%-45% of the MCS syndrome telephone samples attributed psychiatric treatment to MCS syndrome or to an associated chemical exposure or illness, whereas none of those in the general population did so. In the case of the telephone-interviewed MCS syndrome subjects, we subtracted from the total number of subjects who had received psychiatric treatment the number of subjects who sought help solely for illness from chemical exposures, illness, and hypersensitivity. We then determined the following estimated percentages of subjects who sought psychiatric help for problems unrelated to physical health: 21.7% of the general sample versus 35% of the SBS-onset MCS syndrome group, 5% of the industrial-onset MCS syndrome group, and 10% of the organophosphate-pesticide-onset MCS syndrome group. Forty percent of the chlorine-dioxide-onset MCS syndrome subjects had sought psychiatric help for unrelated problems, whereas 50% had sought help for MCS syndrome or illness and stress secondary to illness and chemical exposure. In terms of psychiatric treatment for reasons unrelated to illness, the different one another. Collectively, the interviewed MCS syndrome groups that were interviewed over the telephone were not significantly different from one another. Collectively, the interviewed MCS syndrome groups were not significantly different from the general population sample.

The PANAS yielded estimates of positive affect and negative affect during the few weeks preceding the survey. Positive affect scores were relatively similar for the general population sample (mean=34.8) and two MCS syndrome groups (i.e., cases of SBS origin [mean=34.1] and organophosphate pesticide origin [mean=32.2). The MCS syndrome subjects in the industrial-solvent- and chlorine-dioxide-onset samples reported less positive affect (means=28.3 and 26.4, respectively). The negative affect scores of the MCS syndrome samples (means=21.4-24.5) were all at least slightly higher than those of the general population sample (mean=18.5). The general population subjects also showed the highest balance of positive to negative affect (mean=16.3), followed by MCS syndrome subjects in the organophosphate-onset (mean=11.9) and SBS-onset groups (mean=10.5). The industrial-solvent-onset group showed the lowest balance of positive to negative affect (mean=3.8).

In seeking further understanding of the trends observed on the PANAS, we calculated Pearson-product moment correlations between the affect scores and selected psychiatric and illness variables for all subjects interviewed over the telephone. Affect scores were not correlated at a statistically significant level with stress during childhood, personal psychiatric history, or familial psychiatric history. All three affect scores (positive affect, negative affect, balance of positive to negative affect) were correlated at a statistically significant level with number of current symptoms experienced weekly and with number of hours sick per week. Negative affect scores and balance of positive-to-negative affect scores were also associated significantly with total chemical sensitivity score.

Clinical ecologist contact and MCS syndrome: Because MCS syndrome is sometimes considered an "invention" of physicians known as clinical ecologists, we examined data on MCS syndrome subjects interviewed by telephone who had and who had not been in contact with a clinical ecologist. We looked for differences between the two groups with respect to selected variables that represented demographics, general health status, changed tolerances, current illness, and chemical sensitivity. Given that the mixed-onset ecologist-treated and -untreated participants were drawn from the same populations, we compared these two groups. There were only two statistically significant differences between the two groups on the variables examined: the ecologist-treated group had more changes in tolerance and more musculoskeletal complaints. The two groups were not differentiated by indicators of general health, illness, and chemical sensitivity, or by mean number of symptoms attributed to chemical exposures that occurred in each system each week during the preceding 2 months.

Discussion

The MCS syndrome participants who reported four different sensitizing exposures were compared, both with one another and with a general population sample, with respect to self-reported health and mental health history and status variables. The MCS syndrome participants were diverse with respect to gender and education, and prevalence of seeking help from a clinical ecologist also differed among the participants. The five questions that were of interest in this study and our discussion of each follow in the paragraphs below.

Do the Self-Reports of Diverse Samples Alleging MCS Syndrome Resemble One Another?

Despite considerable diversity in SES, education, gender, and reporting of sensitizing exposure, the general health status of the MCS syndrome participants was very similar. Generally, they considered their health status to have changed, and they rated their current health status as fair or poor (i.e., lowest ratings on a five-point scale). Most claimed to have been disabled at some time in their lives for 3 months or more, and the majority described limitations regarding socialization with others. On average, MCS syndrome subjects in all four groups reported being ill 59 to 78 hours per week, with 17-20 symptoms. Sickliness before the onset of MCS syndrome, a characteristic of somatization disorder, was reported only by a minority.

Although we expected congruity among diverse MCS syndrome groups with respect to reported health indices of a general nature, we were more surprised to find similarities in reports pertaining to specific health status measures. Reports of diagnosed autoimmune and thyroid conditions tended to be elevated in three of the four MCS syndrome groups; this finding is not explained easily by the psychosomatic or conditioning theories of MCS syndrome.

Reports of changes in tolerance for natural substances (e.g., allergens, foods), as well as for alcohol, medicines, and odors, were elevated by about the same amount in all four MCS syndrome groups, with most affected subjects reporting two or more such changes in tolerance. Such changed tolerances cannot be explained easily by the conditioning hypothesis of MCS syndrome. The assumption of this hypothesis is that MCS syndrome is caused primarily by generalizing a conditioned response from a "sensitizing exposure" to stimuli with similar odors. Allergens and foods have very different types of odors than synthetic chemicals, the most commonly reported sensitizing event. Medicines have very little odor. Whatever MCS syndrome is, our data suggest that it is not merely a change in chemical odor tolerance.

We were also surprised to find that the organ systems implicated in MCS syndrome by all four groups of subjects were quite consistent. More than 60% of the subjects in each group reported symptoms that implicated all of the following: upper and lower respiratory, gastrointestinal, musculoskeletal, central nervous system (excluding headache), and dermatologic systems; and, in addition, systemic symptoms and headache. Effects on the genitourinary and circulatory systems were reported less consistently. In contrast, genitourinary symptoms are among those associated prominently with psychosomatic illnesses.

If MCS syndrome were primarily psychosomatic, we would expect more diverse symptoms and consistent signs of illness before age 18 years. If MCS syndrome were primarily a conditioned syndrome, we would expect (a) intolerance primarily to chemicals that resembles a "sensitizing" exposure; (b) more individuality of symptomatology (i.e., resembling responses to the "sensitizing" exposure); and fewer signs of chronic illness. In our opinion, neither the psychosomatic nor conditioning model can easily explain the consistency in symptoms, changed tolerances, and recovery times from illness related to exposure and elevated prevalences of thyroid and autoimmune conditions. In summary, our data appeared less consistent with currently formulated psychogenic models than with a biogenic model.

Do Members of the General Population Report Chemical Sensitivity? Is the Chemical Sensitivity Reported in MCS Syndrome Similar to That Reported in the General Population?

The sensitivity reported by members of the general population was mild, even in a subset of subjects who appeared to be particularly sensitive. As a group, general population subjects reported that an average of four less-than-21-minute exposures to chemicals functioned as incitants. General population subjects reported a mean of only one upper respiratory symptom in response to chemical exposures per week; the majority reported that they recovered from chemical exposures within 1 hour. Even when we considered the 15 members of the general population who reported that six or more less-than-21-min exposures made them sick, the pattern was similar: for the majority, few symptoms were involved in the response, responses implicated the upper respiratory system, and clearing occurred within 1 hour. Only one subject in the general population sample reported daily responses to chemical incitants.

In contrast, the MCS syndrome subjects reported that an average of at least 10 less-than-21-minute exposures to chemicals functioned as incitants to illness. The majority of MCS syndrome subjects reported daily illness to chemical exposures, and many indicated that recovery from illness occurred during intervals that exceeded 12 hours. In responses occurring weekly, the MCS syndrome subjects implicated 11 or more symptoms that affected a minimum of 5 organ systems; in addition to upper respiratory, lower respiratory, CNS, musculoskeletal, and gastrointestinal systems, systemic symptoms and headache were commonly implicated in weekly symptom reports.

The general population and MCS syndrome subjects also differed substantially in terms of changed tolerance for allergens, odors, foods, and so forth. Although most members of the general population—including the subset of 15 relatively sensitive subjects—tended to report no changes or a single change in tolerance, 90% or more of each MCS syndrome sample reported two or more changes.

These data suggest that although some level of chemical sensitivity is common in the general population, it appears very different from that reported in MCS syndrome.

Is MCS Syndrome Associated with a Particular Type of Psychiatric History or Status?

Striking psychiatric differences between the general population and the MCS syndrome subjects were not observed in this study. The similarities were pronounced. The majority of MCS syndrome and general population subjects did not report potential indicators of psychiatric illness (i.e., having been sickly as children, a familial psychiatric history, intense long-lasting stresses during childhood, and treatment for psychiatric conditions unrelated to chemical exposure). On a standardized test of affect, the majority of general population and MCS syndrome subjects reported that they experienced a similar degree of positive affect.

A minority of MCS syndrome subjects reported elevated indicators of psychiatric disturbance, compared with general population subjects (i.e., having been sickly as children [consistent with both true sickliness and with somatizing], unusually intense stress during childhood, familial psychiatric histories, and personal psychiatric treatment for conditions unrelated to illness). These findings suggest that in a minority of MCS subjects, psychiatric variables may precede the condition. To what extent, if any, they contribute to the expression of MCS syndrome cannot be deduced from the data collected for this study.

The MCS syndrome subjects exceeded the general population subjects consistently on one psychiatric index used in this study: negative affect scores. Results of correlational analyses suggested that the differences between the groups on affect scores were more related to illness than to psychiatric history. Number of hours sick each week and number of symptoms and systems affected weekly were associated negatively with positive affect scores and were associated positively with negative affect scores, whereas positive and negative affect scores were not correlated significantly with psychiatric history or psychiatric status variables. These correlations are consistent with the hypothesis that the psychopathology observed in case studies of MCS syndrome subjects are sequelae of illness, rather than indications of preexisting psychopathology or evidence of psychogenic causation. The finding of significant correlations between indices of illness and positive and negative affect scores is consistent with the results of other studies that have shown high negative affect scores and low positive affect scores to be correlated with health complaints in college students.[55,56] The lower negative affect scores in the chlorine-dioxide-onset group, compared with the organic-solvent-onset group, may be an effect of their older age; negative affect has been shown to decrease with age.[57] Collectively, these results are supportive of the notions that chronic medical complaints (a) are burdensome, (b) augment negative affect, and (c) decrease positive affect.

Do the Reports of MCS Syndrome Patients of Clinical Ecologists Differ from Reports of Other MCS Syndrome Patients?

Because MCS syndrome is sometimes considered a figment of the clinical ecologist's imagination, we examined reports by MCS syndrome subjects who had and had not been treated by a clinical ecologist. This comparison was restricted to the telephone interview subjects who attributed their sensitivity to either a sick building, organic solvent in industry, or organophosphate pesticide. The ecologist-treated and ecologist-untreated subjects were similar in gender distribution, education, and age. We found only two statistically significant differences between mixed-onset MCS syndrome subjects who had and had not been treated by a clinical ecologist on the variables under study: (1) number of musculoskeletal symptoms attributed to chemical exposure weekly and (2) mean number of changed tolerances. Simple inspection of the data suggested that consistently larger percentages of ecologist-treated subjects (a) reported more illness and more chemical sensitivity, (b) considered their general health to be fair or poor, (c) reported having been disabled, (d) felt sick more hours each week, and (e) experienced more severe chemical sensitivity outcomes. Psychiatric events did not distinguish ecologist-treated and -untreated MCS syndrome subjects.

The chlorine-dioxide-onset MCS syndrome sample was particularly interesting because of its "naivete." None of the members of this group had been seen by a clinical ecologist. None labeled their health condition MCS syndrome, and none appeared to be aware of media coverage of the condition. Nonetheless, the self-reports of this sample were very similar to those of the ecologist-untreated mixed-onset subjects on indices of general illness, changed tolerances for odors, allergens, foods, alcohol and medicine, number of systems represented in illness episodes after chemical incitants, number of brief-duration incitants, and level of illness ensuing from brief duration incitants.

This finding of overall congruence among diverse samples of ecologist-treated and -untreated MCS syndrome subjects provides evidence that MCS syndrome is not a figment of the clinical ecologists' collective imagination.

Limitations of the Study

The selection methods for recruiting cases and controls were not ideal. The 60 MCS syndrome subjects who reported sensitizing exposures from solvents in industry, SBS, or organophosphate pesticides often originated from the referrals of interested physicians or supportive groups. It is certainly possible that group membership and physicians influenced participants' notions of the condition. This hypothesis was not supported, however, by the congruent data on the chlorine-dioxide-gas-exposed subjects, who were not members of a support group; were not being seen by a sympathetic physician; and did not possess an organizing label, "MCS syndrome." The bias inherent in interviewing volunteers from the general population sample probably worked against finding significant differences between the MCS subjects and the general population (i.e., we suspect that some of our general population subjects may have volunteered because of experiencing some degree of chemical sensitivity). Therefore, the differences that we found were all the more striking. Using a systematic approach, the investigators found demographically different samples of subjects who attributed MCS syndrome to diverse "sensitizing" exposures to be very similar to one another in symptom presentation and health characteristics and to be very different from members of the general population. Understanding of this puzzling syndrome will be advanced greatly by further systematic research that explores the basis for the similarities that we observed.

References

1. Ashford NA, Miller CS. *Chemical exposures: low levels and high stakes*. New York: Van Nostrand Reinhold, 1991.

2. Ad Hoc Committee on Environmental Hypersensitivity Disorders. Report to the Province of Ontario, Canada; 1985.

3. Cullen MR. The worker with multiple chemical sensitivities: an overview. *Occup Med* (State Art Rev) 1987; 2:655-61.

4. Nethercott, JR, Davidoff LL, Curbow B, Abbey H. Multiple chemical sensitivities syndrome: toward a working case definition. *Arch Environ Health* 1993; 48:19-26.

5. Mooser SB. The epidemiology of multiple chemical sensitivities (MCS). *Occup Med* (State Art Rev) 1987; 2:663-68.

6. Tabershaw IR, Cooper WC. Sequelae of acute organic phosphate poisoning. *J Occup Med* 1966; 8:5-20.

7. Gyntelberg F, Vesterhauge S, Fog P, et al. Acquired intolerance to organic solvents and results of vestibular testing. *Am J Ind Med* 1986; 9:363-70.

8. Woods JE, Drawny GM, Morey PR. Office worker perceptions of indoor air quality effects on discomfort and performance. In: Seifert B, Esdorn H, Fischer M, Ruden H, Wegner J (Eds), *Indoor Air '87, Proceedings of the 4th International Conference on Indoor Air Quality and Climate*. Berlin: Institute for Water, Soil, and Air Hygiene; 1987.

9. Bardana EJ, Montanaro A. "Chemically sensitive" patients: avoiding the pitfalls. *J Respir Dis* 1989; 10:32-45.

10. Mygind N, Weeke B. Allergic and non-allergic rhinitis. In: Middleton E (Ed), *Allergy Principles and Practice*. St. Louis, MO: Mosby, 1983; 2nd ed; pp 1101-17.

11. Bell IR, Schwartz GE, Peterson JM, Amend D. Self-reported illness from chemical odors in young adults without clinical syndromes or occupational exposures. *Arch Environ Health* 1993; 48:6-13.

12. Bascom R. *Chemical Hypersensitivity Syndrome Study*. Baltimore, MD: State of Maryland, Department of Environment; 1989.

13. Cullen MR, Cherniack MG, Rosenstock L. Medical progress: occupational medicine. *Ann Intern Med* 1988, 322:675-83.

14. Black DW, Rathe A, Goldstein RB. Environmental illness: a controlled study of 26 subjects with "20th century disease." *JAMA* 1990; 64:3166-70.

15. Bolla-Wilson K, Wilson R, Bleecker ML. Conditioning of physical symptoms after neurotoxic exposure. *J Occup Med* 1988; 30:684-86.

16. Dager SJ, Holland JP, Cowley DS, et al. Panic disorder precipitated by exposure to organic solvents in the work place. *Am J Psychiatry* 1987; 144:1056 58.

17. Rosenberg SJ, Freedman MR, Schmaling KB, Rose C. Personality styles of patients asserting environmental illness. *J Occup Med* 1990; 32:678-81.

18. Schottenfeld RS, Cullen MR. Occupation induced post-traumatic stress disorders. *Am J Psychiatry* 1985; 142:198-202.

19. Schusterman D, Balmes J, Cone J. Behavioral sensitization to irritants/odorants after acute overexposures. *J Occup Med* 1988; 30:565-567.

20. Simon GE, Katon WJ, Sparks PJ. Allergic to life: psychological factors in environmental illness. *Am J Psychiatr* 1990; 147:901-06.

21. Staudenmayer HS, Selner JC. Neuropsychophysiology during relaxation in generalized universal "allergic" reactivity to the environment: a comparison study. *J Psychosomat Res* 1990; 34: 259-70.

22. Stewart DE, Raskin J. Psychiatric assessment of patients with "20th century disease" ("total allergy syndrome"). *Can Med Assoc J* 1985; 133:1001-06.

23. Terr Al. Environmental illness: a clinical review of 50 cases. *Arch Intern Med* 1986; 146:145-49.

24. Terr Al. Clinical ecology in the workplace. *J Occup Med* 1989; 31 :257-61.

25. Black DW, Rathe A, Goldstein RB. Measures of distress in 26 "environmentally ill" subjects. *Psychosomatics* 1993; 34:131-38.

26. Brodsky C. "Allergic to everything": a medical subculture. *Psychosomatics* 1983; 24:731 42.

27. Selner JC, Staudenmayer H. The relationship of the environment and food to allergic and psychiatric illness. In: Young SH, Rubin JM, Daman HR (Eds), *Psychobiological Aspects of Allergic Disorders*. New York: Praeger, 1986; pp 102-46.

28. Lum LC. Hyperventilation and pseudo-allergic reactions In: Dukor P, Kallos P, Schlumberger HD, West GB (Eds), *Idiopathic, Food-Induced and Drug-Induced Pseudo-Allergic Reactions. Vol 4: Involvement of Drugs and Chemicals*. Basel, Switzerland: Karger, 1985; pp 106-19.

29. Kahn E, Letz G. Clinical ecology: environmental medicine or unsubstantiated theory? *Ann Intern Med* 1989; 111:104-05.

30. Salvaggio JE. Clinical and immunological approach to patients with alleged environmental injury. *Ann Allergy* 1991; 66:493-503.

31. Bell IR. Neuropsychiatric and biopsychosocial mechanisms in multiple chemical sensitivity: an olfactory-limbic system model. In: Board of Environmental Studies and Toxicology, Commission on Life Sciences, National Research Council. *Multiple Chemical Sensitivities*. Washington, DC: National Academy Press, 1992; pp 89-108.

32. Meggs WJ, Cleveland CH Jr. Rhinolaryngoscopic examination of patients with multiple chemical sensitivity. *Arch Environ Health* 1993, 48:14-18.

33. Broughton A, Thrasher JD, Madison R. Chronic health effects and immunological alterations associated with exposures to pesticides. Comments *Toxicol* 1990; 4(1):59-71.

34. Broughton A, Thrasher JD, Gard Z. Immunological evaluation of four arc welders exposed to fumes from ignited polyurethane (isocyanate) foam: antibodies and immune profiles. *Am J Ind Med* 1988, 13 :463-72.

35. Broughton A, Thrasher JD. Antibodies and altered cell mediated immunity in formaldehyde exposed humans. Comments *Toxicol* 1988, 2:155-74.

36. Galland L. Biochemical abnormalities in patients with multiple chemical sensitivities. *Occup Med* (State Art Rev) 1987; 2:713-20.

37. Levin AS, Byers VS. Environmental illness: a disorder of immune regulation. *Occup Med* (State Art Rev) 1987; 2:669-81.

38. McConnachie PR, Zahalsky AC. Immununological consequences of exposure to pentachlorophenol. *Arch Environ Health* 1991; 46:249-53.

39. Doty RL, Deems DA, Frye RE, Pelberg R, Shapiro A. Olfactory sensitivity, nasal resistance, and autonomic function in patients with multiple chemical sensitivities. *Arch Otolaryngol Head Neck Surg* 1988; 114:1422-27.

40. Thrasher JD, Broughton A, Micevich P. Antibodies and immune profiles of individuals occupationally exposed to formaldehyde: six case reports. *Am J Ind Med* 1988; 14:479-88.

41. Thrasher JD, Madison R, Broughton A, Gard Z. Building-related illness and antibodies to albumin conjugates of formaldehyde, toluene diisocyanate and trimellitic anhydride. *Am J Ind Med* 1989; 15:187-95.

42. Thrasher JD, Wojdani A, Heuser G, Cheung G. Evidence for formaldehyde antibodies and altered cellular immunity in subjects exposed to formaldehyde in mobile homes. *Arch Environ Health* 1987; 42:347-50.

43. Thrasher JD, Broughton A, Madison R. Immune activation and autoantibodies in long-term inhalation to formaldehyde. *Arch Environ Health* 1990; 45(4):217-23.

44. Truss CO. Metabolic abnormalities in patients with chronic Candidiasis. *J Orthomol Psychiatr* 1984; 13:66-93.

45. Ryan CM. Morrow LM, Hodgson M. Cacosmia and neuro-behavioral dysfunction associated with occupational exposure to mixtures of organic solvents. *Am J Psychiatry* 1988; 145:1442-45.

46. McGovern JJ Jr, Lazaroni JA, Hicks MF, Adler JC, Cleary R. Food and chemical sensitivity: clinical and immunologic corre-lates. *Arch Otolaryngol* 1983; 109:292-97.

47. Heuser G, Wojdani A, Heuser S. Diagnostic markers of mul-tiple chemical sensitivity. In: Board on Environmental Studies and Toxicology, Commission on Life Sciences, National Re-search Council. *Multiple Chemical Sensitivities: Addendum to Biologic Markers in Immunotoxicology* Washington, DC: Na-tional Academy Press, 1992; pp 117-38.

48. Callender TJ. Metabolic brain imaging abnormalities in chemically exposed individuals who developed multiple chemical sensitivity syndrome or chronic fatigue syndrome. Paper presented at the 119th Annual Meeting of the American Public Health Association Atlanta, Georgia, November 10-14, 1991. (Session on multiple chemical sensitivity and the envi-ronment. II. Diagnosis and therapy.)

49. Morrow LA, Steinhauer SR, Robin N, Hodgson MJ, Tortora S, Baber S. Neurophysiological and neuropsychological impair-ment following chemical exposure. Paper presented to the In-ternational Neuropsychological Society, San Antonio; 1991.

50. Rea WJ. Study of 100 consecutive patients admitted to the en-vironmental control unit at Northeast Community Hospital in Bedford Texas. Unpublished. Cited in Rea WJ. *Chemical Sen-sitivity* (vols 14). Boca Raton, FL: Lewis Publishers, 1992.

51. Cone JE, Harrison R, Reiter R. Patients with multiple chemi-cal sensitivities: clinical diagnostic subsets among an occupa-tional health clinic population. *Occup Med* (State Art Rev) 1987; 2:721-38.

52. Cone JE, Sult TA. Acquired intolerance to solvents following pesticide/solvent exposure in a building: a new group of workers at risk for multiple chemical sensitivities? *Toxicol Ind Health* 1992; 8:29 40.

53. Watson D, Clark LA, Tellegen A. Development and validation of brief measures of positive and negative affect: the PANAS Scales. *J Person Social Psychol* 1988; 54:1063-70.

54. Rothman KJ. *Modern Epidemiology*. Boston, MA: Little, Brown; 1986.

55. Clark LA, Watson D. Mood and the mundane: relations between daily life events and self-reported mood. *J Person Soc Psychol* 1988; 54:296-308.

56. Watson D. Intraindividual and interindividual analyses of positive and negative affect: their relation to health complaints, perceived stress, and daily activities. *J Person Soc Psychol* 1988; 54:1020-30.

57. Staats S. Variations in expected affect in young and middle-aged adults. *J Genetic Psychol* 1990; 151:429-38.

This study was supported, in part, by grant ES03819 from the National Institute for Environmental Health Sciences and by grant OH07090 from the National Institute of Occupational Safety and Health.

Financial assistance in support of this project was provided, in part, by the Johns Hopkins University Center for Occupational and Environmental Health.

Submitted for publication January 12, 1995; revised; accepted for publication October 5, 1995.

Section 15.3

MCS: Government Findings and Recommendations

Excerpted from *A Report on Multiple Chemical Sensitivity (MCS)*, The Interagency Workgroup on Multiple Chemical Sensitivity, Predecisional Draft, National Institute for Environmental Health Sciences, National Institutes of Health, August 24, 1998.

Overview

The public's concern about chemical exposures has historical origins. Many substances that brought great benefits were later found to have long-term risks. Substances such as lead and asbestos were widely used, and their hazards were only slowly identified. The first recognition of concerns usually occurred in highly exposed populations—frequently in occupational settings—among those with readily definable clinical illnesses. For example, the carcinogenic properties of benzene were first identified by the disproportionate occurrence of acute leukemia among persons in certain occupations.

Populations with particular susceptibilities, especially children, have also served to alert public health officials to the dangers of certain chemical exposures. The hazards associated with exposure to leaded paint were first dramatized by clear signs of poisoning in young children who had high levels of exposure because they had eaten paint chips. Now, after decades of use and widespread environmental contamination, the effects of low doses of lead on children are widely recognized. The health of the public as a whole depends on the vigilant monitoring of such emerging diseases and disabilities, regardless of the extent to which medical science is able to explain their origin.

It is appropriate for public health leadership to work to mitigate illness in persons with disorders that are not yet fully explainable. In so doing, it must be recognized that chemical agents found to be noxious by a significant portion of the population may, and often do, present public health hazards that lead to health concerns such as MCS.

150

Because of the concern for the health and well-being of persons with symptoms of MCS and because MCS presents challenging policy issues, several Federal agencies formed a workgroup in 1995 to review the key scientific literature pertinent to MCS, consider the recommendations from various expert panels on MCS, review past federal actions, and develop technical and policy recommendations.

It is currently unknown whether MCS is a distinct disease entity and what role, if any, the biochemical mechanisms of specific chemicals have in the onset of this condition. The workgroup finds that MCS is currently a symptom-based diagnosis without supportive laboratory tests or agreed-upon clinical manifestations. This dependence on symptom-based diagnosis has resulted in the absence of a uniformly agreed-upon case definition. The workgroup could locate no previously published reports of definite end-organ damage attributable to MCS. However, scientific knowledge changes over time as additional findings are reported; it is therefore important not to lose sight of lessons from the past in which suspected health effects of environmental exposures were verified at a later date through scientific research. A summary of specific findings follows.

Summary Findings

- No single accepted case definition of MCS has been established; proposed definitions all differ in key criteria, and some definitions suggest a broad spectrum of possible symptoms. The validated epidemiologic data required to clarify the natural history, etiology, and diagnosis of MCS are not available.

- Several limitations are found in the design of many published MCS studies. Outcome measures in some studies may be influenced by bias in subject selection, lack of investigator blinding during patient assessment, and inconsistent quality assurance of laboratory determinations. Certain outcome measures (e.g., functional imaging techniques) are investigative research tools and need validation by additional studies.

- The workgroup finds that there are few data on the prevalence of MCS. Only three studies have reported the prevalence of self-reported physician-diagnosed MCS. The prevalence of self-reported physician-diagnosed MCS ranges from published values of 0.2 percent in college students to 4.0 percent in elderly persons and an unpublished value of 6 percent among randomly selected California residents.

- The amount of ongoing MCS-specific research conducted or otherwise supported by the Federal Government is confined to a limited effort by the National Institutes of Health, National Institute of Environmental Health Sciences (NIEHS). Other than the workgroup on MCS, there appears to be no other Federal Government group convened expressly to examine MCS as a medical entity of relevance to occupational and environmental health. Although there is ancillary research at NIEHS, the Department of Veterans Affairs (DVA), and the U.S. Environmental Protection Agency (EPA) concerning the potential relevance of advancing the scientific database on MCS, no federal effort formulates and oversees a collaborative MCS research plan.

- The major recommendations from several expert workshops held since 1990 are still appropriate. These recommendations, if addressed, should advance the public health response to the public's concerns about MCS.

- Information on the fiscal cost of MCS to society is scarce. The fiscal outlay required for or involved in medical diagnosis and treatment of MCS needs additional study.

- Only limited efforts are being made within federal health and environmental agencies to communicate to healthcare providers what is known and not known about MCS; these efforts are primarily being made by the Agency for Toxic Substances and Disease Registry (ATSDR). This lack of education for healthcare providers is accompanied by increasing public concern about MCS.

- Numerous therapies aimed at treating MCS have been identified in the literature; however, no widely accepted protocols are proven to be effective in addressing MCS symptomatology. Therapeutic interventions that claim to effectively address or minimize these impacts need objective study and validation.

- While study and validation of therapeutic interventions continue, the goal of patient care should be to promote health without causing harm.

MCS as a Public Health Priority

The workgroup was aware of the many demands placed on Federal agencies to protect the environment and the public's health. The pressure of constrained budgets and tight personnel ceilings makes it essential that agencies carefully weigh and prioritize research and protective actions directed toward an imposing list of environmental problems.

The workgroup feels compelled, therefore, to comment on MCS in the context of its priority as a national environmental health problem. Three primary circumstances usually characterize an environmental health issue as being of high priority. First, compelling findings from epidemiologic investigations or surveillance systems can portend consequential health problems in human populations. An example is the identification of the nature and extent of lead toxicity in young children through careful epidemiologic investigations. Second, a priority environmental health problem can be identified through clinical reports verified by the medical community. For example, clinical reports of pesticide poisonings helped shape the understanding that contact with certain pesticides can place pesticide applicators at risk. Third, compelling findings from basic biomedical research may identify mechanisms of action that can translate into human health implications. An example is the basic research on the effects of endocrine disrupters and the implications for human reproductive and developmental health. The workgroup commends these criteria for use in developing a strategic plan for MCS.

The workgroup concludes that the subject of MCS is unlikely to receive extensive research support as a single entity. Personnel and budgetary resources are constrained, and Federal agencies are attempting concurrently to evaluate a variety of syndromes that can have disabling symptoms but lack objective clinical or laboratory evidence of disease. Examples include CFS [chronic fatigue syndrome], fibromyalgia, and Persian Gulf War-related illnesses, and diseases diagnosed as chronic subclinical infections.

The workgroup identified the need for an overall strategic plan for these syndromes, including MCS, because of scientific uncertainties and unclear public health relevance that attend each syndrome. The strategic plan should articulate the goals and objectives of the research effort, offer guidance on the priorities and sequence for studies, present the critical elements of study design, and reflect on appropriate resource levels. Those involved in the strategic planning process for research should have a broad range of knowledge and experience and represent a variety of scientific disciplines. Public input should be a vital component of this process.

The workgroup determined that the strategic plan should consider the following recommendations with regard to MCS research:

Research Recommendations for Consideration

- Comprehensive biomedical and clinical research is necessary for a consensus case definition of MCS that can be used in epidemiologic studies and clinical evaluations. This research needs to include the study of individual MCS patients under controlled conditions. The workgroup encourages a directed effort in this area, recognizing that this issue is a matter of policy as well as an issue of research.

- Data on the prevalence of MCS and disability related to MCS remain a key requisite for a more informed prioritization of MCS-directed resources. The workgroup emphasizes the need for data from representative populations selected by valid epidemiologic methods.

- Data on the role of psychosocial factors in MCS need to be gathered. The tools used to obtain this information should be standardized and validated through the use of reference populations, including those with well-established illnesses (e.g., allergies, asthma, porphyria, and pesticide-related illnesses) known or reported to be associated with susceptibility to chemical exposures. Carefully designed studies should be planned to evaluate both the primary and secondary psychological factors in MCS.

- A targeted effort in basic research is needed to explore pathophysiologic mechanisms that might be associated with MCS. The development and refinement of animal models that could help identify biomarkers of susceptibility in humans is particularly important.

- MCS-related research on biomarkers should be directed as quickly as possible toward validation studies in humans. The populations chosen for such studies should have defined health endpoints, including MCS and other conditions (e.g., asthma and autoimmune disorders) in which chemical exposures are suspected contributors.

- Well-coordinated, multicenter studies are encouraged to detect or exclude the subtle effects that may be associated with low exposures and idiosyncratic reactions. Blinded assessment, testable hypotheses, and objective outcome measures are essential to control for experimenter bias. Federal support for MCS-related clinical research will require stringent quality assurance of all tests under study and ongoing review of results by an independent board, such as those established for therapeutic trials.

- Until a consensus case definition is developed, the case definition of MCS used in research studies should be fully operational that is, it must be described in sufficient detail to be reproducible by other investigators seeking to conform or extend published findings.

- Consideration should be given to conducting a project that collects data on MCS-relevant health costs from sources such as states' workers compensation databases, private insurance records, and federal and state health-care programs.

- A process of obtaining direct public input on the research and policy agenda for MCS and enabling public participation in MCS decision making should be established. The workgroup supports the framework for stakeholder involvement developed by the Presidential/Congressional Commission on Risk Assessment and Risk Management (1997). The framework encourages appropriate and feasible stakeholder involvement during all stages of the risk management process. The framework would equally apply to stakeholder involvement in MCS decision making.

- Because there are no widely accepted protocols that have proven to be effective in treating MCS, the therapeutic interventions claimed to be effective need objective study and validation.

- A cross-agency evaluation of federal granting mechanisms should be conducted to ensure that research review systems are appropriate to support basic and applied research on MCS.

Policy Recommendations for Consideration

The scientific literature is currently inadequate to enable determination of the associations between human exposure(s) to chemicals in the environment and the development or exacerbation of MCS. Targeted research would reduce this uncertainty. Increased scientific knowledge about MCS and the role of environmental chemicals will inevitably be put into the context of benefits and risk.

Virtually all chemicals in use convey both benefits and risks. Every technology, no matter how beneficial, can exert a negative impact on some sector(s) of society. Many chemicals have well-established

155

toxicologic and allergenic properties; undoubtedly, others will be found to have adverse effects in the future. Public health leaders and other risk managers have an obligation to ensure that the benefits of technologies justify the risks. The public health vision is health for the entire population. The reality of public health will always involve balancing maximum benefit and minimum harm to the public's health and well-being. Risk managers faced with decisions regarding MCS are offered the following policy recommendations by the workgroup:

- Because of the public health issues and challenges presented by MCS, it is recommended that phased efforts be initiated to conduct the targeted research described in the previous section. A phased approach would make the greatest use of available resources, and at the same time, answer key questions such as prevalence and basic mechanisms of action that would guide follow-up research.

- There is a need to better inform the healthcare community about MCS. Health agencies should consider a focused, limited effort in clinician education and awareness.

- Persons should not be offered ineffective, costly, or potentially dangerous treatments. Appropriate care for well-characterized medical and psychological illnesses should not be withheld or delayed. The ramifications of recommending functional changes in workplace or home settings should be considered carefully. Persons identified as having MCS also need education about what is known and not known about MCS.

- There is need for a continuing effort in interagency coordination, whether through the workgroup or a successor group.

- An overall strategic plan for MCS and related syndromes is needed. The strategic plan should articulate the research effort and offer guidance on communication and education of health care providers and persons experiencing symptoms of MCS.

- The Environmental Health Policy Committee of the Department of Health and Human Services appears to be an appropriate body for overseeing the development of an improved science database on MCS and attendant public health responses.

Chapter 16

Ménière's Disease and Allergies

Little is known about the cause of Ménière's disease, an idiopathic hearing disorder characterized by vertigo, nausea, vomiting, tinnitus, and progressive hearing loss that usually begins between the ages of 20 and 50. Previous research has suggested trauma, viral infections, and autoimmune factors are to blame.

New research presented at the annual meeting of the American Academy of Otolaryngology—Head and Neck Surgery Foundation, in New Orleans, LA, suggests the inner ear may be a target of an allergic reaction that produces the symptoms of this disabling disorder.

Researchers mailed surveys to 1,490 clinic patients diagnosed with Ménière's disease; 734 responded to the survey. Of that number, 42 percent reported having airborne allergies. By comparison, in a control group of 172 randomly-selected adults who visited the same clinic for other otologic disorders, 28 percent had airborne allergies, and typically reported airborne allergy incidence rates range between 14 percent and 20 percent.

In addition, 18 percent of the Ménière's disease patients suspected airborne allergies, compared to 15 percent in the control group. Forty percent had known or suspected food allergies compared to 25 percent of controls.

From "DG DISPATCH—AAO: Allergies May Be Culprit In Disabling Inner Ear Disorder," by Andrew Bowser, September 30, 1999. © 1999 P\S\L Consulting Group. Reprinted by permission. *Doctor's Guide to the Internet* is at http://www.docguide.com.

Ménière's disease patients most commonly reported nasal or sinus congestion (67.8 percent), itching (48.7 percent), runny nose (47.7 percent), and excessive fatigue (39.3 percent).

Dr. M. Jennifer Derebery, of the House Ear Institute in Los Angeles, CA., suggested that Ménière's disease patients might experience a dramatic reduction in severity of ear symptoms when treated with an allergy medication or if they eliminate certain dietary products believed to impact ear problems, such as wheat, milk, corn, eggs, yeast and soy.

Part Three

Food Allergies and Intolerances

Chapter 17

Understanding Food Allergy

Allergies affect the lives of millions of people around the world. Fresh spring flowers, a friend's cat or dog, even the presence of dust can make people itch, sneeze, and scratch almost uncontrollably. But what about that seemingly innocent peanut butter sandwich, glass of milk, or fish fillet?

Almost two percent of Americans have an allergy to these or other foods. Food allergies can be life threatening. Knowledge about food allergies can help save a life.

What is a food allergy?

Food allergy is a reaction of the body's immune system to something in a food or an ingredient in a food—usually a protein. It can be a serious condition and should be diagnosed by a board-certified allergist. A true food allergy (also called "food hypersensitivity") and its symptoms can take many forms.

Which foods cause food allergy?

The eight most common food allergens—milk, eggs, peanuts, tree nuts, soy, wheat, fish and shellfish—cause more than 90 percent of

all food allergic reactions. However, many other foods have been identified as allergens for some people.

What are the symptoms of food allergy?

Symptoms of food allergy differ greatly among individuals. They
can also differ in the same person during different exposures. Allergic reactions to food can vary in severity, time of onset, and may be
affected by when the food was eaten.

Common symptoms of food allergy include skin irritations such as
rashes, hives and eczema, and gastrointestinal symptoms such as
nausea, diarrhea, and vomiting. Sneezing, runny nose, and shortness
of breath can also result from food allergy. Some individuals may experience a more severe reaction called anaphylaxis.

What is anaphylaxis?

Anaphylaxis is a rare but potentially fatal condition in which several different parts of the body experience allergic reactions. These
may include itching, hives, swelling of the throat, difficulty breathing, lower blood pressure, and unconsciousness.

Symptoms usually appear rapidly, sometimes within minutes of
exposure to the allergen, and can be life threatening. Immediate
medical attention is necessary when anaphylaxis occurs. Standard
emergency treatment often includes an injection of epinephrine
(adrenaline) to open up the airway and blood vessels.

Do I have a food allergy?

Of all the individuals who have any type of food sensitivity, most
have food intolerances. Fewer people have true food allergy involving the immune system. According to the National Institutes of
Health, approximately 5 million Americans, (5 to 8% of children and
1 to 2% of adults) have a true food allergy.

What are other reactions or sensitivities to foods called?

Other reactions to foods are called food intolerance and food idiosyncrasy. Food intolerance and food idiosyncrasy reactions are generally localized, temporary, and rarely life threatening, whereas food
allergy can cause life-threatening reactions.

Food intolerance is an adverse reaction to a food substance or additive that involves digestion or metabolism (breakdown of food by

the body) but does not involve the immune system. Lactose intolerance is an example of food intolerance. It occurs when a person lacks an enzyme needed to digest milk sugar. If a person who is lactose intolerant eats milk products, they may experience symptoms such as gas, bloating, and abdominal pain.

Food idiosyncrasy is an abnormal response to a food or food substance. The reaction can resemble or differ from symptoms of true food allergy. Idiosyncratic reactions to food do not involve the immune system. Sulfite sensitivity or sulfite-induced asthma is an example of a food idiosyncrasy that affects small numbers of people in the population. However, sulfite-induced asthma can be potentially life threatening.

Other suspected adverse reactions to foods such as to corn, high fructose corn syrup, and sugar have rarely been demonstrated as true food allergies. Some foods contain a variety of either naturally occurring or added components that can cause a chemical, or drug-like reaction. The "burning" sensation when eating foods like chili peppers is an example of a chemical food reaction.

What should I do if I believe I have an adverse reaction to a certain food?

You should see a board-certified allergist to get a diagnosis. An allergist and dietitian can best help the food-allergic patient manage diet issues with little sacrifice to nutrition or the pleasure of eating.

Making a diagnosis may include:

- A thorough medical history;

- The analysis of a food diary; and

- Several tests including skin-prick tests, RAST tests (blood test), and food challenges (using different foods to test for allergic reactions).

Once a diagnosis is complete, an allergist will help set up a response plan to manage allergic reactions that may occur. A response plan may include taking medication by injection to control allergic reactions.

Am I allergic to food additives?

Probably not. Misconceptions abound regarding allergy to food additives and preservatives. Although some food components have been shown to trigger asthma or hives in certain people, these reactions are not the same as those observed with food.

Many of these additives, including aspartame, monosodium glutamate, and several food dyes have been studied extensively. Scientific evidence shows that they do not cause allergic reactions.

What important information should I and my friends and family know?

Because food allergy can be life threatening, the allergy-producing food must be completely avoided. If you, or someone else, are experiencing a severe food allergic reaction, call 911 (or an ambulance) immediately and execute your response plan.

Most life-threatening allergic reactions to foods occur when eating away from the home. It is important to explain your situation and needs clearly to your host or food server. If necessary, ask to speak with the chef or manager.

The Food and Drug Administration (FDA) requires that ingredients are listed on most food labels. Be sure to look at the listings on labels to determine the presence of the eight major allergens. Since food and beverage manufacturers are continually making improvements, food-allergic persons should read the food label for every product purchased, each time it is purchased.

Many different foods can cause food allergic reactions. However, most reactions to foods are not food allergies but some other type of food sensitivity.

Food sensitivities may be a...

- food allergy,

- food intolerance, or

- food idiosyncrasy.

The eight most common food allergens are milk, eggs, peanuts, tree nuts, soy, wheat, fish, and shellfish.

If you, or someone else, are having a serious allergic reaction to a food... CALL 911! (or call an ambulance).

Chapter 18

Food Allergy and Intolerances

Food allergies or food intolerances affect nearly everyone at some point. People often have an unpleasant reaction to something they ate and wonder if they have a food allergy. One out of three people either say that they have a food allergy or that they modify the family diet because a family member is suspected of having a food allergy. But only about three percent of children have clinically proven allergic reactions to foods. In adults, the prevalence of food allergy drops to about one percent of the total population.

This difference between the clinically proven prevalence of food allergy and the public perception of the problem is in part due to reactions called "food intolerances" rather than food allergies. A food allergy, or hypersensitivity, is an abnormal response to a food that is triggered by the immune system. The immune system is not responsible for the symptoms of a food intolerance, even though these symptoms can resemble those of a food allergy.

It is extremely important for people who have true food allergies to identify them and prevent allergic reactions to food because these reactions can cause devastating illness and, in some cases, be fatal.

"Food Allergy and Intolerances," a fact sheet produced by the National Institute of Allergy and Infectious Diseases (NIAID), January 1999, updated January 19, 2000. Available online at http://www.niaid.nih.gov.

How Allergic Reactions Work

An allergic reaction involves two features of the human immune response. One is the production of immunoglobulin E (IgE), a type of protein called an antibody that circulates through the blood. The other is the mast cell, a specific cell that occurs in all body tissues but is especially common in areas of the body that are typical sites of allergic reactions, including the nose and throat, lungs, skin, and gastrointestinal tract.

The ability of a given individual to form IgE against something as benign as food is an inherited predisposition. Generally, such people come from families in which allergies are common—not necessarily food allergies but perhaps hay fever, asthma, or hives. Someone with two allergic parents is more likely to develop food allergies than someone with one allergic parent.

Before an allergic reaction can occur, a person who is predisposed to form IgE to foods first has to be exposed to the food. As this food is digested, it triggers certain cells to produce specific IgE in large amounts. The IgE is then released and attaches to the surface of mast cells. The next time the person eats that food, it interacts with specific IgE on the surface of the mast cells and triggers the cells to release chemicals such as histamine. Depending upon the tissue in which they are released, these chemicals will cause a person to have various symptoms of food allergy. If the mast cells release chemicals in the ears, nose, and throat, a person may feel an itching in the mouth and may have trouble breathing or swallowing. If the affected mast cells are in the gastrointestinal tract, the person may have abdominal pain or diarrhea. The chemicals released by skin mast cells, in contrast, can prompt hives.

Food allergens (the food fragments responsible for an allergic reaction) are proteins within the food that usually are not broken down by the heat of cooking or by stomach acids or enzymes that digest food. As a result, they survive to cross the gastrointestinal lining, enter the bloodstream, and go to target organs, causing allergic reactions throughout the body.

The complex process of digestion affects the timing and the location of a reaction. If people are allergic to a particular food, for example, they may first experience itching in the mouth as they start to eat the food. After the food is digested in the stomach, abdominal symptoms such as vomiting, diarrhea, or pain may start. When the food allergens enter and travel through the bloodstream, they can cause a drop in blood pressure. As the allergens reach the skin, they can induce hives or eczema, or when they reach the lungs, they may cause asthma. All of this takes place within a few minutes to an hour.

Common Food Allergies

In adults, the most common foods to cause allergic reactions include: shellfish such as shrimp, crayfish, lobster, and crab; peanuts, a legume that is one of the chief foods to cause severe anaphylaxis, a sudden drop in blood pressure that can be fatal if not treated quickly; tree nuts such as walnuts; fish; and eggs.

In children, the pattern is somewhat different. The most common food allergens that cause problems in children are eggs, milk, and peanuts. Adults usually do not lose their allergies, but children can sometimes outgrow them. Children are more likely to outgrow allergies to milk or soy than allergies to peanuts, fish, or shrimp.

The foods that adults or children react to are those foods they eat often. In Japan, for example, rice allergy is more frequent. In Scandinavia, codfish allergy is more common.

Cross Reactivity

If someone has a life-threatening reaction to a certain food, the doctor will counsel the patient to avoid similar foods that might trigger this reaction. For example, if someone has a history of allergy to shrimp, testing will usually show that the person is not only allergic to shrimp but also to crab, lobster, and crayfish as well. This is called cross-reactivity.

Another interesting example of cross-reactivity occurs in people who are highly sensitive to ragweed. During ragweed pollination season, these people sometimes find that when they try to eat melons, particularly cantaloupe, they have itching in their mouth and they simply cannot eat the melon. Similarly, people who have severe birch pollen allergy also may react to the peel of apples. This is called the "oral allergy syndrome."

Differential Diagnoses

A differential diagnosis means distinguishing food allergy from food intolerance or other illnesses. If a patient goes to the doctor's office and says, "I think I have a food allergy," the doctor has to consider the list of other possibilities that may lead to symptoms that could be confused with food allergy.

One possibility is the contamination of foods with microorganisms, such as bacteria, and their products, such as toxins. Contaminated meat sometimes mimics a food reaction when it is really a type of food poisoning.

There are also natural substances, such as histamine, that can occur in foods and stimulate a reaction similar to an allergic reaction. For example, histamine can reach high levels in cheese, some wines, and in certain kinds of fish, particularly tuna and mackerel. In fish, histamine is believed to stem from bacterial contamination, particularly in fish that hasn't been refrigerated properly. If someone eats one of these foods with a high level of histamine, that person may have a reaction that strongly resembles an allergic reaction to food. This reaction is called histamine toxicity.

Another cause of food intolerance that is often confused with a food allergy is lactase deficiency. This most common food intolerance affects at least one out of ten people. Lactase is an enzyme that is in the lining of the gut. This enzyme degrades lactose, which is in milk. If a person does not have enough lactase, the body cannot digest the lactose in most milk products. Instead, the lactose is used by bacteria, gas is formed, and the person experiences bloating, abdominal pain, and sometimes diarrhea. There are a couple of diagnostic tests in which the patient ingests a specific amount of lactose and then the doctor measures the body's response by analyzing a blood sample.

Another type of food intolerance is an adverse reaction to certain products that are added to food to enhance taste, provide color, or protect against the growth of microorganisms. Compounds that are most frequently tied to adverse reactions that can be confused with food allergy are yellow dye number 5, monosodium glutamate, and sulfites. Yellow dye number 5 can cause hives, although rarely. Monosodium glutamate (MSG) is a flavor enhancer, and, when consumed in large amounts, can cause flushing, sensations of warmth, headache, facial pressure, chest pain, or feelings of detachment in some people. These transient reactions occur rapidly after eating large amounts of food to which MSG has been added.

Sulfites can occur naturally in foods or are added to enhance crispness or prevent mold growth. Sulfites in high concentrations sometimes pose problems for people with severe asthma. Sulfites can give off a gas called sulfur dioxide, which the asthmatic inhales while eating the sulfited food. This irritates the lungs and can send an asthmatic into severe bronchospasm, a constriction of the lungs. Such reactions led the U.S. Food and Drug Administration (FDA) to ban sulfites as spray-on preservatives in fresh fruits and vegetables. But they are still used in some foods and are made naturally during the fermentation of wine, for example.

There are several other diseases that share symptoms with food allergies including ulcers and cancers of the gastrointestinal tract. These disorders can be associated with vomiting, diarrhea, or cramping abdominal pain exacerbated by eating.

Gluten intolerance is associated with the disease called gluten-sensitive enteropathy or celiac disease. It is caused by an abnormal immune response to gluten, which is a component of wheat and some other grains.

Some people may have a food intolerance that has a psychological trigger. In selected cases, a careful psychiatric evaluation may identify an unpleasant event in that person's life, often during childhood, tied to eating a particular food. The eating of that food years later, even as an adult, is associated with a rush of unpleasant sensations that can resemble an allergic reaction to food.

Diagnosis

To diagnose food allergy a doctor must first determine if the patient is having an adverse reaction to specific foods. This assessment is made with the help of a detailed patient history, the patient's diet diary, or an elimination diet.

The first of these techniques is the most valuable. The physician sits down with the person suspected of having a food allergy and takes a history to determine if the facts are consistent with a food allergy. The doctor asks such questions as:

- What was the timing of the reaction? Did the reaction come on quickly, usually within an hour after eating the food?

- Was allergy treatment successful? (Antihistamines should relieve hives, for example, if they stem from a food allergy.)

- Is the reaction always associated with a certain food?

- Did anyone else get sick? For example, if the person has eaten fish contaminated with histamine, everyone who ate the fish should be sick. In an allergic reaction, however, only the person allergic to the fish becomes ill.

- How much did the patient eat before experiencing a reaction? The severity of the patient's reaction is sometimes related to the amount of food the patient ate.

- How was the food prepared? Some people will have a violent allergic reaction only to raw or undercooked fish. Complete cooking of the fish destroys those allergens in the fish to which they react. If the fish is cooked thoroughly, they can eat it with no allergic reaction.

- Were other foods ingested at the same time of the allergic reaction? Some foods may delay digestion and thus delay the onset of the allergic reaction.

Sometimes a diagnosis cannot be made solely on the basis of history. In that case, the doctor may ask the patient to go back and keep a record of the contents of each meal and whether he or she had a reaction. This gives more detail from which the doctor and the patient can determine if there is consistency in the reactions.

The next step some doctors use is an elimination diet. Under the doctor's direction, the patient does not eat a food suspected of causing the allergy, like eggs, and substitutes another food, in this case, another source of protein. If the patient removes the food and the symptoms go away, the doctor can almost always make a diagnosis. If the patient then eats the food (under the doctor's direction) and the symptoms come back, then the diagnosis is confirmed. This technique cannot be used, however, if the reactions are severe (in which case the patient should not resume eating the food) or infrequent.

If the patient's history, diet diary, or elimination diet suggests a specific food allergy is likely, the doctor will then use tests that can more objectively measure an allergic response to food. One of these is a scratch skin test, during which a dilute extract of the food is placed on the skin of the forearm or back. This portion of the skin is then scratched with a needle and observed for swelling or redness that would indicate a local allergic reaction. If the scratch test is positive, the patient has IgE on the skin's mast cells that is specific to the food being tested.

Skin tests are rapid, simple, and relatively safe. But a patient can have a positive skin test to a food allergen without experiencing allergic reactions to that food. A doctor diagnoses a food allergy only when a patient has a positive skin test to a specific allergen and the history of these reactions suggests an allergy to the same food.

In some extremely allergic patients who have severe anaphylactic reactions, skin testing cannot be used because it could evoke a dangerous reaction. Skin testing also cannot be done on patients with extensive eczema.

For these patients a doctor may use blood tests such as the RAST and the ELISA. These tests measure the presence of food-specific IgE in the blood of patients. These tests may cost more than skin tests, and results are not available immediately. As with skin testing, positive tests do not necessarily make the diagnosis.

The final method used to objectively diagnose food allergy is double-blind food challenge. This testing has come to be the "gold standard" of allergy testing. Various foods, some of which are suspected of inducing an allergic reaction, are each placed in individual opaque capsules. The patient is asked to swallow a capsule and is then watched to see if a reaction occurs. This process is repeated until all the capsules have been swallowed. In a true double-blind test, the doctor is also "blinded" (the capsules having been made up by some other medical person) so that neither the patient nor the doctor knows which capsule contains the allergen.

The advantage of such a challenge is that if the patient has a reaction only to suspected foods and not to other foods tested, it confirms the diagnosis. Someone with a history of severe reactions, however, cannot be tested this way. In addition, this testing is expensive because it takes a lot of time to perform and multiple food allergies are difficult to evaluate with this procedure.

Consequently, double-blind food challenges are done infrequently. This type of testing is most commonly used when the doctor believes that the reaction a person is describing is not due to a specific food and the doctor wishes to obtain evidence to support this judgment so that additional efforts may be directed at finding the real cause of the reaction.

Exercise-Induced Food Allergy

At least one situation may require more than the simple ingestion of a food allergen to provoke a reaction: exercise-induced food allergy. People who experience this reaction eat a specific food before exercising. As they exercise and their body temperature goes up, they begin to itch, get light-headed, and soon have allergic reactions such as hives or even anaphylaxis. The cure for exercised-induced food allergy is simple—not eating for a couple of hours before exercising.

Treatment

Food allergy is treated by dietary avoidance. Once a patient and the patient's doctor have identified the food to which the patient is sensitive, the food must be removed from the patient's diet. To do this, patients must read lengthy, detailed ingredient lists on each food they are considering eating. Many allergy-producing foods such as peanuts, eggs, and milk, appear in foods one normally would not associate them with. Peanuts, for example, are often used as a protein source and eggs are used in some salad dressings. The FDA requires ingredients in a food to appear on its label. People can avoid most of the things to which they are sensitive if they read food labels carefully and avoid restaurant-prepared foods that might have ingredients to which they are allergic.

In highly allergic people even minuscule amounts of a food allergen (for example, 1/44,000 of a peanut kernel) can prompt an allergic reaction. Other less sensitive people may be able to tolerate small amounts of a food to which they are allergic.

Patients with severe food allergies must be prepared to treat an inadvertent exposure. Even people who know a lot about what they are sensitive to occasionally make a mistake. To protect themselves, people who have had anaphylactic reactions to a food should wear medical alert bracelets or necklaces stating that they have a food allergy and that they are subject to severe reactions. Such people should always carry a syringe of adrenaline (epinephrine), obtained by prescription from their doctors, and be prepared to self-administer it if they think they are getting a food allergic reaction. They should then immediately seek medical help by either calling the rescue squad or by having themselves transported to an emergency room. Anaphylactic allergic reactions can be fatal even when they start off with mild symptoms such as a tingling in the mouth and throat or gastrointestinal discomfort.

Special precautions are warranted with children. Parents and caregivers must know how to protect children from foods to which the children are allergic and how to manage the children if they consume a food to which they are allergic, including the administration of epinephrine. Schools must have plans in place to address any emergency.

There are several medications that a patient can take to relieve food allergy symptoms that are not part of an anaphylactic reaction. These include antihistamines to relieve gastrointestinal symptoms, hives, or sneezing and a runny nose. Bronchodilators can relieve asthma symptoms. These medications are taken after people have inadvertently ingested a food to which they are allergic but are not effective in preventing an allergic reaction when taken prior to eating the food. No medication in any form can be taken before eating a certain food that will reliably prevent an allergic reaction to that food.

There are a few non-approved treatments for food allergies. One involves injections containing small quantities of the food extracts to which the patient is allergic. These shots are given on a regular basis for a long period of time with the aim of "desensitizing" the patient to the food allergen. Researchers have not yet proven that allergy shots relieve food allergies.

Infants and Children

Milk and soy allergies are particularly common in infants and young children. These allergies sometimes do not involve hives and asthma, but rather lead to colic, and perhaps blood in the stool or poor growth. Infants and children are thought to be particularly susceptible to this allergic syndrome because of the immaturity of their immune and digestive systems. Milk or soy allergies in infants can develop within days to months of birth. Sometimes there is a family history of allergies or feeding problems. The clinical picture is one of a very unhappy colicky child who may not sleep well at night. The doctor diagnoses food allergy partly by changing the child's diet. Rarely, food challenge is used.

If the baby is on cow's milk, the doctor may suggest a change to soy formula or exclusive breast milk, if possible. If soy formula causes an allergic reaction, the baby may be placed on an elemental formula. These formulas are processed proteins (basically sugars and amino acids). There are few if any allergens within these materials. The doctor will sometimes prescribe corticosteroids to treat infants with severe food allergies. Fortunately, time usually heals this particular gastrointestinal disease. It tends to resolve within the first few years of life.

Exclusive breastfeeding (excluding all other foods) of infants for the first 6 to 12 months of life is often suggested to avoid milk or soy allergies from developing within that time frame. Such breastfeeding often allows parents to avoid infant-feeding problems, especially if the parents are allergic (and the infant therefore is likely to be allergic). There are some children who are so sensitive to a certain food, however, that if the food is eaten by the mother, sufficient quantities enter the breast milk to cause a food reaction in the child. Mothers sometimes must themselves avoid eating those foods to which the baby is allergic.

There is no conclusive evidence that breastfeeding prevents the development of allergies later in life. It does, however, delay the onset of food allergies by delaying the infant's exposure to those foods that can prompt allergies, and it may avoid altogether those feeding problems seen in infants. By delaying the introduction of solid foods until the infant is 6 months old or older, parents can also prolong the child's allergy-free period.

Controversial Issues

There are several disorders thought by some to be caused by food allergies, but the evidence is currently insufficient or contrary to such claims. It is controversial, for example, whether migraine headaches can be caused by food allergies. There are studies showing that people who are prone to migraines can have their headaches brought on by histamines and other substances in foods. The more difficult issue is whether food allergies actually cause migraines in such people. There is virtually no evidence that most rheumatoid arthritis or osteoarthritis can be made worse by foods, despite claims to the contrary. There is also no evidence that food allergies can cause a disorder called the allergic tension fatigue syndrome, in which people are tired, nervous, and may have problems concentrating, or have headaches.

Cerebral allergy is a term that has been applied to people who have trouble concentrating and have headaches as well as other complaints. This is sometimes attributed to mast cells degranulating in the brain but no other place in the body. There is no evidence that such a scenario can happen, and most doctors do not currently recognize cerebral allergy as a disorder.

Another controversial topic is environmental illness. In a seemingly pristine environment, some people have many non-specific complaints such as problems concentrating or depression. Sometimes this is attributed to small amounts of allergens or toxins in the environment. There is no evidence that such problems are due to food allergies.

Some people believe hyperactivity in children is caused by food allergies. But researchers have found that this behavioral disorder in children is only occasionally associated with food additives, and then only when such additives are consumed in large amounts. There is no evidence that a true food allergy can affect a child's activity except for the proviso that if a child itches and sneezes and wheezes a lot, the child may be miserable and therefore more difficult to guide. Also, children who are on anti-allergy medicines that can cause drowsiness may get sleepy in school or at home.

Controversial Diagnostic Techniques

One controversial diagnostic technique is cytotoxicity testing, in which a food allergen is added to a patient's blood sample. A technician then examines the sample under the microscope to see if white cells in the blood "die." Scientists have evaluated this technique in several studies and have not been found it to effectively diagnose food allergy.

Another controversial approach is called sublingual or, if it is injected under the skin, subcutaneous provocative challenge. In this procedure, dilute food allergen is administered under the tongue of the person who may feel that his or her arthritis, for instance, is due to foods. The technician then asks the patient if the food allergen has aggravated the arthritis symptoms. In clinical studies, researchers have not shown that this procedure can effectively diagnose food allergies.

An immune complex assay is sometimes done on patients suspected of having food allergies to see if there are complexes of certain antibodies bound to the food allergen in the bloodstream. It is said that these immune complexes correlate with food allergies. But the formation of such immune complexes is a normal offshoot of food digestion, and everyone, if tested with a sensitive enough measurement, has them. To date, no one has conclusively shown that this test correlates with allergies to foods.

Another test is the IgG subclass assay, which looks specifically for certain kinds of IgG antibody. Again, there is no evidence that this diagnoses food allergy.

Controversial Treatments

Controversial treatments include putting a dilute solution of a particular food under the tongue about a half hour before the patient eats that food. This is an attempt to "neutralize" the subsequent exposure to the food that the patient believes is harmful. As the results of a carefully conducted clinical study show, this procedure is not effective in preventing an allergic reaction.

Summary

Food allergies are caused by immunologic reactions to foods. There actually are several discrete diseases under this category, and a number of foods that can cause these problems.

After one suspects a food allergy, a medical evaluation is the key to proper management. Treatment is basically avoiding the food(s) after it is identified. People with food allergies should become knowledgeable about allergies and how they are treated, and should work with their physicians.

Chapter 19

Food Allergy Myths and Realities

Do you, or someone you know, shun certain foods because you are "allergic?" Surveys show that nearly one-third of all adults believe they have a food allergy. The following seeks to shed light on such frequently asked questions as: What is a food allergy? How do you know if you have one? What should you do if you have a food allergy? And, if it is not a food allergy, what might it be?

Myth: Lots of people have food allergies.

Reality: "From talking with the public, you might think almost everyone has a food allergy," said Daryl Altman, M.D., Fellow of the American College of Allergy, Asthma and Immunology and researcher at the Allergy Information Services in Long Island, New York. "In surveys, nearly one-in-three American adults indicated he or she was allergic to some food." But in reality, the most conservative estimates indicate two percent of the population in the United States are food allergic. Children are more susceptible than adults to food allergy-up to five percent have some type of food allergy. However, common allergens such as eggs and milk are typically outgrown by age five.

From *Food Insight*, November/December 1997, © 1997 International Food Information Council Foundation (IFIC); reprinted with permission. Write to the International Food Information Council Foundation, 1100 Connecticut Avenue, NW, Suite 430, Washington, DC 20036 or visit http://ificinfo.health.org for more information about food and health.

The eight most common food allergens in people are: Peanuts, tree nuts (for example, almonds, pecans and walnuts), dairy, soy, wheat, eggs, fish, and shellfish (for example, shrimp and crab). Nevertheless, allergies to nearly 175 different types of food have been documented. "These foods are responsible for over 90 percent of serious allergic reactions to food," stated Susan L. Hefle, Ph.D., co-director of the Food Allergy Research and Resource Program at the University of Nebraska-Lincoln.

Myth: A food allergy means I'll just get a runny nose, right?

Reality: No—although food allergy is rare, it is a serious condition and should be diagnosed by a board-certified allergist. Food allergy is a reaction of the body's immune system to a certain component, usually a protein, in a food or ingredient. The reactions can be uncomfortable and mild including vomiting, diarrhea, skin rashes, or runny nose, sneezing, coughing and wheezing, and may occur within hours or days after eating. However, anaphylaxis, a more serious and life-threatening reaction, may occur. Anaphylaxis is a rapidly occurring reaction that often involves hives and swelling, enlarging of the larynx with a choking sensation, wheezing, severe vomiting, diarrhea, and even shock. These symptoms can also occur within minutes, hours, or days. "Food allergic patients should have an anaphylaxis reaction plan worked out ahead of time with their allergist," according to Anne Munoz-Furlong, president and founder of The Food Allergy Network. "The plan should be practiced with family and friends in case of an emergency."

An allergic reaction occurs when a susceptible person is exposed to a specific protein. Because the body perceives this protein (an allergen) as being a threat, it produces a special material—a substance that recognizes allergens—known as Immunoglobulin E (IgE) antibody. A person who has a tendency to develop allergies tends to produce increased amounts of IgE. After the initial exposure to a specific allergen (such as "cat" or "dog" protein) the body reacts to future exposures by creating millions of IgE antibodies. These newly produced IgE antibodies then connect to special blood cells called basophils, and special tissue cells called mast cells. These cells are then "stimulated" to release histamine which causes the allergy symptoms: Itchy watery eyes and nose, scratchy throat, rashes, hives, eczema, and even life-threatening anaphylaxis.

Myth: Any negative reaction to a food is a food allergy.

Reality: Adverse reactions to food can have many causes. If something does not "agree with you," it does not necessarily mean you are

178

allergic to it. Food allergy is a very specific reaction involving the immune system of the body, and it is important to distinguish food allergy from other food sensitivities. Whereas food allergies are rare, food intolerances, which are the other classification of food sensitivities, are more common. Intolerances are reactions to foods or ingredients that do not involve the body's immune system. Intolerance reactions are generally localized, transient, and rarely life threatening with one possible exception—sulfite sensitivity.

"A good example of a food intolerance is lactose intolerance. And, it is extremely important to know the difference between it and a milk allergy," said Robert K. Bush, M.D., University of Wisconsin. He emphasized that, "Whereas lactose intolerance may result in a bloated feeling or flatulence after consuming milk or dairy products, milk allergy can have life-threatening consequences. The milk allergic patient must avoid all milk proteins."

Myth: I think I'm allergic to a food—I just won't eat it, so I don't need to be seen by a doctor.

Reality: Just thinking you are allergic to a food does not mean you have an allergy. To properly diagnose a food allergy or sensitivity the offending substance must be accurately identified. Avoiding a food may deprive you of food choices and important nutrients, and could be dangerous if the allergen is actually different. Diagnosis of a food allergy can be complex, with three major components. The first and most important is involving a board-certified allergist, preferably a food allergy specialist. Second, a history of a specific food causing an allergic reaction is necessary; a food diary can help. Third, an IgE antibodies test, is only useful when combined with the former components, but it does not always pinpoint a food allergy.

Hugh Sampson, M.D., director, Food Allergy Clinic, Mt. Sinai Medical Center, and chair of the American Academy of Allergy, Asthma and Immunology's Adverse Reactions to Foods Committee, emphasized an examination by a board-certified allergist: "Due to many people claiming to have food allergies, many physicians have become "desensitized" to taking their symptoms seriously."

The Double-Blind Placebo-Controlled Food Challenge. This test, considered the "gold standard" for food allergy testing, is performed by a board-certified allergist. The suspected allergen is placed in a capsule or hidden in food, and fed to the patient under strict supervision. Neither the allergist, nor the patient, is aware of which

179

capsule, or food, contains the suspected allergen—hence the name "double-blind." In order for the test to be effective, the patient must also be fed capsules or food which do not contain the allergen to make sure the reaction, if any, being observed is to the allergen and not some other factor—hence the name "placebo-controlled." It is tests of this kind that have enabled allergists to identify the most common allergens, and also to determine what foods, ingredients, and additives do not cause allergic reactions.

Myth: I don't frequently eat food I'm allergic to, so I can eat a little bit for a special occasion.

Reality: Because food allergy can be life threatening, the allergen must be completely avoided—even the most minute amounts. Although an extreme case, a man allergic to shellfish died of anaphylaxis shock after encountering simply the steam from shrimp. It can be fatal to assume a given food environment is safe and not be cautious. A board-certified allergist can help the food allergic patient manage diet issues without sacrificing nutrition or pleasure when eating at and away from home. Since most life-threatening, and sometimes fatal, allergic reactions to foods occur when eating away from home, it is imperative that the food allergic individual or responsible guardian clearly explain the risks of exposure to a certain food or ingredient to food service workers, family, and friends—and always ask before eating.

Myth: With all the ingredients in processed food I can never completely avoid my allergen.

Reality: When purchasing groceries, labels should be read for every product purchased—every time. Although food and beverage manufacturers are often improving and changing their products, changes in ingredients must be listed on ingredient labels.

According to Fred Shank, Ph.D., director of the Center for Food Safety and Applied Nutrition, Food and Drug Administration (FDA), "Foods which contain allergenic substances must be properly labeled or be subject to recall. The FDA supports the activities of independent organizations to inform consumers of these recall activities." The FDA includes on its list of recall substances all eight of the major allergens, so if these substances are present in a food, but not listed on the label, they must be recalled. Additionally, substances which cause non-allergic-based reactions, such as the additives sulfites and tartrazine (FD&AMPC Yellow #5), are on this list. Some individuals have unique sensitivities to these food components which are not allergenic or allergy-causing in nature, but may cause comparably severe reactions.

Sulfiting agents are commonly used to preserve the color of foods, such as dried fruits and vegetables, and to inhibit the growth of microorganisms in fermented foods, like wine. Sulfites can also be found in beer, some fruit drinks, shrimp, and some prepared foods. Although sulfites are safe for the majority of people, for some, they have been found to cause a reaction. For this reason, the FDA requires that when sulfites are added to foods in greater than 10 parts/million (or, 10 sulfite molecules per million molecules) they must be indicated on the label.

Myth: Since I'm allergic to peanuts, I can't eat anything with peanut oil.

Reality: There are many misunderstandings regarding exactly what might stimulate the food allergic reaction. "Virtually all food allergens are proteins," explained Steve L. Taylor, Ph.D., co-director of the Food Allergy Research and Resource Program at the University of Nebraska-Lincoln. "And, the process of refining oil removes the protein which would trigger an allergic reaction." Oils used in processed foods and in cosmetics are highly refined and should pose no problem for the food allergic individual. Yet, caution should be taken with natural, cold pressed, or flavored oils. These oils, as well as oil that has been used to cook peanuts (or another food to which an individual might have an allergy), might contain the protein of the allergen and should be avoided. For example, an individual with a fish allergy should ensure that the oil used to cook his or her food was not first used to fry fish.

Cross contact of foods with those that may present a food allergy problem is poorly understood and not well communicated. Although food processors are well aware of the dangers of cross contact and manage them appropriately, such caution is not always taken in the home, school cafeteria, or restaurant. Although unintentional, the effects can be devastating. For some food allergic individuals, the most minute particle of the allergen can be fatal. Some examples of mishaps that can induce a food allergic reaction include: Plain chocolate brownies are served using the same spatula that was used to serve peanut-containing brownies. French fries are prepared in the same oil used to deep-fry fish.

Myth: I'm allergic to food additives.

Reality: Other common misconceptions regarding food allergy are additives and preservatives. Although some—sulfites and tartrazine— have been shown to trigger asthma or hives in certain people, these reactions do not follow the same pathway observed with food. There are other food additives that have historically been associated with adverse reactions, but because they do not contain proteins or involve the immune system, true allergic pathways cannot be used to explain the reported reactions. In addition, many of these additives, includ- ing monosodium glutamate, aspartame, and most food dyes have been studied extensively, and the results show little scientific evidence exists to suggest they cause any reaction at all.

Myth: "Tell me about my corn allergy."

Reality: There are those suspected food allergies that are so rare that their existence is questioned. The most common of these are corn and chocolate "allergy," and there are several probable explanations for adverse reactions. Even though many people claim to be allergic to them, allergists can rarely demonstrate allergy to corn or choco- late in double-blind, placebo-controlled food challenges.

Corn "allergy" is often associated with a reaction to another aller- genic substance. In some cases soy-allergic individuals may react to products containing corn. Occasionally corn is carried, handled, or stored in the same containers used for soy. Although only minute resi- dues of soy may remain, this can be enough to cause an allergic reac- tion in highly sensitive people.

Chocolate "allergy" is also thought to be extremely rare, and though some are truly chocolate-allergic, most who complain of symptoms have irreproducible reactions. Possibly the reactions are due to an- other ingredient found in the chocolate product being consumed.

Conclusion

Food allergy is certainly nothing to be taken lightly. Although its prevalence appears to be increasing, overreaction, self-diagnosis and incorrect assumptions only lead to skepticism of physicians and food service workers—obviously, a less-than-ideal situation for the truly allergic individual. It is vitally important to leave the diagnosis of a food allergy to a board-certified allergist.

Chapter 20

Manifestations of Food Allergy

Adverse reactions to foods may be toxic or nontoxic.[1] Toxic reactions are not related to individual sensitivity but occur in anyone who ingests a sufficient quantity of tainted food. Examples of toxic reactions include reactions to histamine in scombroid fish poisoning or to bacterial toxins in food poisoning. In contrast, non-toxic adverse reactions to food depend on individual susceptibility and are either non-immune-mediated—i.e., food intolerance (Table 20.1), or immune-mediated—i.e., food allergy. This chapter focuses on the clinical manifestations of food allergy.

Allergic Reactions

Allergic reactions to food are either IgE [immunoglobulin E]-mediated or non-IgE-mediated (Table 20.2). The role of IgE-mediated reactions in food allergy is well established. Persons who are genetically predisposed to atopy [hypersensitive to environmental allergens] produce specific IgE antibodies to certain proteins to which they are exposed.[2] These antibodies bind to mast cells and other cells in body tissues and to basophils circulating in the blood stream. When a food protein is ingested, the IgE recognizes it on the surface of these cells; mediators (e.g., histamine) are released, and symptoms occur. The symptoms of IgE-mediated reactions typically involve the skin, respiratory system, and gastrointestinal tract.[3] The pathogenesis of non-IgE-mediated reactions in food allergy is not as clearly defined, but T cells and macrophages most likely play a role. Illnesses caused by these non-IgE-mediated immunologic responses to food affect the same organ systems that the IgE-mediated forms affect.

Skin

Urticaria. The skin is a common target organ for allergic responses to food. Acute urticaria is characterized by pruritic, transient, erythematous raised lesions, sometimes accompanied by localized swelling (angioedema). Food allergy accounts for up to 20 percent of cases of acute urticaria[4] and is mediated by IgE specific to food protein. Lesions usually occur within one hour after ingestion of or contact with the causal food. Because only 1.4 percent of cases of chronic or persistent urticaria (i.e., lasting more than six weeks) are caused

Table 20.1. Some Conditions Related to Food Intolerance (nonimmunologic adverse reactions to food)

Gastrointestinal disorders	Metabolic disorders
Structural abnormalities: hiatal hernia, pyloric stenosis, Hirschsprung's disease, tracheoesophageal fistula	Galactosemia
	Phenylketonuria
	Pharmacologic-related conditions
Disaccharidase deficiencies: lactase, sucrase-isomaltase complex, glucose-galactose complex	Jitteriness (caffeine)
	Pruritus (histamine)
	Headache (tyramine)
Pancreatic insufficiency: cystic fibrosis	Disorientation (alcohol)
	Psychologic disorders
Gallbladder disease	Neurologic disorders
Peptic ulcer disease	Gustatory rhinitis
Malignancy	Auriculotemporal syndrome (facial flush from tart food)

by food allergy,[5] a search for a causative food in the initial evaluation of this condition is not generally warranted.

Atopic Dermatitis. Atopic dermatitis usually begins in early infancy and is characterized by a typical distribution (face, scalp, and extremities), extreme pruritus, and a chronic and relapsing course. This inflammatory skin condition is frequently associated with allergic disorders (e.g., asthma and allergic rhinitis) and with a family history of allergy.[6] Evidence suggests that IgE-mediated food allergy plays a pathogenic role in atopic dermatitis, particularly in children,[6] although non-IgE-mediated food allergy has also been implicated.[7] Clinical studies using double-blind, placebo-controlled food challenges have shown that 37 percent of children with moderate atopic dermatitis have food allergy.[8] By contrast, 6 to 8 percent of infants and children in the general population are allergic to some type of food.[9]

Table 20.2. Food Allergy: Target Organs and Disorders

Target organ	IgE-mediated disorder
Skin	Urticaria and angioedema Atopic dermatitis
Gastrointestinal tract	Oral allergy syndrome Gastrointestinal "anaphylaxis" Allergic eosinophilic gastroenteritis
Respiratory tract	Asthma Allergic rhinitis
Multisystem	Food-induced anaphylaxis Food-associated, exercise-induced anaphylaxis
Target organ	Non-IgE-mediated disorder
Skin	Atopic dermatitis Dermatitis herpetiformis
Gastrointestinal tract	Proctocolitis Enterocolitis Allergic eosinophilic gastroenteritis Enteropathy syndrome Celiac disease
Respiratory tract	Heiner syndrome

Dermatitis Herpetiformis. Dermatitis herpetiformis is a chronic papulovesicular skin disorder in which lesions are distributed over the extensor surfaces of the elbows, knees and buttocks.[10] The disorder is associated with a specific non-IgE-mediated immune sensitivity to gluten (a protein found in wheat, barley, oat and rye). Although dermatitis herpetiformis is related to celiac disease, patients often appear to have no associated gastrointestinal problems. The rash abates with the elimination of gluten from the diet.

Gastrointestinal Tract

The gastrointestinal tract is another common target organ for IgE-mediated reactions to foods. Symptoms of gastrointestinal "anaphylaxis" occur shortly after the ingestion of an implicated food and include nausea, vomiting, abdominal pain and diarrhea.

Oral Allergy Syndrome. The oral allergy syndrome is characterized by pruritus and edema of the oral mucosa occurring after the ingestion of certain fresh fruits and vegetables.[11] The symptoms rarely progress beyond the mouth. The reaction occurs primarily in patients with allergic sensitivity to pollens and is caused by IgE antibodies directed toward cross-reacting proteins found in pollens, fruits and vegetables.[11] Patients with birch-pollen hay fever may have symptoms of oral allergy syndrome after ingesting hazelnut, apple, carrot, and celery, whereas patients with IgE sensitivity to ragweed pollen may react to melons (e.g., watermelon or cantaloupe) and banana. Interestingly, patients are usually able to ingest cooked forms of the foods without symptoms because the responsible allergens are destroyed in the heating process. It is crucial to differentiate the symptoms of oral allergy syndrome from the early symptoms of a systemic reaction to food.

Celiac Disease. A number of immunologic reactions to food proteins are not mediated by IgE. Celiac disease presents over a period of months with steatorrhea, flatulence, and weight loss. Hyper-sensitivity to gluten causes the disease, and the characteristic diagnostic feature is extensive flattening of villi in a biopsy specimen taken from the jejunal mucosa.

Allergic Eosinophilic Gastroenteritis. Although allergic eosinophilic gastroenteritis is an IgE-mediated disease in some patients, about one half of patients do not exhibit specific IgE antibody to foods. Patients with allergic eosinophilic gastroenteritis have severe reflux, postprandial abdominal pain, vomiting, early satiety, and diarrhea. The diagnosis is suggested by the presence of inflammation and significant eosinophilic infiltration of the esophagus, stomach, or small intestine. Treatment with a strict avoidance diet using an elemental formula is efficacious in some patients.[12]

Infantile Proctocolitis. The symptoms of infantile proctocolitis are limited to the lower gastrointestinal tract and are of short duration. The ingestion of the responsible food (usually cow's-milk protein or breast milk from mothers who are consuming cow's milk) provokes diarrhea with blood in the stool, but anemia rarely occurs.

Food Protein-Induced Enterocolitis and Enteropathy. Patients with enterocolitis induced by food protein are often diagnosed in infancy and present with profuse vomiting and diarrhea. When severe, these symptoms may lead to lethargy, dehydration, and hypotension (often mimicking bacterial sepsis). The symptoms may be complicated by acidosis. The enterocolitis resolves with elimination of the responsible protein, most often cow's milk or soy.[13,14]

Patients may also have more indolent food protein-induced gastrointestinal symptoms that are induced by milk, soy, egg, wheat, rice, chicken, or fish. These patients, classified as having food protein-induced enteropathy, do not typically experience colitis, and they have a lower incidence of emesis (30 percent) than patients with enterocolitis (90 percent).[15]

The role of IgE-mediated or non-IgE-mediated food protein sensitivity in cases of infantile colic[16] and inflammatory bowel disease[17] remains controversial. Although failure to thrive in infants may be associated with malabsorption resulting from food allergy, a restrictive diet imposed by the family can also result in poor growth. This factitious food allergy was diagnosed in 5 percent of children with failure to thrive who were referred to an academic allergy program.[18]

Respiratory Tract

Rhinitis. The upper respiratory tract can be a target of IgE-mediated food allergy. Symptoms may include nasal congestion, rhinorrhea, sneezing, and pruritus. The prevalence of food-induced allergic rhinitis, even among patients referred to allergy clinics, appears to be less than 1 percent, although 25 to 80 percent of patients with documented IgE-mediated food allergy have nasal symptoms during oral food challenges.[19]

Gustatory rhinitis is rhinorrhea caused by spicy foods. This is not an immunologic reaction; it is mediated by neurologic mechanisms.[20]

Asthma. Food-induced asthma is an IgE-mediated illness that may result from the ingestion of a causative food or from the inhalation of vapors released during cooking or in occupational settings. The prevalence of food-related asthma in the general population is unknown, but this illness has been found to occur in 6.7 percent of children with asthma, 11 percent of children with atopic dermatitis, and 24 percent of children with a history of food-induced wheezing.[21] The prevalence of food-induced wheezing in adults with asthma is less than 2 percent.[22]

Heiner Syndrome. An example of a non-IgE-mediated adverse pulmonary response to food is Heiner syndrome. This uncommon syndrome of infancy is characterized by an immune reaction to cow's-milk proteins with precipitating antibody (IgG) to cow's-milk protein resulting in pulmonary infiltrates, pulmonary hemosiderosis, anemia, recurrent pneumonia, and failure to thrive.

Anaphylaxis

Anaphylaxis refers to a dramatic multiorgan reaction associated with IgE-mediated hypersensitivity. Fatal food-related anaphylaxis appears to be more common in patients with underlying asthma.[23] Patients who experienced fatal or nearly fatal food-induced anaphylaxis were unaware that they had ingested the incriminated food, had almost immediate symptoms, and experienced a delay in receiving adrenaline therapy. In about one half of the patients, a period of quiescence preceded the respiratory decompensation. The foods most often responsible for food-induced anaphylaxis are peanuts, tree nuts (walnut, almond, pecan, cashew, hazel nut, Brazil nut, etc.), and shellfish.[23]

Food-associated, exercise-induced anaphylaxis occurs in two forms.[24] Anaphylaxis may occur when exercise follows the ingestion of a particular food to which IgE-mediated sensitivity is usually demonstrable (e.g., celery) or, less commonly, may occur after the ingestion of any food. Ingestion of the incriminated food with exercise or exercise without ingestion of the food does not result in symptoms.

Controversies and Food Allergies

The relationship of food allergy to a number of clinical entities remains controversial. Food allergy may play a role in a minority of patients with migraine headaches,[25] although the pharmacologic activity of chemicals found in some foods (i.e., tyramine in cheeses) is more often responsible.

The role of food allergy in childhood behavior disorders is also controversial. A small subset of children with behavior disorders may be affected by food dyes, but no convincing evidence shows that food allergy plays a direct role in these disorders.[26] Unfortunately, unreliable information in the lay press and the use of unconventional and unproven methods, such as "provocation-neutralization,"[27] for diagnosing and treating behavior disorders can divert the patient's family from more useful treatments. On the other hand, in children with behavior disorder who also have bona fide allergies, treatment to relieve the symptoms of asthma, atopic dermatitis, and hay fever should be pursued.

Diagnosis

Initial Evaluation. An evaluation is warranted in patients who have the common clinical manifestations of food allergy. The initial evaluation, beginning with a thorough history and physical examination, must consider a broad differential diagnosis, including metabolic disorders, anatomic abnormalities, malignancy, pancreatic insufficiency, nonimmunologic adverse reactions to foods, and many other disorders that could lead to similar symptoms. Allergic reactions to substances other than foods (e.g., animal dander, molds, dust) must also be considered. Once food allergy is identified as a likely cause of symptoms, confirmation of the diagnosis and identification of the implicated food(s) can proceed.

In patients with acute reactions such as acute urticaria or anaphylaxis, the history may clearly implicate a particular food. In patients with chronic disorders such as atopic dermatitis or asthma, it is more difficult to pinpoint causal food(s). Virtually any food protein can cause a reaction; however, only a small number of foods account for more than 90 percent of adverse food reactions, and most patients are sensitive to fewer than three foods.[3,28] In children, the most common foods causing reactions are egg, milk, peanuts, soy, wheat, tree nuts, and fish.[3,28] Adults most often react to peanuts, tree nuts, fish, and shellfish.[29]

Prick-Puncture Skin Testing. In the evaluation of IgE-mediated food allergy, specific tests can help to identify or exclude responsible foods. One method of determining the presence of specific IgE antibody is prick-puncture skin testing. While the patient is not taking anti-histamines, a device such as a bifurcated needle or a lancet is used to puncture the skin through glycerinated extract of a food and also through appropriate positive (histamine) and negative (salineglycerin) control substances. A local wheal-and-flare response indicates the presence of food-specific IgE antibody, with a wheal diameter of more than 3 mm indicating a positive response.

Prick skin tests are most valuable when they are negative because the negative predictive value of these tests is very high (over 95 percent).[30,31] Unfortunately, the positive predictive value is on the order of only 50 percent.[30,31] Thus, a positive skin test in isolation cannot be considered proof of clinically relevant hypersensitivity, whereas a negative test virtually rules out IgE-mediated food allergy to the food in question.

Intradermal allergy skin tests with food extracts give an unaccept-ably high false-positive rate and therefore should not be used.[31] The protein in commercial extracts of some fruits and vegetables is prone to degradation, so fresh extracts of these foods are more reliable.[32]

In Vitro Testing (RAST). In vitro tests for specific IgE (radio-allergosorbent tests [RAST]) are more practical than prick skin tests for food allergy screening in the primary care office setting. As with skin tests, a negative result on RAST testing is very reliable in rul-ing out an IgE-mediated reaction to a particular food, but a positive result has a low positive predictive value. In vitro tests for IgE are generally less sensitive than skin tests; however, when highly sensi-tive assays are used, the levels of food-specific IgE antibody correlate with clinical reactivity to certain foods (e.g., milk, egg, peanuts, fish).[33] Because most patients with food allergy are sensitive to only a few foods[3,28] and a small number of foods are responsible for most reac-tions,[3,28] it is usually inappropriate to test for allergies to an exten-sive number of foods. In the context of a detailed history, selective testing is more likely to reveal causal foods. Measurement of immu-noglobulin G4 (IgG4) antibody, provocation-neutralization, cyto-toxicity, applied kinesiology, and other unproved methods are not useful.[34]

When patients have a history suggestive of food-related illness and tests for IgE antibody to the food are positive, the first course of ac-tion is to eliminate the food from the diet. Further testing is usually not needed in patients with severe, acute reactions. However, if symp-toms are chronic (atopic dermatitis, asthma) and/or many foods are implicated, diagnostic oral food challenges may be necessary.

Oral Food Challenges. Double-blind, placebo-controlled food challenges are considered the gold standard for diagnosing food allergy.[3,30,35] The procedure is labor intensive but can be modified for an office setting.[35] Patients avoid the suspected food(s) for at least two weeks, antihistamine therapy is discontinued according to the elimination half-life of the specific medication, and doses of asthma medications are reduced as much as possible. After intravenous access is obtained, graded doses of either a challenge food or a placebo food are administered. The food is hidden either in another food or in opaque capsules.

Medical supervision and immediate access to emergency medications, including epinephrine, antihistamines, steroids, and inhaled beta agonists, and equipment for cardiopulmonary resuscitation are required because reactions can be severe. During the challenge, patients are assessed frequently for changes in the skin, gastrointestinal tract, and respiratory system. Challenges are terminated when a reaction becomes apparent, and emergency medications are given as needed. Patients are also observed for delayed reactions. If allergy to only a few foods is suspected, single-blind or open challenges may be used to screen for reactivity.

Negative challenges are always confirmed with open feeding of a larger, meal-sized portion of the food. Oral challenges should usually not be performed in patients with a clear history of reactivity or a severe reaction. A general approach to the diagnosis of food allergy is shown in Table 20.3.

Challenges in Non-IgE-Mediated Allergy. It is more difficult to diagnose non-IgE-mediated reactions (e.g., allergic eosinophilic gastroenteritis, enterocolitis) and to pinpoint specific causative foods because no specific laboratory tests are used to identify these illnesses. In some situations (e.g., allergic eosinophilic gastroenteritis), a biopsy may be required to establish the diagnosis. Elimination diets with gradual reintroduction of foods and supervised oral food challenges are often necessary to identify the causal foods. Care must be taken because symptoms from, for example, enterocolitis syndrome, can be severe and even shock can ensue.[13]

Another diagnostic difficulty occurs when food additives (coloring and flavoring agents and preservatives) are implicated in reactions. Certain additives have been documented to cause the same types of reactions as those caused by IgE-mediated responses (i.e., asthma, urticaria, atopic dermatitis) but with a much lower prevalence.[36,37] Because these reactions generally are not mediated by IgE, diagnosis requires trials of food elimination and oral challenge tests.

Table 20.3. General Approach to the Diagnosis of Food Allergy

I. Obtain a detailed history and perform a complete physical examination

    A. Formulate suspicion of food allergy based on history and physical findings

    B. Rule out other causes of symptoms

II. Evaluate for IgE-mediated food allergy with skin prick-puncture tests or radioallergosorbent tests

    A. Tests are negative

        1. Reintroduce the food to the diet

        2. If the patient has a history of significant reaction or a non-IgE-mediated reaction is suspected, reintroduce the food to the diet in a physician-supervised or challenge setting

    B. Tests are positive

        1. Eliminate food

        2. If the patient has multiple sensitivities or an unclear history, perform open or single-blind food challenges

            a. If the challenge test is negative, reintroduce food

            b. If the challenge test is positive, challenge

                (1) Eliminate foods (if only a few foods)

                (2) If multiple foods are implicated, consider double-blind, placebo-controlled food challenges

                    (a) If the challenge is positive, eliminate food

                    (b) If the challenge is negative, reintroduce food

III. Diagnosis established

    A. Educate patient about treatment and avoidance

    B. Re-evaluate at appropriate intervals if tolerance is likely

Treatment

In addition to medical management of the manifestations of food allergy (e.g., topical therapy for atopic dermatitis, inhaled medication for asthma), food allergy is treated by dietary elimination of the offending food(s). Immunotherapy ("allergy shots") has not proved practical,[38] except when pollens are responsible for the symptoms of oral allergy syndrome.[39]

The elimination of food proteins is a difficult task. In a milk-free diet, for example, patients must be instructed not only to avoid all obvious milk products but also to read food product ingredient labels for key words that may indicate the presence of cow's-milk protein, including "casein," "whey," "lactalbumin," "caramel color," and "nougat." When vague terms such as "high protein flavor" or "natural flavorings" are used, it may be necessary to call the manufacturer to determine if the offending protein, such as milk protein, is an ingredient.

Patients and parents must also be made aware that the food protein, as opposed to sugar or fat, is the ingredient being eliminated. For example, lactose-free milk contains cow's milk-protein, and many egg substitutes contain chicken-egg proteins. Conversely, peanut oil and soy oil generally do not contain the food protein unless the processing method is one in which the protein is not completely eliminated (as with cold-pressed or "extruded" oil).

Elimination of a particular food can be tricky. For example, a spatula used to serve cookies both with and without peanut butter can contaminate the peanut-free cookie with enough protein to cause a reaction. Similarly, contamination can occur when chocolate candies without peanuts are processed on the same equipment used for making peanut-containing candy. Hidden ingredients can also cause a problem. For example, egg white may be used to glaze pretzels, or peanut butter may be used to seal the ends of egg rolls.

The Food Allergy Network (telephone: 1-800-929-4040) is a lay organization that provides educational materials to assist families, physicians, and schools in the difficult task of eliminating allergenic foods and in approaching the treatment of accidental ingestions. When multiple foods are eliminated from the diet, it is prudent to enlist the aid of a dietitian in formulating a nutritionally balanced diet.

In addition to eliminating the offending food, an emergency plan must be in place for the treatment of reactions caused by accidental ingestion. Injectable epinephrine and an oral antihistamine should always be readily available to treat patients at risk for severe reactions.

Prompt administration of epinephrine at the first signs of a severe reaction must be emphasized because delayed administration has reportedly been associated with fatal and near-fatal food allergic reactions.[23] Caregivers must be taught the indications for the use and administration of epinephrine and antihistamine medications.

Final Comment

Fortunately, young children often lose their sensitivity to most of the common allergenic foods (egg, milk, wheat, soy) in a few years, particularly with avoidance of the foods.[40] However, positive skin tests may persist despite the development of clinical tolerance. Serial diagnostic food challenges over time are often helpful in managing these food-allergic children. Unfortunately, sensitivity to certain foods, such as peanuts, tree nuts, fish, and shellfish, is rarely lost, and sensitivity persists into adulthood.

The author thanks Hugh A. Sampson, M.D., for a thoughtful review of the manuscript. The author's work is supported in part by the Jaffe Institute for Food Allergy, Mount Sinai School of Medicine, New York, N.Y.

References

1. Bruijnzeel-Koomen C, Ortolani C, Aas K, Bindslev-Jensen C, Bjorksten B, Moneret-Vautrin D, et al. Adverse reactions to food. *Allergy* 1995;50:623-35.

2. Geha RS. Regulation of IgE synthesis in humans. *J Allergy Clin Immunol* 1992;90:143-50.

3. Bock SA, Atkins FM. Patterns of food hypersensitivity during sixteen years of double-blind, placebo-controlled food challenges. *J Pediatr* 1990;117:561-7.

4. Sehgal VN, Rege VL. An interrogative study of 158 urticaria patients. *Ann Allergy* 1973;31:279-83.

5. Champion RH. Urticaria: then and now. *Br J Dermatol* 1988;119:427-36.

6. Sampson HA. Atopic dermatitis. *Ann Allergy* 1992;69:469-79.

7. Isolauri E, Turjanmaa K. Combined skin prick and patch testing enhances identification of food allergy in infants with atopic dermatitis. *J Allergy Clin Immunol* 1996;97(1 Pt 1):9-15.

8. Eigenmann PA, Sicherer SH, Borkowski TA, Cohen BA, Sampson HA. Prevalence of IgE-mediated food allergy among children with atopic dermatitis. *Pediatrics* 1998;101(3 Pt 1):E8.

9. Bock SA. Prospective appraisal of complaints of adverse reactions to foods in children during the first 3 years of life. *Pediatrics* 1987;79:683-8.

10. Fry L, Seah PP. Dermatitis herpetiformis: an evaluation of diagnostic criteria. *Br J Dermatol* 1974;90:137-46.

11. Ortolani C, Ispano M, Pastorello E, Bigi A, Ansaloni R. The oral allergy syndrome. *Ann Allergy* 1988;61(6 Pt 2):47-52.

12. Kelly KJ, Lazenby AJ, Rowe PC, Yardley JH, Perman JA, Sampson HA. Eosinophilic esophagitis attributed to gastroesophageal reflux: improvement with an amino-acid based formula. *Gastroenterology* 1995;109:1503-12.

13. Powell GK. Food protein-induced enterocolitis of infancy: differential diagnosis and management. *Compr Ther* 1986;12(2):28-37.

14. Sicherer SH, Eigenmann PA, Sampson HA. Clinical features of food protein-induced enterocolitis syndrome. *J Pediatr* [in press].

15. Walker-Smith JA. Food sensitive enteropathies. *Clin Gastroenterol* 1986;15:55-69.

16. Sampson HA. Infantile colic and food allergy: fact or fiction? *J Pediatr* 1989;115:583-4.

17. Enzer NB, Hijmans JC. Ulcerative colitis beginning in infancy. *J Pediatr* 1963;63:437-40.

18. Roesler TA, Barry PC, Bock SA. Factitious food allergy and failure to thrive. *Arch Pediatr Adolesc Med* 1994;148:1150-5.

19. Sampson H, Eigenmann PA. Allergic and non-allergic rhinitis: Food allergy and intolerance. In: Mygind N, Naclerio R, eds. *Allergic and non-allergic rhinitis*. Copenhagen: Munksgaard, 1997.

20. Raphael G, Raphael MH, Kaliner M. Gustatory rhinitis: a syndrome of food-induced rhinorrhea. *J Allergy Clin Immunol* 1989;83(1):110-5.

21. Sicherer SH, Sampson HA. The role of food allergy in childhood asthma. *Immunol Allergy Clin North Am* 1998;18(1):49-60.

22. Onorato J, Merland N, Terral C, Michel FB, Bousquet J. Placebo-controlled double-blind food challenge in asthma. *J Allergy Clin Immunol* 1986;78:1139-46.

23. Sampson HA, Mendelson LM, Rosen JR. Fatal and near-fatal anaphylactic reactions to food in children and adolescents. *N Engl J Med* 1992;327:380-4.

24. Romano A, Di Fonso M, Giuffreda F, Quaratino D, Papa G, Palmieri V, et al. Diagnostic work-up for food-dependent, exercise-induced anaphylaxis. *Allergy* 1995;50:817-24.

25. Weber RW, Vaughan TR. Food and migraine headache. *Immunol Allergy Clin North Am* 1991; 11:831-41.

26. National Institutes of Health Consensus Development Panel. Conference statement: defined diets and childhood hyperactivity. *Am J Clin Nutr* 1983;37:161-5.

27. Jewett D, Fein G, Greenberg MH. A double-blind study of symptom provocation to determine food sensitivity. *N Engl J Med* 1990;323:429-33.

28. Sampson HA, McCaskill CC. Food hypersensitivity and atopic dermatitis: evaluation of 113 patients. *J Pediatr* 1985;107:669-75.

29. Metcalfe DD. Food allergy in adults. In: Metcalfe DD, Sampson HA, Simon RA, eds. *Food allergy: adverse reactions to foods and food additives.* Cambridge, Mass.: Blackwell Science, 1997:183-92.

30. Sampson HA, Albergo R. Comparison of results of skin tests, RAST, and double-blind, placebo-controlled food challenges in children with atopic dermatitis. *J Allergy Clin Immunol* 1984;74:26-33.

31. Bock SA, Lee WY, Remigio L, Hoist A, May CD. Appraisal of skin tests with food extracts for diagnosis of food hypersensitivity. *Clin Allergy* 1978;8:559-64.

32. Ortolani C, Ispano M, Pastorello EA, Ansaloni R, Magri GC. Comparison of results of skin prick tests (with fresh foods and

commercial food extracts) and RAST in 100 patients with oral allergy syndrome. *J Allergy Clin Immunol* 1989;83:683-90.

33. Sampson HA, Ho DG. Relationship between food-specific IgE concentrations and the risk of positive food challenges in children and adolescents. *J Allergy Clin Immunol* 1997;100:444-51.

34. Terr Al, Salvaggio JE. Controversial concepts in allergy and clinical immunology. In: Bierman CW, Pearlman DS, Shapiro GG, Busse WW, eds. *Allergy, asthma, and immunology from infancy to adulthood.* 3d ed. Philadelphia: Saunders, 1996:749-60.

35. Bock SA, Sampson HA, Atkins FM, Zeiger RS, Lehrer S, Sachs M, et al. Double-blind, placebo-controlled food challenge (DBPCFC) as an office procedure: a manual. *J Allergy Clin Immunol* 1988;82:986-97.

36. Fuglsang G, Madsen C, Halken S, Jorgensen M, Ostergaard PA, Osterballe O. Adverse reactions to food additives in children with atopic symptoms. *Allergy* 1994;49:31-7.

37. Schwartz HJ. Asthma and food additives. In: Metcalfe DD, Sampson HA, Simon RA, eds. *Food allergy: adverse reactions to foods and food additives.* 2d cd. Cambridge: Blackwell Science, 1997:411-8.

38. Nelson HS, Lahr J, Rule R, Bock A, Leung D. Treatment of anaphylactic sensitivity to peanuts by immunotherapy with injections of aqueous peanut extract. *J Allergy Clin Immunol* 1997;99(6 Pt 1):744-51.

39. Kelso JM, Jones RT, Tellez R, Yunginger JW. Oral allergy syndrome successfully treated with pollen immunotherapy. *Ann Allergy Asthma Immunol* 1995;74:391-6.

40. Bock SA. The natural history of food sensitivity. *J Allergy Clin Immunol* 1982;69:173-7.

—by Scott H. Sicherer

About the Author

Scott H. Sicherer, M.D., is assistant professor of pediatrics in the Department of Pediatrics, Division of Pediatric Allergy/Immunology, at Mount Sinai Hospital, New York, N.Y. Dr. Sicherer received his medical degree from Johns Hopkins University School of Medicine, Baltimore. He completed a residency in pediatrics at Mount Sinai Hospital, where he served as chief resident. Dr. Sicherer also completed a fellowship in pediatric allergy/immunology at Johns Hopkins Hospital.

Chapter 21

Risky Food Allergies Are Rare

Do you start itching whenever you eat peanuts? Does seafood cause your stomach to churn? Symptoms like these cause millions of Americans to suspect they have a food allergy.

But true food allergies affect a relatively small percentage of people: Experts estimate that only 2 percent of adults, and from 2 to 8 percent of children, are truly allergic to certain foods. Food allergy is different from food intolerance, and the term is sometimes used in a vague, all-encompassing way, muddying the waters for people who want to understand what a real food allergy is.

"Many people who have a complaint, an illness, or some discomfort attribute it to something they have eaten. Because in this country we eat almost all the time, people tend to draw false associations between food and illness," says Dean Metcalfe, M.D., head of the Mast Cell and Physiology Section at the National Institute of Allergy and Infectious Diseases.

Allergy and Intolerance—Different Problems

The difference between an allergy and an intolerance is how the body handles the offending food. In a true food allergy, the body's immune system recognizes a reaction-provoking substance, or allergen, in the food—usually a protein—as foreign and produces antibodies

"Food Allergies Rare but Risky," originally published in *FDA Consumer,* May 1994, U.S. Food and Drug Administration Publication No. (FDA) 94-2279. Reviewed and revised by David A. Cooke, M.D. January 24, 2001.

to halt the "invasion." As the battle rages, symptoms appear throughout the body. The most common sites are the mouth (swelling of the lips), digestive tract (stomach cramps, vomiting, diarrhea), skin (hives, rashes or eczema), and the airways (wheezing or breathing problems). People with allergies must avoid the offending foods altogether.

Cow's milk, eggs, wheat, and soy are the most common sources of food allergies in children. Allergists believe that infant allergies are the result of immunologic immaturity and, to some extent, intestinal immaturity. Children sometimes outgrow the allergies they had as infants, but an early peanut allergy may be lifelong. Adults are usually most affected by tree nuts, fish, shellfish, and peanuts.

Food intolerance is a much more common problem than allergy. Here, the problem is not with the body's immune system, but, rather, with its metabolism. The body cannot adequately digest a portion of the offending food, usually because of some chemical deficiency. For example, persons who have difficulty digesting milk (lactose intolerance) often are deficient in the intestinal enzyme lactase, which is needed to digest milk sugar (lactose). The deficiency can cause cramps and diarrhea if milk is consumed. Estimates are that about 80 percent of African-Americans have lactose intolerance, as do many people of Mediterranean or Hispanic origin. It is quite different from the true allergic reaction some have to the proteins in milk. Unlike allergies, intolerances generally intensify with age.

Dangerous Dishes

For people with true food allergies, the simple pleasure of eating can turn into an uncomfortable—and sometimes even dangerous— situation. For some, food allergies cause only hives or an upset stomach; for others, one bite of the wrong food can lead to serious illness or even death.

Food intolerance may produce symptoms similar to food allergies, such as abdominal cramping. But while people with true food allergies must avoid offending foods altogether, people with food intolerance can often eat some of the offending food without suffering symptoms. The amount that may be eaten before symptoms appear is usually very small and varies with each individual.

When Food Additives Are a Problem

Over the years, people have reported to the U.S. Food and Drug Administration (FDA) adverse reactions to certain food additives, including aspartame (a sweetener), monosodium glutamate (a flavor enhancer), sulfur-based preservatives, and tartrazine, also known as FD&C Yellow No. 5 (a food color). The federal Food, Drug, and Cosmetic Act requires that FDA ensure the safety of all substances added to foods, but individual health conditions sometimes cause problems with certain additives.

Aspartame

After reviewing scientific studies, FDA determined in 1981 that aspartame was safe for use in foods. In 1987, the General Accounting Office investigated the process surrounding FDA's approval of aspartame and confirmed the agency had acted properly. However, FDA has continued to review complaints alleging adverse reactions to products containing aspartame. To date, FDA has not determined any consistent pattern of symptoms that can be attributed to the use of aspartame, nor is the agency aware of any recent studies that clearly show safety problems.

Carefully controlled clinical studies show that aspartame is not an allergen. However, certain people with the genetic disease phenylketonuria (PKU), those with advanced liver disease, and pregnant women with hyperphenylalanine (high levels of phenylalanine in blood) have a problem with aspartame because they do not effectively metabolize the amino acid phenylalanine, one of aspartame's components. High levels of this amino acid in body fluids can cause brain damage. Therefore, FDA has ruled that all products containing aspartame must include a warning to phenylketonurics that the sweetener contains phenylalanine.

Monosodium Glutamate

Monosodium glutamate (MSG) has been used for many years in home and restaurant foods, and in processed foods. People sensitive to MSG may have mild and transitory reactions when they eat foods that contain large amounts of MSG (such as would be found in heavily flavor-enhanced foods). Because MSG is commonly used in Chinese cuisine, these reactions were initially referred to as "Chinese restaurant syndrome." Most of these reactions are not believed to be true food allergies. Rather, some individuals do appear to have an unusual reaction to MSG, but it is not allergic, and it is not life-threatening.

FDA believes that MSG is a safe food ingredient for the general population. It is regarded by the agency as among food ingredients that are "generally recognized as safe." FDA has studied adverse reaction reports and other data concerning MSG's safety. The agency also has an ongoing contract with the Federation of American Societ- ies for Experimental Biology to re-examine the scientific data on possible adverse reactions to glutamate in general. MSG must be declared on the label of any food to which it is added.

Sulfites

Of all the food additives for which FDA has received adverse reaction reports, the ones that most closely resemble true allergens are sulfur-based preservatives. Sulfites are used primarily as antioxidants to prevent or reduce discoloration of light-colored fruits and vegetables, such as dried apples and potatoes, and to inhibit the growth of microorganisms in fermented foods such as wine.

Though most people don't have a problem with sulfites, they are a hazard of unpredictable severity to people, particularly asthmatics, who are sensitive to these substances. FDA uses the term "allergic-type responses" to describe the range of symptoms suffered by these individuals after eating sulfite-treated foods. Responses range from mild to life-threatening.

FDA's sulfite specialists say scientists, at this time, are not sure how the body reacts to sulfites. To help sulfite-sensitive people avoid problems, FDA requires the presence of sulfites in processed foods to be declared on the label, and prohibits the use of sulfites on fresh produce intended to be sold or served raw to consumers.

FD&C Yellow No. 5

Color additives must go through the same safety approval process as food additives. But one color, FD&C Yellow No. 5 (listed as tartrazine on medicine labels), may prompt itching or hives in a small number of people.

Since 1980 (for drugs taken orally) and 1981 (for foods), FDA has required all products containing Yellow No. 5 to list it on the labels so sensitive consumers could avoid it. (As of May 8, 1993, food labels must list all certified colors as part of the requirements of the Nutrition Labeling and Education Act of 1990.)

True Allergies

Heredity may cause a predisposition to have allergies of any type, and repeated exposure to allergens starts sensitizing those who are susceptible. Some experts believe that, rarely, a specific allergy can be passed on from parent to child. Several studies have indicated that exclusive breast-feeding, especially with maternal avoidance of major food allergens, may deter some food allergies in infants and young children. (Smoking during pregnancy can also result in the increased possibility that the baby will have allergies.) Most patients who have true food allergies have other types of allergies, such as dust or pollen, and children with both food allergies and asthma are at increased risk for more severe reactions.

Life-Threatening Reactions

The greatest danger in food allergy comes from anaphylaxis, a violent allergic reaction involving a number of parts of the body simultaneously. Like less serious allergic reactions, anaphylaxis usually occurs after a person is exposed to an allergen to which he or she was sensitized by previous exposure (that is, it does not usually occur the first time a person eats a particular food). Although any food can trigger anaphylaxis (also known as anaphylactic shock), peanuts, tree nuts, shellfish, milk, eggs, and fish are the most common culprits. As little as one-fifth to one-five-thousandth of a teaspoon of the offending food has caused death.

Anaphylaxis can produce severe symptoms in as little as 5 to 15 minutes, although life-threatening reactions may progress over hours. Signs of such a reaction include: difficulty breathing, feeling of impending doom, swelling of the mouth and throat, a drop in blood pressure, and loss of consciousness. The sooner that anaphylaxis is treated, the greater the person's chance of surviving. The person should be taken to a hospital emergency room, even if symptoms seem to subside on their own.

There is no specific test to predict the likelihood of anaphylaxis, although allergy testing may help determine what a person may be allergic to and provide some guidance as to the severity of the allergy. Experts advise people who are susceptible to anaphylaxis to carry medication, such as injectable epinephrine, with them at all times, and to check the medicine's expiration date regularly. Doctors can instruct patients with allergies on how to self-administer epinephrine. Such prompt treatment can be crucial to survival.

Injectable epinephrine is a synthetic version of a naturally occurring hormone also known as adrenaline. For treatment of an anaphylactic reaction, it is injected directly into a thigh muscle or vein. It works directly on the cardiovascular and respiratory systems, causing rapid constriction of blood vessels, reversing throat swelling, relaxing lung muscles to improve breathing, and stimulating the heartbeat.

Т̲п̲д̲п̲д̲п̲т̲п̲т̲п̲ т̲п̲т̲п̲т̲п̲т̲п̲т̲п̲ f̲п̲ т̲т̲т̲т̲т̲т̲т̲т̲т̲ home use comes in two forms: a traditional needle and syringe kit known as Ana-Kit®, or an automatic injector system known as Epi-Pen®. Epi-Pen's automatic injector design, originally developed for use by military personnel to deliver antidotes for nerve gas, is described by some as "a fat pen." The patient removes the safety cap and pushes the automatic injector tip against the outer thigh until the unit activates. The patient holds the "pen" in place for several seconds, then throws it away.

While Epi-Pen delivers one premeasured dosage, the Ana-Kit provides two doses. Which system a patient uses is a decision to be made by the doctor and patient, taking into account the doctor's assessment of the patient's individual needs.

Advice from Study

Hugh A. Sampson, M.D., and colleagues at Johns Hopkins University School of Medicine in Baltimore, MD., published a study of anaphylactic reactions in children in the August 6, 1992, issue of the *New England Journal of Medicine*. The study involved 13 children who had severe allergic reactions to food: Six died, and seven nearly died. Among the study's conclusions:

- Asthma, a disease with allergic underpinnings, was common to all children in the study.

- Epinephrine should be prescribed and kept available for those with severe food allergies.

- Children who have an allergic reaction should be observed for three to four hours after a reaction in a medical center capable of dealing with anaphylaxis.

Finding the Forbidden

Because there is no "cure" for food allergies other than strict avoidance of an offending food, one of the biggest problems those with food allergies face is verifying whether a forbidden product is contained in a particular food. For example, in Sampson's study, all six deaths occurred because either the child or the parent was unaware the food contained a substance to which the child was allergic. Munoz-Furlong says the Nutrition Labeling and Education Act, which requires more complete food labeling, should greatly help people with food allergies to avoid dangerous foods.

"The new labeling changes will make it easier for the consumer to readily identify things they could be allergic to," says Linda Tollefson, D.V.M., chief of the epidemiology branch at FDA's Center for Food Safety and Applied Nutrition. "Before this law was passed, true allergens were required to be on the label, but the exceptions were standardized foods, which will now have to list all ingredients."

According to Elizabeth J. Campbell, director of the center's division of programs and enforcement policy, the principle underlying standardized foods originally was that people basically knew what was in various foods.

"Originally, food standards were adopted to ensure uniformity. If you saw a product labeled mayonnaise, food standardization meant it had to be mayonnaise. People used to know what was in mayonnaise; nowadays they have to be told that mayonnaise contains both eggs and oil," Campbell says. "Years ago, when the law was first written to provide for standards of identity for certain foods, it only required that optional ingredients be declared. The new law stipulates that all ingredients in standardized foods must be declared."

Campbell believes that once the labeling is in place, consumers will have the information they need to make correct food choices. "In most cases, ingredients have to be labeled simply because they are ingredients, not because they are unsafe," she stresses. "For those with food allergies, I think it is more of a patient education problem."

Food additives, such as sulfites and certain colors, can also cause problems for people sensitive to them.

"If you have a food allergy, you really have to alter your life," Tollefson says. "You have to really read labels, and really be careful about what you eat."

Steve Taylor, Ph.D., a professor and head of Department of Food Science and Technology at the University of Nebraska in Lincoln, says the biggest problem for people with food allergies is restaurant food. Historically, restaurants have been regulated by local heath departments and have not had to label foods.

"For many restaurants, labeling of food products they serve would cause horrendous problems...what about chalkboard menus? How would you include all the ingredients? Enforcement would be a nightmare," he admits.

But steps are being taken to better educate restaurant employees. The Food Allergy Network and The American Academy of Allergy and Immunology, along with the National Restaurant Association, recently produced a pamphlet on food allergies, which has been distributed to 30,000 members of the association. The brochure explains what restaurants can do to help customers who need to avoid certain foods, defines anaphylaxis, and advises employees on what to do if food allergy incidents occur.

John A. Anderson, M.D., director of the Allergy and Immunology Training Program at Henry Ford Hospital in Detroit, says changes in food habits may be responsible for the feeling some physicians have that food allergies may be on the rise.

"You could make a case for the fact that we are introducing peanuts, in the form of peanut butter, to people at a very young age, which would affect the prevalence rate for people who are sensitive to that allergen," he notes. "In Japan, where they use more soy, there is a higher prevalence of soy allergy. My feeling is that as soy, a cheap protein supplement, is put in a lot of commercial foods you will see an increase in the rate sensitivity worldwide."

Metcalfe say that if food allergies are rising, it is due to more common use of foods that tend to be allergenic. He cites milk as a source of protein supplement in many prepared foods, and points out that people are eating more exotic seafood and more fish.

"But it's important to remember that the majority of people with true food allergies are allergic to three or fewer foods," Metcalfe says.

Other than advising anyone with a known or suspected severe food allergy to carry and know how to self-administer epinephrine, there is no treatment for food allergy other than to eliminate the offending food. But Metcalfe is optimistic about the future.

"I don't think it is likely a drug will be found to prevent food allergies. But I do think within 10 years we will see allergy shots available for some of the more common food allergies, because we are learning to identify and purify food allergens. I think we will see some development of immunotherapy for food allergies," he says.

Food Allergies and Biotechnology

People with food allergies have expressed the concern that new varieties of food, developed through the new techniques of biotechnology (such as gene splicing), may introduce allergens not found in the food before it was altered.

FDA addressed this concern in its 1992 biotechnology policy statement and said it will regulate whole foods developed through biotechnology by applying the same rigorous safety standards as for all other foods. The agency is taking steps to ensure that foods developed though biotechnology do not pose any new risks for consumers.

Under the new policy guidelines, a protein copied by genetic engineering from a food commonly known to cause an allergic reaction is presumed to be allergenic unless clearly proven otherwise. Any food product of biotechnology that contains such proteins must list the allergen on the label.

Labeling would not be required if the manufacturer could demonstrate that the allergen was not transferred. For example, if a food company were to breed potatoes containing a genetically engineered soy protein (to which some people might be allergic), the labeling on the potatoes would have to disclose the presence of the soy protein. But labeling would not be required if scientific data clearly showed that the protein had been changed and no longer contained the soy allergen.

To ensure that FDA has state-to-the-art information for its food biotechnology policy, the agency sponsored a scientific conference in the spring of 1994 to discuss what makes a substance a food allergen.

How to Cope

Anne Munoz-Furlong, who founded The Food Allergy Network for people with food allergies in 1991 after struggling to deal with her own child's allergies, comments: "My youngest daughter was diagnosed with milk and egg allergies when she was 9 months old, nine years ago. We tried to lead a life around her restricted diet. For example, we had Jell-O mold for her first birthday because I didn't know it was possible to create a cake without milk or eggs. I knew there must be other families struggling with the same issue."

What should you do if you suspect you have a food allergy?

The Food Allergy Network's Anne Munoz-Furlong suggests keeping a food diary as a first step, writing down everything you eat or drink for a one- or two-week period. Note any symptoms and how long it took for such symptoms to develop.

But Furlong and other experts agree that those who suspect food allergies also need to be evaluated by a physician with intensive specialty training in allergy and immunology. Be sure to discuss what diagnostic and treatment plan is anticipated, and the costs.

Ask if the tests have been proven effective by accepted standards of scientific evaluation.

"Go to a board-certified physician who is an allergy expert," advises Paul C. Turkeltaub, M.D., associate director of the division of allergenic products and parasitology at FDA's Center for Biologics Evaluation and Research. Be very wary of claims of food allergy to explain chronic, common complaints."

The diagnosis of food allergy requires a careful history, physical exam, appropriate exclusion diet, and diagnostic test to rule out other conditions. Tests can include direct allergy skin tests, blood tests, or "elimination and challenge" tests for suspected foods.

The most accurate kind of test is a controlled challenge test, often done in "blind" or "double-blind" fashion to eliminate psychological factors. In a blind challenge, the patient is given either a sample of the food, without being told what it is, or a placebo, an inert substance used as a control in the test. The observer (a doctor or assistant), however, knows what the substance is. Both patient and observer record any symptoms of allergic reaction. In a double-blind challenge, neither the patient nor the observer knows if the patient is given the food (allergen) or the placebo.

In recent years, unproven tests such as "food cytotoxic blood tests" and "sublingual provocation food testing" have been promoted as supposed "diagnostic" tools to detect food allergies. FDA believes that food cytotoxic blood tests are not supported by well-controlled studies and clinical trials.

In food cytotoxic testing, a test tube of blood is taken from the patient. The white cells (leukocytes) are mixed with plasma and sterile water and placed on microscope slides coated with dried extracts of a particular food. The reaction of the cells is then examined under a microscope; if they change shape, disintegrate, or collapse—or the person examining them says they do—the patient is supposedly allergic to that particular food. Test results may be interpreted by a "nutritional counselor" working on commission, who recommends vitamins and minerals (often available on site) that the patient needs to correct his or her "allergic condition." But FDA and other experts emphasize there is no evidence that such tests are valid in diagnosing food allergies.

Sublingual provocation food testing dates back to 1944. The test consists of placing three drops of an allergenic extract under a patient's tongue and waiting 10 minutes for any symptoms to appear. When the doctor is satisfied he has determined the cause of the symptoms, he administers a "neutralizing" dose, which is usually three drops of a diluted solution of the same allergenic extract. The symptoms are then expected to disappear in the same sequence in which they appeared. Advocates claim that if the neutralizing dose is given before a challenge test (for instance, eating a meal containing the offending food), the person will not have symptoms.

But after careful study of existing data, The American Academy of Allergy and Immunology says no controlled clinical studies demonstrate either diagnostic or therapeutic effects of sublingual provocation food testing. The academy concludes that use of the tests should be reserved for experiments in well-designed trials.

If you are diagnosed with a food allergy, scrutinize food labels to detect potential sources food allergens. When eating out, ask about ingredients if you are unsure about a particular food; ask to talk to the manager of the restaurant about ingredients in specific dishes.

Keep epinephrine with you and know how to administer it. If you do experience a reaction, seek medical attention immediately, even if the symptoms are mild or seem to subside. Mild symptoms may be followed 10 to 60 minutes later by the onset of severe problems.

Chapter 22

Preparing for Dinner Guests with Food Allergies

Just when you think you've thought of everything for your dinner party—food, flowers, music, guests who will enjoy each other—something comes along to remind you that feeding a group of people may present special challenges. In this case, it might be the unexpected food allergy of a guest's date. If only you'd thought to mention that shrimp would be the main course.

Avoiding the above scenario isn't too difficult. It's mostly a matter of communicating with the guests and knowing how to handle certain food allergy issues in the kitchen. This is important because, although an unexpected food allergy situation is inconvenient for the cook, it can be dangerous for the food-allergic guest.

A Food Allergy Primer for the Non-Allergic

Although it may seem that nearly everyone has an allergy to some food or another, in reality true food allergies are quite rare, affecting only 2 to 2.5 percent of the adult population. Food allergies are more common among infants (4 to 6 percent of the population) and children (1 to 2 percent). Many infants outgrow allergies.

"Guess Who's Coming to Dinner?" from *Food Insight*, July/August 2000, © 1997 International Food Information Council Foundation (IFIC); reprinted with permission. Write to the International Food Information Council Foundation, 1100 Connecticut Avenue, NW, Suite 430, Washington, DC 20036 or visit http://ificinfo.health.org for more information about food and health.

There are two types of sensitivities to foods: those that involve the immune system (immunological) and those that don't (non-immunological). All true food allergies are immunological in nature, while non-immunological reactions include a wide variety of adverse food reactions. Here are the basic facts about food allergies, and how they differ from other food sensitivities.

What makes it an allergy?

A true food allergy is a reaction of the body's immune system to something in a food or a food ingredient (virtually always a protein). When a susceptible person is exposed to this protein (called the allergen), the body mistakenly interprets the protein as foreign and produces antibodies to fight it. With repeated exposures to the offending food protein, the body continues to mount its "defense," so that at some point consuming the allergenic food triggers the release of histamine and other powerful chemicals which cause common allergy symptoms.

The most severe food allergy reaction is called anaphylaxis. This infrequent, yet potentially fatal, response to a food allergen involves several different body systems and results in a number of symptoms instead of the usual one or two seen with a typical food allergy. An anaphylactic reaction can progress quickly from the mild symptom stage—where the individual experiences an itchy tongue or mouth, throat tightening, and wheezing—to the life-threatening stage of cardiac

Table 22.1. Food Allergy Symptoms

• Skin symptoms	Swelling, hives, eczema/atopic dermatitis (skin rash)
• Gastrointestinal symptoms	Abdominal cramps, nausea, vomiting, diarrhea
• Respiratory symptoms	Runny nose, asthma/difficulty breathing, tightening of the throat
• Oral symptoms	Itching, swelling and hives in the mouth, palate and tongue
• Systemic symptoms	Anaphylactic shock (severe shock involving several body systems)

arrest and shock. Immediate medical attention is necessary, and treatment usually includes an injection of epinephrine. "Although they are rare, anaphylactic reactions which are fatal most often occur when the allergic individual is eating away from home and inadvertently consumes the offending food, fails to recognize the reaction quickly, and there is a delay in epinephrine administration," explains Susan Hefle, Ph.D., co-director of the Food Allergy Research and Resource Program and assistant professor of food science at the University of Nebraska at Lincoln.

Food Sensitivities

Non-immunological food reactions, while not true allergies, can produce symptoms similar to those of a food allergy. This can be confusing to people who suffer from them and is probably one reason why people are quick to say they have a food "allergy" when in fact they may just have a food sensitivity or intolerance of some sort. Food sensitivities are rarely life threatening and the symptoms tend to be more localized. Lactose intolerance, where the body lacks the enzyme to break down the milk sugar, lactose, is one example of a non-immunological food reaction. Idiosyncratic food reactions, where the cause is unknown, also don't involve the immune system. One example of a food idiosyncrasy is sulfite-induced asthma, which is estimated to affect about 1.7 percent of all asthmatics, according to Hefle. "Some idiosyncratic reactions, such as a connection between food colors and hyperactivity have been disproved through scientific research, while still others, such as monosodium glutamate (MSG) sensitivity remain unproved," adds Hefle.

Common Causes of Food Allergy

Amazingly, over 160 food allergens have been identified—but only a handful of them account for more than 90 percent of the food allergies in the United States. Most food ingredients (such as aspartame, MSG, food colors, high fructose corn syrup, and sugar) are not food allergens. Food oils, such as peanut oil or soybean oil are generally highly refined, rendering them free of allergenic proteins. In fact, research has shown that people with allergies to the oil's originating food (such as peanut or soybean) do not react to commercially refined and processed oils—the most commonly used oils. Cold-pressed oils, such as various nut oils, can still contain allergenic proteins, which may trigger an allergic reaction in a sensitive individual.

Table 22.2. Common Food Allergies

In Infants: Cow's milk, eggs, peanuts, tree nuts (almond, walnut, hazelnut, Brazil nut, etc.), soybeans, wheat

In Adults: Peanuts, crustacea (shrimp, crab, lobster, crawfish), tree nuts,
fish

Tips for Hosts: Coping with Food-Allergic Guests

Granted, most of the responsibility for avoiding food allergens rests
with the person who has the allergy, and one would expect that a life-
threatening food allergy would be acknowledged by the individual
when he or she is invited to a dinner party. However, a little planning and preparation can eliminate the need for dealing with a food
allergy situation altogether.

Here are some recommendations:

- Ask about food sensitivities when inviting guests and let your
  guests know what you plan to serve when inviting them. Knowing what you may be dealing with is half the battle. If a guest
  insists he or she is allergic to a food or ingredient which isn't a
  known food allergen (and may instead be just a sensitivity)
  don't get into a debate, simply offer to change the menu.

- Invite guests far enough ahead of time so that the menu can be
  revised, if necessary.

- Practice safe food handling methods during both the preparation and serving of foods.

Sometimes one can't avoid serving a common food allergen, even
when an individual has alerted you to the existence of an allergy. In
these cases, it's still possible to have a reaction-free event, but careful cooking and serving is necessary. According to Hefle, measures to
take include:

- Avoiding cross contact by not sharing utensils, food containers,
  cutting boards and serving dishes. For example, simply wiping
  off a knife used for a child's peanut butter sandwich, and then
  using the same knife to spread mustard on a peanut-allergic
  child's cheese sandwich is not adequate for preventing a possible

214

allergic reaction. A separate, clean knife, cutting board and plate should be used.

- Avoiding using the same cooking oil for both allergenic and non-allergenic foods. Food allergens can survive home cooking temperatures—even when deep-frying. If frying fish and chips, for example, two separate batches of hot oil should be used, as well as separate utensils and serving platters.

- Avoiding "creative" recipe formulation— "secret ingredients" can be dangerous. Many times a food-allergic individual doesn't expect a food allergen to be present in a dish, and will unwittingly consume it only to suffer later. For example, if you know a guest has an allergy to seafood, you should tell him that bottled Asian fish sauce has been used in the salad dressing.

With a few questions and some attention to planning and preparation, both you and your guests can have an enjoyable dinner.

Chapter 23

Food Allergies in Children

In the United States, the foods most commonly responsible for allergic reactions in children are milk, eggs, and peanuts. About 20 percent of the population worldwide can be considered allergic, or atopic, meaning that such persons have a familial tendency to react in an allergic fashion when exposed to common proteins. A child whose parents or close relatives have allergies is not born with allergies but has a tendency to become allergic to specific proteins on repeated exposure.

Foods are among the first new proteins in a child's experience and thus can cause allergic reactions. A greater proportion of infants are allergic to foods than are older children or adults. In time, allergic children tend to become sensitized to agents in the home, such as house dust mites, animals, or cockroaches, because of constant exposure. Only later do these children react to seasonal aeroallergens such as tree, grass or weed pollens, or outdoor mold spores.

Recent consumer surveys have shown that the American public believes food allergies are common.[1] From 13 to 17 percent of respondents to these surveys said that one or more of their family members suffered from food allergies.

Surveys among mothers of young infants in Denver have indicated that more than 20 percent of their infants had allergic symptoms associated with certain foods.[2] However, when these foods were eliminated from the diet for a short period and then reinstituted, no reaction occurred in the majority of cases. Double-blind, placebo-controlled food challenge trials suggest that the prevalence of true allergy during the first three years of life is no more than 8 percent. In controlled studies among newborns, the prevalence of milk protein reactions involving both allergy and intolerance is approximately 2 percent.[3] Food reactions are estimated to occur in 1 to 2 percent of older children and adults.[4]

Natural History of Food Allergy in Children

The majority of true food allergies in children—that is, allergies to milk, eggs, wheat, or soy—last for only a brief period in the child's lifetime. Clinical tolerance usually develops within a few years of the diagnosis of allergy, despite the continued presence of serum IgE antibodies to the allergenic food.[5] How quickly a child who is allergic to milk or eggs begins to tolerate these foods often depends on the severity of the initial reaction. Children who have a systemic reaction initially develop clinical tolerance for the allergenic food later than do children whose first allergic reaction is contact urticaria around the mouth or simple generalized hives.[6] Newly reintroduced foods are better tolerated if they are mixed with other foods or are processed. Thus, small amounts of eggs in bakery products are better tolerated than scrambled eggs, and milk is best reintroduced as cheese or yogurt, rather than scrambled eggs or a glass of whole milk.

The natural history of allergies to other foods, such as peanuts, is different.[7] Individuals who become allergic to peanuts have been found to be just as clinically allergic 14 years later. Therefore, foods that have been closely associated with systemic anaphylaxis, at any age, present a lifelong risk. In addition to peanuts, these foods include tree nuts (almonds, Brazil nuts, cashews, filberts, pecans, pistachios, walnuts), fish, shellfish (especially crab, crayfish, prawns, shrimp and lobster), and seeds (such as sesame and caraway).

Pathogenesis

IgE, the immunoglobulin class responsible for allergic antibodies, is present in both allergic and non-allergic children. Allergic children, however, are more likely to produce more IgE allergen-specific antibodies than normal children. Once formed, these IgE antibodies affix to tissue mast cells on body surfaces such as the skin, the gastrointestinal tract or the sinopulmonary tract, ready to react when the allergic child is reexposed to even a small amount of allergen, such as a food protein to which the IgE antibodies are directed.

On reexposure to the allergen, the mast cells release performed mediators (such as histamine or chemotactic factors) or cause other mediators (prostaglandins and leukotrienes, for example) to be formed in the tissue around the mast cells. These mediators are responsible collectively for producing the signs and symptoms of an immediate allergic reaction.

The chemotactic factors released by the mast cells attract other cells, such as eosinophils, into the area of the allergic reaction. These cells release another round of mediators, which prolong the allergic reaction. This is a form of allergic inflammation, called the late-phase allergic reaction. In most cases, a biphasic clinical reaction occurs, immediately followed by a late-phase reaction.

Regardless of the type of allergy, the usual symptoms of true allergic reactions range from hives to generalized systemic anaphylaxis, which is life-threatening. Allergic reactions also include symptoms that involve the upper airway and the eyes (e.g., hay fever), the lower airway (e.g., asthma), the skin (e.g., urticaria, atopic dermatitis) or the gastrointestinal tract (e.g., vomiting, blood in the stool, diarrhea). Generalized hives resulting from a bee sting are the same as those produced by a reaction to penicillin or by ingestion of a peanut. Symptoms must conform to an allergic pattern. Patients who present with other kinds of symptoms (such as behavior problems, headache, or muscular aches or pains) may be allergic, but these symptoms are not usually caused by allergy.

Diagnosis of Food Allergies

Adverse reactions to foods associated with symptoms that are clearly allergic in nature are generally IgE-mediated. To confirm the suspicion of allergy, the physician usually skin-tests the child with commercial or fresh food extract, using the epicutaneous (prick or puncture), immediate-reacting method to determine the presence of food-specific IgE antibodies.[8] Laboratory in vitro analysis of food-specific IgE antibodies is sometimes helpful but is less sensitive than the skin test.[9] This method of testing, however, is safe and would be appropriate in a child with a history of life-threatening systemic allergic-like reactions (i.e., anaphylaxis). In this situation, food allergy is likely to produce a positive result.

If the direct, epicutaneous skin test gives a negative result or, in the case of anaphylaxis, the in vitro IgE antibody test is negative, an

IgE-mediated (allergic) reaction can almost always be ruled out as the cause of the presenting symptoms, especially if the foods of concern are milk, eggs or peanuts.[9] In the case of suspected food-related anaphylaxis, a presumptive diagnosis of food allergy is adequate in most clinical situations.[10] A history consistent with an allergic reaction to a food commonly associated with anaphylaxis, coupled with evidence of in vitro IgE food-specific antibodies or a positive in vivo skin test, is sufficient for a presumptive diagnosis.

In research situations with less serious systemic reactions, particularly when food allergy is questionable, direct food challenges may be important to verify the relationship between a given set of symptoms and a food, even in the presence of a positive food skin test or in vitro

Table 23.1. Confirming the Suspicion of True Allergy (IgE Reactions)

Method	Comments
Immediate-reacting IgE skin test	Good screen for allergy. Virtually rules out allergy. A positive result indicates likelihood of allergy (50% with milk, eggs and peanuts, plus other "anaphylactically associated" foods).
In vitro test for allergen-specific IgE antibodies	Appropriate test in cases of life-threatening anaphylaxis. A negative result usually rules out allergy, but the test is less sensitive than skin testing. A positive result is usually obtained in anaphylaxis and is helpful for a presumptive diagnosis of allergy.
Food challenge	Only method to confirm the suspicion of food reaction regardless of mechanism (allergy or otherwise).
Open challenge	Usually sufficient in most clinical situations.
Double-blind, placebo-controlled food challenge	"Gold standard." Necessary in research studies and in all unclear clinical situations.
Diagnostic food diet/diary and home challenges	Possibly helpful when reactions are not life-threatening.

test.[11] In clinical situations, open food challenges are usually sufficient, but to be absolutely sure about a food, a double-blind, placebo-controlled challenge is necessary. The methods of such testing have been standardized as an office procedure.[11,12] In the case of an infant with hives caused by eggs or milk, after a few years of avoidance, rechallenge with these foods is more safely carried out in the office or the hospital than at home. Diet diaries and short-term elimination diets followed by home food challenge may be helpful when a child has had non-life-threatening symptoms thought to be related to food ingestion.[10]

Management of Food Allergy in Children

If food anaphylaxis is suspected, the food in question should be strictly avoided until some tests for confirmation have been performed. If a presumptive or confirmed diagnosis of food allergy with anaphylaxis is made, the food should be avoided indefinitely.[9] In case of accidental exposure to the food, the parent or caretaker should be prepared to use epinephrine for emergency treatment and then take the child to the emergency room of the nearest hospital. The physician must make this clear to the parents when food anaphylaxis is first suspected in the child.

The most convenient epinephrine devices to use at home or school are the auto-injectors: EpiPen® or Epi-EZ-Pen® (0.3 mg of epinephrine 1:1,000) and, for the child under age six, Epi-Pen Jr.® or Epi-EZ-Pen Jr.® (0.15 mg of epinephrine 1:2,000). An alternative is an epinephrine syringe from an emergency kit such as AnaKit®.

For the infant with gastrointestinal symptoms caused by either milk allergy or milk intolerance, casein hydrolysate (cow's milk) formulas such as Nutramigen, Progestimil, or Alimentum are the best-tolerated substitutes available.[13] Whey hydrolysate (cow's milk) preparations are not appropriate in this situation since allergic reactions have occurred in infants proved to be allergic to whole cow's milk protein.[14] Neocate (an amino acid-based formula) is safe for the severely milk-allergic infant who cannot use a casein hydrolysate formula.[15]

According to new data, soy-based infant formulas are not appropriate substitutes for the majority of infants with gastrointestinal symptoms in response to milk, either from allergy or from intolerance. However, soy infant formulas may be helpful in the management of some children who experienced milk-induced urticaria or systemic anaphylaxis reactions.[16]

221

Whey hydrolysate, casein hydrolysate, and soy-based preparations have been used as initial formulas in infants born to highly allergic parents to help prevent the early onset of food-induced allergic symptoms. Whey or casein hydrolysate formulas have been found superior to soy formulas in this situation.[16,17] Breastfeeding or the use of a casein hydrolysate formula plus a one- to two-year delay in the introduction of frequently allergenic solid foods has been found to prevent symptoms of

Table 23.2. Dietary Management of Adverse Reactions to Foods (continued on next page).

Problem	Infant feeding or child diet
Anaphylaxis due to true food allergy	Breast feeding, with maternal avoidance of offending foods Casein hydrolysate (cow's milk-based) formula Amino acid-based formula Soy protein-based formula
Prevention of food allergy symptoms for the first two years of life in an atopic family	Breastfeeding Casein hydrolysate formula Whey hydrolysate formula
Infant colic	Casein hydrolysate formula Soy protein-based formula Breast feeding, with maternal avoidance of offending foods
Behavior problems in children	Dietary manipulation

Problem	Comment
Anaphylaxis due to true food allergy	The preferred alternative formula for all infants with gastrointestinal symptoms is a casein hydrolysate preparation, such as Nutramigen (Mead Johnson), Progestimil (Mead Johnson), or Alimentum (Ross). Whey hydrolysate formula,

food allergy for the first two years of life[18,19] (see Table 23.2). However, these dietary restrictions did not prevent other respiratory allergies (e.g., allergic rhinitis, asthma) at two and seven years of age.[18,19]

Food allergen immunotherapy has only been attempted experimentally. Although the results to date have not been encouraging, this approach may be an option in the future, especially in cases of foods that are not easily avoided for a lifetime.

Table 23.2. Dietary Management of Adverse Reactions to Foods (continued from previous page).

Problem	Comment (continued)
	such as Good Start (Carnation), is not appropriate, because some children with milk allergy react. Neocate (Scientific Hospital Systems), an amine acid-based formula, is less palatable. Soy-based formula, such as ProSoBee (Mead Johnson), is helpful in some infants who cannot tolerate casein hydrolysate, or who have urticaria or eczema alone.
Prevention of food allergy symptoms for the first two years of life in an atopic family	Breastfeeding or hydrolysate formulas do prevent food allergy symptoms (e.g., urticaria, atopic dermatitis) for the first two years of life but do not prevent respiratory allergy at two and seven years in controlled studies. Soy-based formula is generally not helpful in preventing food allergy symptoms in the first two years of life.
Infant colic	Colic is a problem in the first four months of life and is self-limited. Increased parental attention or motion may help. No studies confirm improvement with a whey hydrolysate formula.
Behavior problems in children	A diet devoid of artificial colors may be helpful in a small percentage of children with attention-deficit disorder. Sugar avoidance has no effect on behavior problems. Allergen avoidance is probably of no benefit in behavior problems.

Special Clinical Situations

The Child with Food Anaphylaxis

Until 1988, death from an allergic reaction to food was considered rare.[22] Now, following a two-year survey of emergency room visits in Colorado,[23] the risk of a serious reaction to food in the U.S. population is estimated at one per year per 250,000 persons. In a recent study conducted in three U.S. urban areas,[24] a total of six children and adolescents were reported to have died of food anaphylaxis, and seven others nearly died of an allergic reaction to food ingestion. All of these individuals were severely allergic and had asthma and allergic rhinitis in addition to food allergy. All knew that they were allergic to a specific food, such as peanuts, nuts, crab, milk, or eggs. All ate the allergenic food accidentally in situations where a small amount of the food was disguised in a prepared product such as cookies or cake (40 percent), in a restaurant meal (30 percent), or in a candy (15 percent). In 12 of the 13 cases (92 percent), the food was ingested in a public place, such as a restaurant or school cafeteria. This study stresses that food-induced anaphylaxis can be minimized by diligent allergen avoidance and greater attention to the severity of clinical symptoms. In addition, prompt administration of epinephrine is recommended.

In the 13 cases described in this report, the difference between survival and death seemed to be directly related to the time at which epinephrine was administered. All of the deaths occurred in individuals who did not receive epinephrine within one hour of the initial ingestion of the food.

Physicians should identify which children under their care are at risk for life-threatening reactions to a food. A history of asthma is important, not because it is associated with a higher incidence of anaphylaxis from a food, but because an asthmatic child is more likely to experience a serious systemic reaction should a food reaction occur.

Lifelong avoidance of even small amounts of a food is very difficult, especially when the food is concealed in a prepared or commercial product.[25] Particularly challenging is the problem of the child who goes to school, and eats at restaurants, cafeterias, fairs, and parties. In a restaurant, the food servers cannot be relied on to describe the exact content of the salad dressing or the soup. At school, the teacher often has not been trained to administer epinephrine in an emergency situation. It is difficult to protect the allergic child from exposure to other children's food when they want to share lunch with their friends.

It is also difficult to keep the allergic child from contact with pro-scribed foods during parties. Both parents and teachers need to be prepared not only to try to prevent unwanted food exposures, but also to manage situations in which the severely allergic child is exposed to and begins to react to a food[26] (see Table 23.3).[27]

The 'Fussy' Baby Who Seems Allergic to Milk-Based Formula

The term "food-allergic" is often applied to individuals who react in an undesired manner to a given dietary exposure, regardless of the reason.[28] Allergists, however, use this term to describe those with true allergic reactions, usually of the IgE-mediated type. Infants who are truly allergic to milk should be switched from a conventional milk protein-based formula to a casein hydrolysate formula. Most "fussy" babies have colic, and colic symptoms can be attributed to allergy in only 10 to 15 percent of cases.[29]

About 20 percent of all infants have colic during the first four months of life, regardless of the formula used or the mother's diet if the child is breastfeeding.[30] Many controlled studies have indicated that colic is not related to diet, and that "fussiness" is better controlled through increased parental attention or motion than through formula changes.[31] It is not uncommon, however, for parents to switch colicky infants from a conventional cow's milk formula to a soy protein or whey hydrolysate formula, neither of which is recommended for the truly milk-allergic infant with gastrointestinal symptoms.[13,14,16,17]

At least one study suggests that such a dietary change can be help-ful. A 1982 double-blind study compared the effects of soy and cow's milk-based infant formulas on the duration of colic in otherwise nor-mal term infants in Denmark.[32] Colic symptoms decreased in 18 per-cent of the infants while on soy formula, whereas 29 percent of a control group receiving conventional cow's milk formula improved spontaneously. Of the infants given a casein hydrolysate formula, 53 percent improved. Thus, this study provides some support for a trial substituting soy or casein hydrolysate formula in infants with gas-trointestinal symptoms apparently due to milk intolerance.

In clinical situations, a dietary switch to a soy formula (the usual choice in the United States) could be expected to result in a decrease in symptoms about 50 percent of the time, with about 20 percent of the reduction due to the soy formula and the other 30 percent to spon-taneous improvement. Switching to a casein hydrolysate formula would be expected to produce even better results: about 50 percent relief of symptoms from use of the formula, plus approximately 30 percent spontaneous improvement.[32] However, casein hydrolysate formula is more expensive and less palatable than any released formula. Controlled studies using a whey hydrolysate formula for colic control have not been published.

The validity of these dietary manipulations has been criticized, and the effect of the diet, if helpful at all in colic, appears to be temporary.[33] Recently, the issue of diet manipulation for infant colic has been revisited by Hill and colleagues in Australia.[34] Both breastfed and formulated infants were studied for one week. The mothers of the breastfed infants were switched to a milk-free diet, and breastfeeding was continued. The formula-fed babies were switched to a casein hydrolysate formula (Progestimil). Infants in the control group remained on their original feeding regimens. No statistical difference was noted

Table 23.3. Management Tips for the Highly Food-Allergic Child (continued on next page)

Patient Information

Food Allergy Network
10400 Eaton Place
Suite 107
Fairfax, VA 22030-2208
Toll Free: 800-929-4040
Phone: 703-691-3179
Website: http://www.foodallergy.org

> NOTE: The Network publishes an informative newsletter and sends out regular warnings about commercial food products containing unwanted food proteins. The Network also offers a kit to help educate school officials and teachers about dealing with food anaphylaxis issues.

Specific Foods

Aerosolized allergens	Most exposures to foods occur through the oral route. However, in the case of fish, crab, shrimp, eggs, and beans, the allergic patient also may be exposed to aerosolized allergens. An example is the fish-allergic person who can easily react to such allergens in a room where fish is being fried, either at home or at a seafood restaurant.

in the response of the breastfed versus the formula-fed babies; 57 percent of the breastfed infants and 65 percent of the formula-fed infants improved as evidenced by an average 25 percent decrease in colic distress. In the control group, however, 38 percent of the breastfed infants and 50 percent of the formula-fed infants also improved, without a dietary change.

The gist of this discussion is that dietary manipulation during colic may be helpful, if for no other reason than it gives the parents something safe to do while waiting for spontaneous disappearance of the colic. Why a change to soy or casein hydrolysate formula should reduce colic symptoms is unclear, but it is unlikely that an allergic phenomenon is involved. The different size and composition of the dietary protein particles as they are presented to the infant's gastrointestinal tract may be important. Elimination of allergenic types of food in

Table 23.3. Management Tips for the Highly Food-Allergic Child (continued from previous page)

Egg allergy	Although measles, mumps, rubella, and influenza vaccines contain a minute amount of egg, most egg-allergic individuals can tolerate these vaccines without problems. Some allergic reactions have been due to gelatin in the vaccines.[27] As a rule of thumb, "If you can eat a food containing egg, the vaccine should offer no problem." However, if the history is questionable, it is safest to perform a skin test using the vaccine in dilute amounts and then administer the vaccine under controlled conditions followed by a two-hour wait.
Fish allergy	The major allergen responsible for fish allergy is found in all fresh and saltwater fish species; however, most fish-allergic individuals can tolerate canned tuna.
Milk "allergy"	Often commercial foods containing cow's milk protein are labeled "casein," "caseinate," "whey" or "milk solids."
Peanut allergy	The peanut is in the legume family (peas, beans, soy, peanut), not the nut family. Most individuals allergic to peanuts, however, can tolerate peas, beans, and soy, even though they are also legumes. Some peanut oils are safe. Others, however, especially those that are cold pressed, contain peanut allergen and should be avoided.

the diet of a breastfeeding mother probably would not decrease colic symptoms in the infant, although temporary elimination of cow's milk by the mother may be helpful,[35,36] since ingested cow's milk proteins can be easily identified in breast milk.[37]

The Parent Who Blames Food Allergy for Abnormal Behavior

The Allergic Attention Fatigue Syndrome

In 1922, Shannon[38] linked behavior problems in children—such as hyperactivity, sleeplessness, and anxiety, alternating with periods of listlessness and fatigue—with allergic reactions to foods. This phenomenon, termed the "allergic attention fatigue syndrome," was popularized by Rowe[39] in the 1950s and Crook[40] in the 1970s.

This hypothesis was advanced more than 50 years ago, but no well-designed clinical trial, using double-blind, placebo-controlled methods, has ever shown a relationship between these types of behavior symptoms and food ingestion.[9] Nevertheless, within the past 20 years, some physicians have continued to popularize the concept in the lay literature. These physicians have used unproved diagnostic and therapeutic techniques, such as provocation and neutralization, in an attempt to verify such relationships and treat the assumed condition.[41]

It is not surprising that parents seeking explanations for their child's abnormal behavior are misled when they read books on the subject or hear discussions on television talk shows.

Attention-Deficit Disorder with Hyperkinesis

In 1975, Feingold published a book in which he stated that 30 to 50 percent of cases of attention-deficit disorder (ADD) with hyperactivity were due to natural dietary salicylates and artificial food colors and flavors. He never mentioned allergy as a mechanism for this reaction, but was often misquoted.

Extensive studies of children with ADD using the Kaiser Permanente (KP) diet, which is devoid of artificial colors, preservatives, and natural salicylates, as well as dietary challenges with food colors, would indicate that only 2 percent of children with ADD would benefit from such dietary manipulation.[42]

Controlled studies involving a group of children with ADD, all of whom had benefited from methylphenidate (Ritalin) use, were performed using a special, controlled learning test.[43] Children with ADD were blindly challenged with either a cocktail containing dyes, particularly yellow #5 (tartrazine), or a placebo. The children with ADD given the placebo made progressively fewer errors on learning tests as the same questions were repeated over time. The children given the dye cocktail made an increasing number of errors over time. These results were interpreted as indicating that the dye produced a drug-like effect in children with ADD.[4] The KP diet has not been found helpful in children with behavior problems other than those with ADD.[42]

The popularity of the Feingold theories and use of the KP diet in ADD have declined but, even now, parents with children who have behavior abnormalities are often led to believe that dietary components, including allergens and food additives, may influence their child's behavior.[44]

Sugar Allergy

The term "sugar allergy" refers to the notion that high quantities of refined sugars in the diet may cause or aggravate hyperactivity, and aggressive or inappropriate behavior.[45] The sugar allergy theory has been tested in blind, placebo-controlled studies, and sugar has not been found to increase activity either in normal children or in already hyperactive children.[46-48] In some situations, sugar has actually been found to have a "calming effect," as in a study comparing the effects of sucrose with those of aspartame in a group of juvenile delinquents.[47,49]

Although the concept of sugar allergy is not as popular as it was in the1980s, it still appears in the lay literature and is believed by many parents. Since it is not harmful to restrict refined sugar content in the diet, efforts to debunk this popular belief may not be necessary, unless parents become fixated on this idea and avoid appropriate conventional therapy and psychological support for their child.

Final Comment

True food allergies are usually only a problem in infants and young children. However, a small group of highly allergic children are at risk for repeated, life-threatening anaphylaxis from re-exposure to foods such as peanuts, fish, tree nuts, shellfish, and seeds, as well as milk and eggs. The family physician needs to support families and teachers in avoiding exposure of these children to unwanted foods and in treating reactions should exposure occur. An infant formula change for the colicky baby may help reduce gastrointestinal symptoms, but the problem is generally self limited. Behavior problems in children should not be attributed to allergic reactions, and a diet free of refined sugars, or dyes and preservatives cannot be expected to improve behavior, even in children with ADD.

References

1. Altman DR, Chiaramonte LT. Public perception of food allergy. *J Allergy Clin Immunol* 1996;97:1247-51.

2. Bock SA. Prospective appraisal of complaints of adverse reactions to foods in children during the first 3 years of life. *Pediatrics* 1987;79:683-8.

3. Host A, Halken S. A prospective study of cow milk allergy in Danish infants during the first 3 years of life. Clinical course in relation to clinical and immunological type of hypersensitivity reaction. *Allergy*1990;45:587-96.

4. Jansen JJ, Kardinaal AF, Huijbers G, Vlieg-Boerstra BJ, Martens BP, Ockhuizen T. Prevalence of food allergy and intolerance in the adult Dutch population. *J Allergy Clin Immunol* 1994;93:446-56.

5. Sampson HA, Scanlon SM. Natural history of food hypersensitivity in children with atopic dermatitis. *J Pediatr* 1989; 115:23-7.

6. Bock SA. The natural history of adverse reactions to foods. *N Engl Reg Allergy Proc* 1986;7(6):504-10.

7. Bock SA, Atkins FM. The natural history of peanut allergy *J Allergy Clin Immunol* 1989;83:900-4.

8. Rosen JP, Selcow JE, Mendelson LM, Grodofsky MP, Factor JM, Sampson HA. Skin testing with natural foods in patients suspected of having food allergies: is it a necessity? *J Allergy Clin Immunol* 1994;93:1068-70.

9. Sampson HA, Albergo R. Comparison of results of skin tests, RAST, and double-blind, placebo-controlled food challenges in children with atopic dermatitis. *J Allergy Clin Immunol* 1984;74:26-33.

10. Anderson JA. Allergic reactions to foods. *Crit Rev Food Sci Nutr* 1996;36(Suppl):S19-S38.

11. Sampson HA, Metcalfe DD. Food allergies. *JAMA* 1992;268: 2840-4.

12. Bock SA, Sampson HA, Atkins FM, Zeiger RS, Lehrer S, Sachs M, et al. Double-blind, placebo-controlled food challenge (DBPCFC) as an office procedure: a manual. *J Allergy Clin Immunol* 1988;82:986-97.

13. Schwartz RH. IgE-mediated allergic reactions to cow's milk. *Immunol Allergy Clin North Am* 1991;11:717-41.

14. Businco L, Cantani A, Longhi MA. Anaphylactic reactions to a cow's milk whey protein hydrolysate (Alfa-Re Nestle) in infants with cow's milk allergy. *Am Allergy* 1989;62:333-5.

15. Sampson HA, James JM, Bernhisel-Broadbent J. Safety of an amino acid-derived infant formula in children allergic to cow milk. *Pediatrics* 1992;90:463-5.

16. Soy-protein formulas: recommendations for use in infant feeding. *Pediatrics* 1983;72:359-63.

17. Chandra RK, Singh G, Shridhara B. Effect of feeding whey hydrolysate, soy and conventional cow milk formulas on incidence of atopic disease in high risk infants. *Ann Allergy* 1989;63:102-6.

18. Zeiger RS, Heller S, Mellon MH, Forsythe AB, O'Connor RD, Hamburger RN, et al. Effect of combined maternal and infant food-allergen avoidance on development of atopy in early infancy: a randomized study *J Allergy Clin Immunol* 1989; 84:7289 [Published erratum appears in *J Allergy Clin Immunol* 1989;84(5 Pt 1):677].

19. Zeiger RS, Heller S. The development and prediction of atopy in high-risk children: follow up at age seven years in a prospective randomized study of combined maternal and infant food allergen avoidance. *J Allergy Clin Immunol* 1995;95:1179-90.

20. Oppenheimer JJ, Nelson HS, Bock SA, Christensen F, Leung DY. Treatment of peanut allergy with rush immunotherapy. *J Allergy Clin Immunol* 1992;90:256-62.

21. Sampson HA. Food allergy and the role of immunotherapy [Editorial]. *J Allergy Clin Immunol* 1992;90:151-2.

22. Yunginger JW, Sweeney KJ, Sturner WQ, Giannandrea LA, Tiegland JD, Brat M, et al. Fatal food-induced anaphylaxis. *JAMA* 1988;260:1450-2.

23. Bock SA. The incidence of severe adverse reactions to food in Colorado. *J Allergy Clin Immunol* 1992; 90(4 Pt 1):683-5.

24. Sampson HA, Mendelson L, Rosen JR Fatal and near-fatal anaphylactic reactions to food in children and adolescents. *N Engl J Med* 1992;327:380-4.

25. Steinman HA. "Hidden" allergens in foods. *J Allergy Clin Immunol* 1996;98:241-50.

26. Committee report from the Adverse Reactions to Food Committee of the American Academy of Allergy and Immunology. The treatment in school of children who have food allergies. *J Allergy Clin Immunol* 1991;87:749-51.

27. Sakaguchi M, Nakayama T, Inouye S. Food allergy to gelatin in children with systemic immediate-type reactions, including anaphylaxis, to vaccines. *J Allergy Clin Immunol* 1996;98(6 Pt 1):1058-61.

28. Anderson JA. The establishment of common language concerning adverse reactions to foods and food additives. *J Allergy Clin Immunol* 1986;78(1 Pt2):140-4.

29. Sampson HA. Infantile colic and food allergy: fact or fiction?[Editorial]. *J Pediatr* 1989;115:583-4.

30. Thomas DW, McGilligan K, Eisenberg LD, Lieberman HM, Rissman EM. Infantile colic and type of milk feeding. *Am J Dis Child* 1987;141:451-3.

31. Hewson P, Oberklaid F, Menahem S. Infant colic, distress, and crying. *Clin Pediatr* 1987;26:69-76.

32. Lothe L, Lindberg T, Jackobsson I. Cow's milk formula as a cause of infantile colic: a double-blind study. *Pediatrics* 1982;70:7-10.

33. Forsyth BW. Colic and the effect of changing formulas: a double-blind, multiple-crossover study. *J Pediatr* 1989;115:521-6.

34. Hill DJ, Hudson IL, Sheffield LJ, Shelton MJ, Menahem S, Hosking CS. A low allergen diet is a significant intervention in infantile colic: results of a community-based study. *J Allergy Clin Immunol* 1995;96(6 Pt 1):886-92.

35. Jakobsson I, Lindberg T. Cow's milk protein causes infantile colic in breast-fed infants: a double-blind crossover study. *Pediatrics* 1983;71:268-71.

36. Evans RW, Fergusson DM, Allardyce RA, Taylor B. Maternal diet and infantile colic in breast-fed infants. *Lancet* 1981; 1(8234):1340-2.

37. Axelsson I, Jakobsson I, Lindberg T, Benediktsson B. Bovinebeta-lactoglobulin in the human milk. A longitudinal study during the whole lactation period. *Acta Paediatr Scand* 1986;75:702-7.

38. Shannon WR. Neuropathic manifestations in infants and children as a result of anaphylactic reactions to foods contained in their diet. *Am J Dis Child* 1922;24:89-94.

39. Rowe AH. Allergic toxemia and fatigue. *Ann Allergy* 1950;8:72-9.

40. Crook WG. Nervous-system symptoms, emotional behavior, and reaming problems. The allergic tension fatigue syndrome. In: *Your allergic child*. New York: Medcom Press, 1973:62-3.

41. Goldberg BJ, Kaplan MS. Controversial concepts and techniques in the diagnosis and management of food allergies. *Immunol Allergy Clin North Am* 1991;11:863-84.

42. Lipton MA, Mayo JR Diet and hyperkinesis—an update. *J Am Diet Assoc* 1983;83:132-4.

43. Swanson JM, Kinsbourne M. Food dyes impair performance of hyperactive children on a laboratory learning test. *Science* 1980;207:1485-7.

44. Kaplan BJ, McNicol J, Conte RA, Moghadam HK. Dietary replacement in preschool-aged hyperactive boys. *Pediatrics* 1989;83:7-17.

45. Prinz RJ, Roberts WA, Hantman E. Dietary correlates of hyperactive behavior in children. *J Consult Clin Psychol* 1980;48:760-9.

46. Milich R, Wolraich ML, Lindgren S. Sugar and hyperactivity: a critical review of empirical findings. *Clin Psychol Rev* 1980,0 197-51 9

47. 'Kruesi MJ, Rapoport JL. Diet and human behavior: how much do they affect each other? *Ann Rev Nutr* 1986;6:113-30.

48. Mahan LK, Chase M, Furukawa CT, Sulzbacher S, Shapiro GG, Pierson WE, et al. Sugar "allergy" and children's behavior. *Ann Allergy* 1988;61:453-8.

49. Bachorowski JA, Newman JP, Nichols SL, Gans DA, Harper AE, Taylor SL. Sucrose and delinquency: behavioral assessment. *Pediatrics* 1990;86:244-53.

—by John A. Anderson

About the Author

John A. Anderson, M.D. is head of the division of allergy and clinical immunology at Henry Ford Hospital and Medical Centers, Detroit, and professor of pediatrics at Case Western University School of Medicine, Cleveland. Dr. Anderson graduated from the University of Illinois College of Medicine, Chicago, where he also completed an internship and the first year of a pediatrics residency. He completed a two-year residency in pediatrics at the U.S. Naval Hospital National Naval Medical Center, Bethesda, Md., and a fellowship in allergy and immunology at Children's Hospital of D.C., Washington, D.C. He is a member of the speaker's bureaus of the following companies: Glaxo Wellcome Inc., Hoechst Marion Roussel, Pfizer Inc. and Rhone-Poulenc Rorer.

Chapter 24

Peanut and Tree Nut Allergy

Chapter Contents

Section 24.1

Prevalence of Peanut and Tree Nut Allergy in America

From "Peanut and Tree Nut Allergy Affects Three Million Americans," *Doctor's Guide to the Internet*, April 12, 1999; © 1999 P\S\L Consulting Group, Inc. Reprinted by permission. *Doctor's Guide to the Internet* is at http://www.docguide.com.

Researchers from New York, Virginia, and Arkansas report in the *Journal of Allergy and Clinical Immunology* (April 1999) that peanut and/or tree nut (such as walnut, almond, and cashew) allergy affects about three million Americans or 1.1 percent of the population.

The prevalence of this allergy in the general population was unknown until now, despite the seriousness and recent attention given to peanut and tree nut allergy with controversy over banning peanuts from schools and airplanes. In addition, the study suggests many affected are not seeking an evaluation by a physician and many do not have epinephrine available for emergency use.

To measure the prevalence of peanut and tree nut allergy, the research team conducted a nationwide, cross-sectional, random digit dial telephone survey using a standardized questionnaire. A total of 4,374 households participated, resulting in data from 12,032 people. Peanut or tree nut allergy was reported by 164 individuals.

Researchers excluded those that did not meet the study's criteria, which required a typical food allergy reaction to have occurred within one hour of consumption (hives, angioedema, wheezing, throat tightness, vomiting, or diarrhea). The remaining 118 subjects reported having allergic reactions to at least one organ system (skin, respiratory, or gastrointestinal systems) and 45 percent of these subjects reported having more than five reactions in their lifetime.

Of the 118 respondents, only 53 percent saw a physician for the condition and only seven percent had self-injectable epinephrine available at the time of the interview. Researchers note two unique findings brought forth by this study. Previous reports indicate that between 20 and 34 percent of patients are allergic to both peanuts and tree nuts. However, only four adults (.02 percent) reported being allergic to both peanuts and tree nuts in this study, suggesting that allergy to both peanuts and tree nuts may not be as common in the general population as compared to rates previously reported by allergic patients' physicians.

Secondly, these allergies were more common in adults than in children, despite the fact that the general prevalence of food allergy is greater in children. Considering that peanut and tree nut allergies are usually not outgrown, there may be a greater representation among adults because that population has accumulated affected individuals.

"This study is a milestone in the understanding of food allergy," said Anne Munoz-Furlong, founder of The Food Allergy Network. "For years, reporters and others have wondered how many people are affected by these potentially life-threatening food allergies. Many believed it was only a small portion of the population that was affected, and therefore no one should care.

"This study indicates that peanut and tree nut allergy involves a significant number of people. Peanuts and tree nuts are the leading cause of severe or fatal food-allergic reactions."

There is no cure for food allergy. Avoidance of the food is critical. However, reactions to these foods commonly occur when the individual is away from home. In almost all cases, the individual thought they were eating a safe food.

"Anyone who serves food to others should be aware of the potential seriousness of food-allergic reactions and make every effort to disclose the ingredients in foods they serve," Munoz-Furlong added.

Quick administration of epinephrine, the medication of choice for managing an anaphylactic, or severe, reaction is critical. It is worrisome that the study shows a significant number of patients did not carry epinephrine, even though 81 percent experienced breathing problems or generalized reactions.

"Accidents are never planned. Individuals with an allergy to peanuts or tree nuts who have been prescribed epinephrine, available as EpiPen® or AnaKit®, should be sure to carry it with them at all times. They should report any allergic reactions to their doctor for follow-up."

The Food Allergy Network (FAN) is a national non-profit organization whose mission is to increase public awareness about food allergy and anaphylaxis, provide education, and advance research.

Section 24.2

Some Young Children May Out Grow Peanut Allergy

Like children who develop allergies to cow's milk or eggs, a proportion of young children who develop a sensitivity to peanuts early in life seem to grow out of their reactions as they get older, says a report in the *British Medical Journal* (April 1998).

Based on findings from research, by Dr. John Hourihane, from the Institute of Child Health, and colleagues conducted at the University of Southampton and South Manchester University Hospitals, the authors stress that children who seem to have a peanut allergy should be evaluated by a specialist food allergy unit, as the allergy may not be as severe as initially thought.

The study recruited 15 children with resolved peanut allergy (resolvers) and 15 with persistent allergy (persisters). The main outcome measure was the reaction on challenge with peanut, serum total and peanut specific IgE concentrations.

The researchers found that the groups had a similar median age at first reaction to peanut (11 months, range five to 38) and similar symptoms. Allergy to other foods was less common in resolvers (two of 15) than persisters (nine of 15).

On skin prick testing with peanut all 13 resolvers tested but only three of 14 persisters had a weal of less than 6 mm. Total and peanut specific IgE concentrations did not differ much between the groups.

The researchers said appropriately trained clinicians must be prepared to challenge pre-school children with peanut as some will be tolerant despite a history of reactions to peanut and a positive skin prick test with peanut. Pre-school children whose apparent peanut allergy is refuted by food challenge show allergy to other foods less often than those in whom peanut allergy persists. The size of weal on skin prick testing to peanut predicts reactivity but not severity on peanut challenge.

The authors cite previous research which suggests that changes in dietary habits of the British population towards vegetarianism and the increasing use of peanut butter as a snack food may be linked to a recently observed decrease in the age of onset of peanut allergy.

Chapter 25

Is It a Milk Allergy or Lactose Intolerance?

Chapter Contents

Section 25.1

Milk Allergy: Common Questions

From the Dairy Farmers of Ontario website at http://www.milk.org,
January 2001; reprinted with permission.

This information has been designed to help you understand the
difference between lactose intolerance and milk allergy, answer some
of your questions, and provide you with dietary tips. For more complete information, speak to your doctor and/or consult a dietitian. But
do keep in mind, milk products are an important part of a healthy,
nutritious diet.

If you, a member of your family, or someone you know has difficulty consuming milk and/or milk products and you suspect either
lactose intolerance or a milk allergy, discuss the matter with your
doctor. Do not depend on this information for a diagnosis. Some of the
same symptoms can be caused by other conditions.

Possible Symptoms of a Milk Allergy

- Skin rash
- Diarrhea and/or constipation
- Bronchitis
- Blood in stool

Who Is Affected?

- 1–8% of infants.
- Very rare among adults

What Is the Cause?

- Allergic reaction to the protein in milk and milk products.

How Long Will It Last?

- Usually not past 3 years of age.

Diagnosis and Treatment

- Do not self diagnose. See your doctor or dietitian. Treatment involves replacing milk and milk products in the diet.

Other Common Questions

What is a milk allergy?

An allergy to cows' milk is an allergic reaction to the protein found in milk. The condition is rare, occurring in only 1 to 8 percent of infants, and even less often in adults. The majority of people allergic to cows' milk are also allergic to goats' milk. Breastfed infants tend to be less likely to develop such a sensitivity while children of parents who have allergies tend to be more likely to develop this sensitivity.

I think my infant may be allergic to milk. What should I do?

Don't try to diagnose this condition by yourself. The same symptoms can indicate a number of other problems. Typical symptoms normally appear by one month of age and may include skin rash, vomiting, diarrhea, and bronchitis. Consult your doctor.

What kind of treatment will my infant need?

Once your child has been properly diagnosed as having a milk allergy, you can relax. After removing milk from the diet and substituting a commercial formula free of cows' milk, symptoms usually subside within a few days.

What about breastfeeding?

For many mothers, breastfeeding is the feeding of choice and indeed the best way to provide your child with the nutrients necessary for healthy growth. In some rare cases, though, an infant may react to the milk in the mother's diet. If you think your infant may be reacting to the milk in your diet, it is important to consult a dietitian.

What if my child is older and no longer breastfeeding or on formula?

Milk contains many essential nutrients that are difficult to replace in a growing child's diet. Some studies have also indicated that infants with a milk allergy tend to have sensitivities to proteins found in other foods. Nutrition counseling is essential to ensure an adequate diet.

When will my child be able to drink milk again?

Most milk sensitive children outgrow their allergy to milk before the age of 3. After the age of 1 or 2, consult your doctor about introducing milk back into the diet. Milk products form one of the four important food groups in Canada's Food Guide to Healthy Eating and should be reintroduced into your child's diet as soon as possible. This is usually done under professional supervision.

Section 25.2

Lactose Intolerance: Common Questions

From the Dairy Farmers of Ontario website at http://www.milk.org, January 2001; reprinted with permission.

Possible Symptoms

- Stomach bloating
- Cramps
- Gas
- Diarrhea

Who Is Affected?

- Most common in adults from Africa, Asia, the Orient, or Native North Americans.
- Less common in children

What Is the Cause?

- Digestive system's inability to break down the milk sugar (lactose) in milk and milk products.

How Long Will It Last?

- Primary lactose intolerance is permanent.
- Secondary lactose intolerance can be caused by a number of ailments and is usually temporary.

Diagnosis and Treatment

- See your doctor or dietitian. There are several methods of coping without eliminating milk products from the diet.

Other Common Questions

I thought I had developed a milk allergy, and now my doctor tells me I just have a lactose intolerance. What is a lactose intolerance anyway?

Allergies to milk are very rare, especially in adults. A lactose intolerance, on the other hand, is not uncommon, especially among people from Asia, African and the Orient or in Native North Americans.

Lactose is a natural sugar in milk and milk products which is normally broken down in the body. Individuals who are lactose intolerant cannot digest this sugar properly. The results can be stomach cramps, bloating and diarrhea.

What's the difference between primary lactose intolerance and secondary lactose intolerance?

The symptoms of primary lactose intolerance usually first appear in older children and adults. Those with primary lactose intolerance seem to be unable to digest the sugar in milk properly. Secondary lactose intolerance on the other hand, is often temporary and can be caused by an illness or condition that affects the digestive system (e.g., "food poisoning"). It gradually disappears when you get over the illness.

Should I give up milk and milk products for good?

Not only is it not necessary, it's not a good idea. Adults, as well as children, need the nutrients milk and milk products provide to stay healthy. There are usually lots of ways you can enjoy these without feeling any discomfort at all. Experimentation is the key to discovering your own level of tolerance. Here are some useful tips:

- Drink smaller amounts of milk at one time and spread it evenly throughout the day. For example, try half a glass instead of a full glass.

- Drink milk with other foods, not on an empty stomach.

- Whole milk may be better tolerated than skim milk since it is digested more slowly than skim milk.

- Products like yogurt, cheese and ice cream may be better tolerated.

- Check the dairy case in your grocery store for ready to use lactose reduced milk such as Lacteeze or Lactaid. Ask your grocer to order it if it is not on the shelf.

- Tablets or drops are also available to help digest the sugar in milk and milk products. The tablets are eaten before taking any milk or milk products and the drops are added to milk 24 hours before drinking. Both are usually available at your drugstore.

Section 25.3

Coping with Lactose Intolerance

From NIH Publication No. 98-2751, 1998.

What Is Lactose Intolerance?

Lactose intolerance is the inability to digest significant amounts of lactose, the predominant sugar of milk. This inability results from a shortage of the enzyme lactase, which is normally produced by the cells that line the small intestine. Lactase breaks down milk sugar into simpler forms that can then be absorbed into the bloodstream. When there is not enough lactase to digest the amount of lactose consumed, the results, although not usually dangerous, may be very distressing. While not all persons deficient in lactase have symptoms, those who do are considered to be lactose intolerant.

Common symptoms include nausea, cramps, bloating, gas, and diarrhea, which begin about 30 minutes to 2 hours after eating or drinking foods containing lactose. The severity of symptoms varies depending on the amount of lactose each individual can tolerate.

Some causes of lactose intolerance are well known. For instance, certain digestive diseases and injuries to the small intestine can reduce the amount of enzymes produced. In rare cases, children are born without the ability to produce lactase. For most people, though, lactase deficiency is a condition that develops naturally over time. After about the age of 2 years, the body begins to produce less lactase. However, many people may not experience symptoms until they are much older.

Between 30 and 50 million Americans are lactose intolerant. Certain ethnic and racial populations are more widely affected than others. As many as 75 percent of all African-Americans and Native Americans and 90 percent of Asian-Americans are lactose intolerant. The condition is least common among persons of northern European descent.

How Is Lactose Intolerance Diagnosed?

The most common tests used to measure the absorption of lactose in the digestive system are the lactose tolerance test, the hydrogen breath test, and the stool acidity test. These tests are performed on an outpatient basis at a hospital, clinic, or doctor's office.

The lactose tolerance test begins with the individual fasting (not eating) before the test and then drinking a liquid that contains lactose. Several blood samples are taken over a 2-hour period to measure the person's blood glucose (blood sugar) level, which indicates how well the body is able to digest lactose.

Normally, when lactose reaches the digestive system, the lactase enzyme breaks down lactase into glucose and galactose. The liver then changes the galactose into glucose, which enters the bloodstream and raises the person's blood glucose level. If lactose is incompletely broken down the blood glucose level does not rise, and a diagnosis of lactose intolerance is confirmed.

The hydrogen breath test measures the amount of hydrogen in the breath. Normally, very little hydrogen is detectable in the breath. However, undigested lactose in the colon is fermented by bacteria, and various gases, including hydrogen, are produced. The hydrogen is absorbed from the intestines, carried through the bloodstream to the lungs, and exhaled. In the test, the patient drinks a lactose-loaded beverage, and the breath is analyzed at regular intervals. Raised levels of hydrogen in the breath indicate improper digestion of lactose. Certain foods, medications, and cigarettes can affect the test's accuracy and should be avoided before taking the test. This test is available for children and adults.

The lactose tolerance and hydrogen breath tests are not given to infants and very young children who are suspected of having lactose intolerance. A large lactose load may be dangerous for very young individuals because they are more prone to dehydration that can result from diarrhea caused by the lactose. If a baby or young child is experiencing symptoms of lactose intolerance, many pediatricians simply recommend changing from cow's milk to soy formula and waiting for symptoms to abate.

If necessary, a stool acidity test, which measures the amount of acid in the stool, may be given to infants and young children. Undigested lactose fermented by bacteria in the colon creates lactic acid and other short-chain fatty acids that can be detected in a stool sample. In addition, glucose may be present in the sample as a result of unabsorbed lactose in the colon.

How Is Lactose Intolerance Treated?

Fortunately, lactose intolerance is relatively easy to treat. No treatment exists to improve the body's ability to produce lactase, but symptoms can be controlled through diet.

Young children with lactase deficiency should not eat any foods containing lactose. Most older children and adults need not avoid lactose completely, but individuals differ in the amounts of lactose they can handle. For example, one person may suffer symptoms after drinking a small glass of milk, while another can drink one glass but not two. Others may be able to manage ice cream and aged cheeses, such as cheddar and Swiss but not other dairy products. Dietary control of lactose intolerance depends on each person's learning through trial and error how much lactose he or she can handle.

For those who react to very small amounts of lactose or have trouble limiting their intake of foods that contain lactose, lactase enzymes are available without a prescription. One form is a liquid for use with milk. A few drops are added to a quart of milk, and after 24 hours in the refrigerator, the lactose content is reduced by 70 percent. The process works faster if the milk is heated first, and adding a double amount of lactase liquid produces milk that is 90 percent lactose free. A more recent development is a chewable lactase enzyme tablet that helps people digest solid foods that contain lactose. Three to six tablets are taken just before a meal or snack.

Lactose-reduced milk and other products are available at many supermarkets. The milk contains all of the nutrients found in regular milk and remains fresh for about the same length of time or longer if it is super-pasteurized.

How Is Nutrition Balanced?

Milk and other dairy products are a major source of nutrients in the American diet. The most important of these nutrients is calcium. Calcium is essential for the growth and repair of bones throughout life. In the middle and later years, a shortage of calcium may lead to thin, fragile bones that break easily (a condition called osteoporosis). A concern, then, for both children and adults with lactose intolerance, is getting enough calcium in a diet that includes little or no milk.

In 1997, the Institute of Medicine released a report recommending new requirements for daily calcium intake. How much calcium a person needs to maintain good health varies by age group. Recommendations from the report are listed in Table 25.1.

In planning meals, making sure that each day's diet includes enough calcium is important, even if the diet does not contain dairy products. Many nondairy foods are high in calcium. Green vegetables, such as broccoli and kale, and fish with soft, edible bones, such as

Table 25.1. Calcium Recommendations

Age group	Amount of calcium to consume daily in milligrams (mg)
0-6 months	210 mg
6-12 months	270 mg
1-3 years	500 mg
4-8 years	800 mg
9-18 years	1,300 mg
19-50 years	1,000 mg
51-70 years	1,200 mg
Pregnant and nursing women	
under 19	1,300 mg
over 19	1,000 mg

salmon and sardines, are excellent sources of calcium. To help in planning a high-calcium and low-lactose diet, Table 25.2 lists some common foods that are good sources of dietary calcium and shows about how much lactose the foods contain.

Recent research shows that yogurt with active cultures may be a good source of calcium for many people with lactose intolerance, even though it is fairly high in lactose. Evidence shows that the bacterial

Table 25.2. Calcium and Lactose in Common Foods

Food	Calcium Content*	Lactose Content**
Vegetables		
Brocoli (cooked), 1 cup	94-177 mg	0
Chinese cabbage (bok choy, cooked), 1 cup	158 mg	0
Collard greens (cooked), 1 cup	148-357 mg	0
Kale (cooked), 1 cup	94-179 mg	0
Turnip greens (cooked), 1 cup	194-249 mg	0
Dairy Products		
Ice cream/ice milk, 8 oz.	176 mg	6-7 g
Milk (whole, low-fat, skim, buttermilk), 8 oz.	291-316 mg	12-13 g
Processed cheese, 1 oz.	159-219 mg	2-3 g
Sour cream, 4 oz.	134 mg	4-5 g
Yogurt (plain), 8 oz.	274-415 mg	12-13 g
Fish/Seafood		
Oysters (raw), 1 cup	226 mg	0
Salmon, with bones (canned), 3 oz.	167 mg	0
Sardines, 3 oz.	371 mg	0
Shrimp (canned), 3 oz.	98 mg	0
Other		
Molasses, 2 tbsp	274 mg	0
Tofu (processed with calcium salts), 3 oz.	225 mg	0

*Nutritive value of foods. Values vary with methods of processing and preparation.

**Derived from *Lactose Intolerance: A Resource Including Recipes,* Food Sensitivity Series, American Dietetic Association, 1991.

cultures used in making yogurt produce some of the lactase enzyme required for proper digestion.

Clearly, many foods can provide the calcium and other nutrients the body needs, even when intake of milk and dairy products is limited. However, factors other than calcium and lactose content should be kept in mind when planning a diet. Some vegetables that are high in calcium (Swiss chard, spinach, and rhubarb, for instance) are not listed in Table 25.2 because the body cannot use their calcium content. They contain substances called oxalates, which stop calcium absorption. Calcium is absorbed and used only when there is enough vitamin D in the body. A balanced diet should provide an adequate supply of vitamin D. Sources of vitamin D include eggs and liver. However, sunlight helps the body naturally absorb or synthesize vitamin D, and with enough exposure to the sun, food sources may not be necessary.

Some people with lactose intolerance may think they are not getting enough calcium and vitamin D in their diet. Consultation with a doctor or dietitian may be helpful in deciding whether any dietary supplements are needed. Taking vitamins or minerals of the wrong kind or in the wrong amounts can be harmful. A dietitian can help in planning meals that will provide the most nutrients with the least chance of causing discomfort.

Watch Out for Hidden Lactose

Although milk and foods made from milk are the only natural sources, lactose is often added to prepared foods. People with very low tolerance for lactose should know about the many food products that may contain lactose, even in small amounts. Food products that may contain lactose include:

- Bread and other baked goods
- Processed breakfast cereals.
- Instant potatoes, soups, and breakfast drinks.
- Margarine.
- Lunch meats (other than kosher)
- Salad dressings.
- Candies and other snacks
- Mixes for pancakes, biscuits, and cookies.

Some products labeled nondairy, such as powdered coffee creamer and whipped toppings, may also include ingredients that are derived from milk and therefore contain lactose.

Smart shoppers learn to read food labels with care, looking not only for milk and lactose among the contents but also for such words as whey, curds, milk by-products, dry milk solids, and nonfat dry milk powder. If any of these are listed on a label, the item contains lactose.

In addition, lactose is used as the base for more than 20 percent of prescription drugs and about 6 percent of over-the-counter medicines. Many types of birth control pills, for example, contain lactose, as do some tablets for stomach acid and gas. However, these products typically affect only people with severe lactose intolerance.

Summary

Even though lactose intolerance is widespread, it need not pose a serious threat to good health. People who have trouble digesting lactose can learn which dairy products and other foods they can eat without discomfort and which ones they should avoid. Many will be able to enjoy milk, ice cream, and other such products if they take them in small amounts or eat other food at the same time. Others can use lactase liquid or tablets to help digest the lactose. Even older women at risk for osteoporosis and growing children who must avoid milk and foods made with milk can meet most of their special dietary needs by eating greens, fish, and other calcium-rich foods that are free of lactose. A carefully chosen diet (with calcium supplements if the doctor or dietitian recommends them) is the key to reducing symptoms and protecting future health.

Chapter 26

Is It Celiac Disease or a Food Allergy?

Individuals with certain food sensitivities can occasionally be misdiagnosed and told they have a true food allergy. This is sometimes the case with celiac disease (also called celiac sprue), which is an immune reaction to wheat gluten (an amino acid chain that provides structure in grains).

According to Roger L. Gebhard, M.D., professor of medicine at the University of Minnesota's Veterans Administration Hospital, "Celiac sprue is not a true food allergy, but a genetic disease that is characterized by damage to the mucosal lining of the small intestine." The highest incidence of the disease occurs primarily in Ireland, where approximately one-in-three hundred people is affected.

Finger-like projectiles or villi are part of the normal lining of the small intestine, and they help to increase the amount of surface available for the absorption of nutrients (such as protein, carbohydrate, fat, vitamins and minerals). In celiac sprue, the villi in the lining of the small intestine are lost and the surface flattens. The amount of surface available for nutrient absorption decreases resulting in malnutrition. Thus, the small intestine can be affected in part or in whole, and the more small intestine that is involved, the more severe the symptoms.

From "Celiac Sprue," *Food Insight*, May/June 1999. © 1999 International Food Information Council Foundation; reprinted with permission. Write to the International Food Information Council Foundation, 1100 Connecticut Avenue, NW, Suite 430, Washington, DC 20036 or visit http://ificinfo.health.org for more information about food and health.

Symptoms of celiac sprue vary depending on the severity of the disease and how much of the small intestine is affected. Symptoms can occur at any time during the life span—many individuals who suffer as young children may have the disease reappear during their third or even fourth decade in life. Diarrhea may be frequent and accompanied by dehydration and loss of minerals. Patients with sprue may develop anemia (lack of iron or folate), osteoporosis (lack of calcium and vitamin D), and easy bruising. Weight loss is also common due to malnutrition, but some individuals may maintain weight since celiac sprue patients generally have healthy appetites.

Avoidance of dietary gluten is the best treatment for celiac sprue patients. Persons must strictly adhere to a gluten-free diet and avoid gluten in wheat, rye, barley, and oats. Since currently there is no cure, the most effective treatment of celiac sprue patients, along with avoidance, is good nutrition.

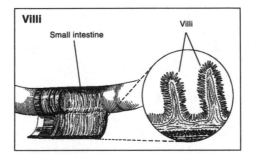

Figure 26.1. *Villi, located in the small intestine, help absorb nutrients as food is digested. (Illustration from* Digestive Diseases Dictionary, *National Digestive Diseases Information Clearinghouse, National Institute of Diabetes and Digestive and Kidney Diseases (NIDDK), NIH Pub. No 97-5750.)*

Chapter 27

Wheat Allergy

What is wheat allergy?

Wheat allergy refers specifically to adverse reactions involving immunoglobulin E (IgE) antibodies to one or more protein fractions of wheat, including albumin, globulin, gliadin and glutenin (gluten). The majority of IgE-mediated reactions to wheat involve the albumin and globulin fractions. Gliadin and gluten may also induce IgE-mediated reactions rarely.

Allergic reactions to wheat may be caused by ingestion of wheat-containing foods or by inhalation of flour containing wheat (baker's asthma).

How common is wheat allergy?

There are no accurate figures for prevalence of wheat allergy. Clinical experience suggests that wheat allergy is relatively uncommon. However, it may be more common in certain subgroups, for example wheat allergy is responsible for occupational asthma in up to 30% of individuals in the baking industry.

What are the symptoms of wheat allergy?

Allergic reactions to wheat (IgE-antibody mediated) usually begin within minutes or a few hours after eating or inhaling wheat. The

"Wheat Allergy," by Dr C. Motala; Copyright: Allergy Society of South Africa; reprinted with permission. This information sheet is obtainable from: ALLSA, P.O. Box 88, Observatory, 7935, Cape Town, R.S.A.

more common symptoms involve the skin (urticaria, atopic eczema, angioedema) gastrointestinal tract (oral allergy syndrome, abdominal cramps, nausea, and vomiting) and the respiratory tract (asthma or allergic rhinitis). IgE-mediated reactions to gliadin or gluten can cause urticaria, angioedema, or life-threatening anaphylaxis in association with exercise. Other gluten-containing cereals (rye, oats, and barley) may also cause these symptoms due to cross-reactivity of the allergens.

How is wheat-allergy diagnosed?

The diagnosis may be easy if a person always has the same reaction after eating wheat-containing food or eats wheat infrequently. But more often the diagnosis is difficult because wheat is a staple food. Diagnosis usually entails clinical evaluation (medical history, family

Table 27.1. Identifying wheat in food products.

Label ingredients that indicate the presence of wheat proteins

- Bread crumbs
- Bran
- Cereal extract
- Couscous
- Cracker meal
- Enriched flour
- Gluten
- High-gluten flour, high-protein flour
- Semolina wheat
- Vital gluten
- Wheat bran, wheat germ, wheat gluten, wheat malt, wheat starch
- Whole wheat flour

Label ingredients that may indicate the presence of wheat protein

- Gelatinized starch
- Hydrolyzed vegetable protein
- Modified food starch, modified starch
- Natural flavoring
- Soy sauce
- Starch
- Vegetable gum, vegetable starch

history, food history) supported by appropriate laboratory tests (RAST, skin prick-testing). Elimination-challenge testing remains the most reliable method of diagnosis.

How is wheat allergy treated?

Avoidance of wheat and wheat-containing foods is the first step in the treatment of wheat allergy. However, because wheat is a staple food product, wheat elimination diets are particularly difficult for a patient and his/her family to maintain. Children on wheat-restricted diets are severely limited in their selection of foods. Alternatives may be found in special health shops. Treatment must be supervised by a dietician—who provides wheat-free recipes and ensures nutritionally adequate diet. Wheat allergic patients who have sensitivity to gluten (or gliadin) should avoid other gluten containing cereals such as oats, rye and barley.

Chapter 28

Soy Allergies

Soy, also referred to as soya, soy bean, or glycine max, is among the main foods that produce reactions worldwide—mostly, but not exclusively, in infants.

It is not completely certain which specific component of soy is responsible for reactions, but at least 15 allergenic proteins have been identified.

Soy allergy is more prevalent in infants. The median age at which the allergy manifests is 3 months, but the majority outgrow it by the age of two. Although adults do suffer from this allergy, it is rare.

The way soy foods are processed can affect allergenicity. All soy products may not cause reactions. Some fermented soy foods may be less allergenic than raw soy beans. Soybean oil, which does not contain protein, may not produce symptoms. It just depends on the individual.

Symptoms of Soy Allergy

The reported symptoms of soy bean allergy include: acne, angioedema, rhinitis, anaphylaxis, asthma, atopic dermatitis, bronchospasm, cankers, colitis, conjunctivitis, diarrhea, diffuse small bowel disease, dyspnea, eczema, enterocolitis, fever, hypotension, itching, laryngeal edema, lethargy, pollinosis, urticaria, vomiting, and wheezing.

Cross Reactivity

Those [who are allergic] to soy beans may also cross react to certain foods, such as peanuts, green peas, chick peas, lima beans, string beans, wheat flour, rye flour, and barley flour.

Soy Terms and Products

A great many foods already in your kitchen cupboard contain products that contain some type of soy food. Listed below are the terms associated with soy foods:

- **Hydrolyzed vegetable protein (HVP)** is a protein obtained from any vegetable, including soy beans that is a flavor enhancer that can be used in soups, broths, sauces, gravies, flavoring and spice blends, canned and frozen vegetables, meats and poultry.

- **Lecithin** is extracted from soybean oil and is used in foods that are high in fats and oils to promote stabilization, antioxidation, crystallization, and spattering control. It is used as an emulsifier in chocolate. Most infant formulas contain soy lechithin.

- **Miso**, used to flavor soups, sauces, dressings, marinades and pâtés, is a rich, salty condiment made from soy beans and a grain such as rice.

- **Mono-diglyceride**, another soy derivative, is used for emulsion in many foods.

- **Monosodium glutamate (MSG)** may contain hydroylzed protein which is often made from soy.

- **Natto**, more easily digested than whole soy beans, is made of fermented and cooked whole soy beans.

- **Natural flavors**, listed on ingredient labels may be a soy derivative.

- **Soy cheese**, a substitute for sour cream or cream cheese, is made from soy milk.

- **Soy fiber** whether okara, soy bran, and soy isolate fiber are used as food ingredients.

- **Soy flour**, whether natural, defatted, and lecithinated, is made from finely ground roasted soy beans. They are often used to give a protein boost to recipes.

- **Soy grits**, made from toasted coarsely cracked soy beans, is used as a flour substitute.

- **Soy meal** and soy oil are used in a number of industrial products, including inks, soaps, and cosmetics.

- **Soy milk** is used alone or can be made into soy yogurt, soy cheese, or tofu.

- **Soy oil**, the natural oil extracted from whole soy beans, is the most widely used oil in the United States. It accounts for more than 75 percent of the total vegetable fats and oils intake. Soy oil is used to make most margarines, Crisco and other vegetable shortenings, prepared pasta sauces, Worcestershire sauce, salad dressings, mayonnaise, canned tuna, dry lemonade mix, and hot chocolate mix. Most commercial baked goods like breads, rolls, cakes, cookies, and crackers contain soy oil. Some prepackaged cereals are also made with soy oil.

- **Soy protein** can be labeled as soy protein concentrate, isolated soy protein, textured soy protein (TSP), and textured soy flour (TSF). Textured soy flour is widely used as a meat extender. Most soup bouillons contain some form of soy protein. Many meat alternatives contain soy protein or tofu.

- **Soy sauces**, the most common being Tamari (a by-product of making miso), Shoyu (a blend of soy beans and wheat), and Teriyaki (with added sugar, vinegar, and spices), are dark brown liquids made from soy beans that have undergone a fermenting process.

- **Soy yogurt**, made from soy milk, is an easy substitute for sour cream or cream cheese. Non dairy frozen desserts are made from soy milk or soy yogurt.

- **Tempeh**, a traditional Indonesian food, is a chunky, tender soybean cake.

- **Tofu**, also known as soybean curd, is a soft cheese-like food made by curdling fresh hot soy milk with a coagulant. It is a bland product that easily absorbs the flavors of other ingredients with which it is cooked. When mixed with other ingredients it can simulate various kinds of meat.

- **Vegetable oil**, a generic term, is usually 100 percent soy oil or a blend of soy oil and other oils.

- **Vegetable protein** is often the term used for soy protein.

- **Vitamin E** contains soy bean oil.

If you are [allergic] to soy, it is best to read all ingredient labels, and if in doubt, contact the manufacturer of the product before purchasing it.

Chapter 29

Seafood Allergies

The third leading cause of food allergy (after eggs and milk) is seafood, which includes both fish and shellfish.

Who Is Affected?

Populations that consume or process large quantities of seafood tend to have the highest prevalence of seafood allergy. For instance, shrimp allergy is more common in the southern United States while fish allergy is more common in Spain and the Scandinavian countries.

Factory workers who work in seafood-processing industries are highly affected, as well as fishermen and restaurant workers. Up to 30 percent of these workers have occupational asthma, contact dermatitis, or eczema.

Fish allergies are more common in children, whereas shellfish allergies seem be more prevalent in adults. Some breastfed infants have been sensitized to cod via their mother's milk. These allergies do not usually go away or diminish with age. These allergies usually last a lifetime with the reactions becoming more severe with each subsequent exposure.

Fish Allergy

It is estimated that about 22 percent of all populations suffer from a fish allergy. The fish commonly known to cause allergic reactions include cod, salmon, trout, herring, sardines, bass, orange roughy, swordfish, halibut, and tuna.

Severe asthmatic attacks can be triggered by the smell of fish in a sensitive person. Even anaphylactic shock has been reported after eating foods cooked in reused cooking oil, or when utensils and containers have been used earlier for cooking fish.

Shellfish Allergy

The shellfish commonly known to cause allergic reactions include shrimp, crab, crayfish, lobster, oysters, clams, scallops, mussels, squid, and snails.

Shrimp is usually associated with seafood allergies. Those allergic to shrimp often suffer from respiratory allergy. Crab is also a potent allergen. Shrimp, lobster, and [crayfish] contain common major allergens, making cross reactivity between shrimp and crab, and lobster and [crayfish] possible.

Symptoms

The manifestations of fish and shellfish allergies can include those of a classic food allergy. The more common symptoms include skin, stomach, or respiratory problems. More specifically they can include nasal congestion, hives, itching, swelling, wheezing or shortness of breath, nausea, upset stomach, cramps, heartburn, gas, diarrhea, lightheadedness, or fainting.

Reactions usually appear within 2 hours after ingestion, inhaling cooking vapors, or handling of seafood. However, it has been reported the reactions can be delayed as long as 24 hours.

Keep in mind, "Fish and shellfish spoil easily," says James T. Li, M.D., a specialist in allergies, asthma and immunology at Mayo Clinic, Rochester, MN. "In some cases, spoiled fish can contain histamine, a substance that causes hives and flushing. If someone eats the spoiled fish, they can have symptoms similar to an allergic reaction. But this is actually a type of food poisoning."

Preventative Tips

Seafood allergies have no effective preventive treatment other than patient education and complete avoidance.

Food labels need to be read carefully because highly processed foods may contain hidden fish or shellfish. For example, the basis for imitation crab, lobster, and shrimp is pollock. It can also be used in beef and pork substitutes as part of hot dogs, ham, and pizza toppings. Also, fish skin is used to clarify some coffees and wines.

If you suffer from seafood allergies, educate and inform others about your sensitivity. Be sure to wear a medic alert tag and carry an adrenaline kit in case of anaphylactic shock.

Chapter 30

Sulfites: Safe for Most, Dangerous for Some

It wasn't a special occasion—or even a fancy restaurant—but Karen, 37, will never forget that meal:

My boyfriend and I were at a hamburger joint, and I had a burger and fries. About 10 minutes after we finished eating, my throat began to itch. I grabbed my [asthma] inhaler but I could feel my throat constricting. I couldn't breathe and started to panic. When I passed out, my boyfriend flagged down a passing police car. The officer radioed for an ambulance, and I was rushed to the hospital. I was revived with a massive dose of epinephrine to counteract the reaction caused by the sulfite solution the potatoes had been soaked in before frying.

I know enough to stay away from wine, shrimp and other foods that contain sulfites, and take note whenever I don't feel right after eating something. But I never expected french fries to be sulfited. I've had allergic reactions to sulfites before, but this time I came close to dying.

I was angry that this happened to me. I felt powerless—I was careful and knowledgeable, and yet I couldn't protect myself. Who ever heard of a lethal french fry? Afterward, I refused to

From "Sulfites: Safe for Most, Dangerous for Some," by Ruth Papazian in *FDA Consumer*, December 1996. *FDA Consumer* is produced by the U.S. Food and Drug Administration.

eat out in restaurants for almost two years, and I still can't visit people or go on vacation without knowing there is a hospital nearby.

The Food and Drug Administration estimates that one out of a hundred people is sulfite-sensitive, and that 5 percent of those who have asthma, like Karen (who asked that her last name not be used), are also at risk of suffering an adverse reaction to the substance. "By law, adverse reactions to drugs must be reported to FDA by doctors or pharmaceutical companies. But with sulfites and other food ingredients, reporting is voluntary so it's difficult to say just how many people may be at risk," cautions FDA consumer safety officer JoAnn Ziyad, Ph.D.

Complicating matters, scientists have not pinpointed the smallest concentration of sulfites needed to provoke a reaction in a sensitive or allergic person. FDA requires food manufacturers and processors to disclose the presence of sulfiting agents in concentrations of at least 10 parts per million, but the threshold may be even lower. The assay used to detect the level of sulfites in food is not sensitive enough to detect amounts less than 10 ppm in all foods (that's 1 part sulfite to 100,000 parts of food—the equivalent of a drop of water in a bathtub) so that's what the regulation has to be based on, explains Ziyad.

"The most rapid reactions occur when sulfites are sprayed onto foods or are present in a beverage, but the most severe reactions occur when sulfites are constituents of the food itself," says Ron Simon, M.D., head of Allergy, Asthma and Immunology at Scripps Clinic and Research Foundation in La Jolla, California.

A person can develop sulfite sensitivity at any point in life, and no one knows what triggers onset or the mechanism by which reactions occur. "Doctors believe that asthmatics develop difficulty breathing by inhaling sulfite fumes from treated foods," notes Dan Atkins, M.D., a pediatrician at the National Jewish Center for Immunology and Respiratory Medicine in Denver, Colorado. He says that in a severe reaction an overwhelming degree of bronchial constriction occurs, causing breathing to stop. This can lead to lack of oxygen reaching the brain, heart, and other organs and tissues and, possibly, a fatal heart rhythm irregularity.

"We now know that asthmatics who have more severe symptoms and are dependent on corticosteroids, such as prednisone or methylprednisolone, are especially prone to sulfite sensitivity and are most at risk of having a severe reaction," notes Atkins. But it's a chicken-and-egg situation, notes Simon: "We don't know which comes first, the asthma or the sulfite sensitivity, because some people's first experience with asthma is a sulfite reaction, and as their asthma becomes more severe they eventually become steroid-dependent."

Sulfite sensitivity can be tricky to diagnose. Karen went to an internist and two pulmonary specialists without getting to the bottom of her problem.

"People who do experience adverse reactions to sulfites know that it's something they ate, but might not know what that something is," says Atkins. "I'll ask a patient complaining of an adverse reaction what he or she ate and drank when it occurred. If beer or wine doesn't seem to be the problem, I tend to dismiss sulfite sensitivity. But if I think sulfites may be the culprit, I'll do a challenge [a type of allergy test in which a small amount of the suspect substance is administered in a capsule or in a drink and the patient is monitored to see whether there is a reaction]."

If a person develops hives after ingesting sulfites, the doctor will do a prick test (a small concentration of sulfite is placed on the skin, which is then pricked; the test is positive if a welt develops on the spot). "People who have positive skin tests to sulfites are likely to be allergic to the additive, rather than have a sensitivity. These people, who are usually not asthmatic, are most at risk of anaphylactic shock, [a life-threatening reaction]," says Simon.

Regulatory Status in Flux

Sulfur-based preservatives, or sulfites, have been used around the world for centuries to:

- inhibit oxidation ("browning") of light-colored fruits and vegetables, such as dried apples and dehydrated potatoes
- prevent melanosis ("black spot") on shrimp and lobster
- discourage bacterial growth as wine ferments
- "condition" dough
- bleach food starches
- maintain the stability and potency of some medications.

When the Federal Food, Drug, and Cosmetic Act was amended in 1958 to regulate preservatives and other food additives, FDA considered sulfites to be generally recognized as safe (GRAS). But when FDA reevaluated their safety and proposed to affirm the GRAS status of sulfiting agents in 1982, the agency received numerous reports from consumers and the medical community regarding adverse health reactions. In response, FDA contracted with the Federation of American Societies for Experimental Biology (FASEB) to examine the link between sulfites and reported health problems that ranged from chest tightness or difficulty breathing to hives to fatal anaphylactic shock.

In 1985, FASEB concluded that sulfites are safe for most people, but pose a hazard of unpredictable severity to asthmatics and others who are sensitive to these preservatives. Based on this report, FDA took the following regulatory actions in 1986:

- Prohibited the use of sulfites to maintain color and crispness on fruits and vegetables meant to be eaten raw (for instance, restaurant salad bars or fresh produce in the supermarket).

- Required companies to list on product labels sulfiting agents that occur at concentrations of 10 ppm or higher, and any sulfiting agents that had a technical or functional effect in the food (for instance, as a preservative) regardless of the amount present. (This labeling requirement was extended to standardized foods, such as pickles and bottled lemon juice, in 1993.)

FDA requires that the presence of sulfites be disclosed on labels of packaged food (although manufacturers need not specify the particular agent used). This information will be included in the ingredient portion of the label, along with the function of the sulfiting agent in the food (for instance, a preservative).

When food is sold unpackaged in bulk form (as with a barrel of dried fruit or loose, raw shrimp at the fresh fish counter), store managers must post a sign or some other type of labeling that lists the food's ingredients on the container or at the counter so that consumers can determine whether the product was treated with a sulfiting agent.

In 1987, FDA proposed to revoke the GRAS status of sulfiting agents on "fresh" (not canned, dehydrated or frozen) potatoes intended to be cooked and served unpackaged and unlabeled to consumers (french fries, for example), and issued a final ruling to this effect in 1990. However, the rule was held null and void in 1990 after a protracted court battle in which the "fresh" potato industry prevailed on procedural grounds.

This legal setback notwithstanding, "the agency continues to have concerns about the safety of sulfiting agents, and plans further action to protect the consumer," notes Ziyad. Steps the agency is considering include establishing maximum residual levels for specific foods and additional labeling rules.

"The ultimate goal of sulfite regulation is to make sure that there is no higher level of sulfite residues in food than is absolutely necessary and to encourage the use of substitutes for sulfites in food processing," says Ziyad.

Sniffing Out Sulfites

Since 1985, FDA's Adverse Reaction Monitoring System has been tracking reactions to sulfites. Over a 10-year period, 1,097 such cases have been reported. However, thanks to regulatory action taken by FDA over the years, coupled with increased consumer savvy, the number of reported sulfite-related health incidents has been dropping steadily. In 1995, just six cases were reported.

FDA banned the use of sulfites on fruits and vegetables that are to be eaten raw (as with a salad bar)—and the vast majority of those in the food service industry honor the prohibition—but consumers who are sulfite-sensitive "shouldn't take anything for granted," says Ziyad.

Current FDA regulations do not require managers of food service establishments to disclose whether sulfites were used in food preparation. "Consumers continually request FDA to extend the regulation to include food service establishments because either waiters and other staff members didn't know whether the food was treated with sulfites, or gave erroneous information," notes Ziyad. "FDA's position on the issue has been that consumers who see sulfites listed on the label of a packaged food should be able to deduce that the same food sold in a food service establishment would also contain sulfites," she explains.

In addition, sulfites are still found in a variety of cooked and processed foods (including baked goods, condiments, dried and glacéed fruit, jam, gravy, dehydrated or pre-cut or peeled "fresh" potatoes, molasses, shrimp, and soup mixes) and beverages (such as beer, wine, hard cider, fruit and vegetable juices, and tea).

Since sulfites are added to so many foods, someone who is sensitive to the additive must not assume that a food is safe to eat, says Atkins. He recommends these measures to avoid sulfites when buying unlabeled foods at the deli or supermarket and ordering at a restaurant:

- If the food is packaged, read the label. If it is being sold loose or by the portion, ask the store manager or waiter to check the ingredient list on the product's original bulk-size packaging.

- Avoid processed foods that contain sulfites, such as dried fruits, canned vegetables, maraschino cherries, and guacamole. If you want to eat a potato, order a baked potato rather than hash browns, fries, or any dish that involves peeling the potato first.

- If you have asthma, have your inhaler with you when you go out to eat. Similarly, if you've experienced a severe reaction to sulfites in the past (such as breaking out in hives), carry an antihistamine and make sure you have handy a self-administering injectable epinephrine, such as EpiPen®, so that if you have a reaction you can stabilize your condition until you get to an emergency room.

"It takes some doing, but you can take steps to minimize your contact with sulfites if you are diagnosed with asthma or sulfite sensitivity," says Ziyad. "But you may not even know you have a problem with sulfites until a reaction occurs. Undiagnosed people are at risk because even if they know that sulfites can cause adverse reactions, they often don't associate sulfites with their own health problems," says Ziyad.

"Regulations can go a long way towards protecting people, but there's no substitute for knowledge."

Chapter 31

Monosodium Glutamate (MSG)

Monosodium glutamate (MSG) is used as a flavor enhancer in a variety of foods prepared at home, in restaurants, and by food processors. Its use has become controversial in the past 30 years because of reports of adverse reactions in people who've eaten foods that contain MSG. Research on the role of glutamate—a group of chemicals that includes MSG—in the nervous system also has raised questions about the chemical's safety.

Studies have shown that the body uses glutamate, an amino acid, as a nerve impulse transmitter in the brain and that there are glutamate-responsive tissues in other parts of the body, as well. Abnormal function of glutamate receptors has been linked with certain neurological diseases, such as Alzheimer's disease and Huntington's chorea. Injections of glutamate in laboratory animals have resulted in damage to nerve cells in the brain. Consumption of glutamate in food, however, does not cause this effect. While people normally consume dietary glutamate in large amounts and the body can make and metabolize glutamate efficiently, the results of animal studies conducted in the 1980s raised a significant question: Can MSG and possibly some other glutamates harm the nervous system? A 1995 report from the Federation of American Societies for Experimental Biology (FASEB), an independent body of scientists, helps put these safety concerns into perspective and reaffirms the Food and Drug

"FDA and Monosodium Glutamate (MSG)," FDA Backgrounder, BG 95-16, U.S. Food and Drug Administration, August 31, 1995; reviewed and revised by David A. Cooke, M.D. February 3, 2001.

Administration's belief that MSG and related substances are safe food ingredients for most people when eaten at customary levels.

The FASEB report identifies two groups of people who may develop a condition the report refers to as "MSG symptom complex." One group is those who may be intolerant to MSG when eaten in a large quantity. The second is a group of people with severe, poorly controlled asthma. These people, in addition to being prone to MSG symptom complex, may suffer temporary worsening of asthmatic symptoms after consuming MSG. The MSG dosage that produced reactions in these people ranged from 0.5 grams to 2.5 grams.

What Is MSG?

MSG is the sodium salt of the amino acid glutamic acid and a form of glutamate. It is sold as a fine white crystal substance, similar in appearance to salt or sugar. It does not have a distinct taste of its own, and how it adds flavor to other foods is not fully understood. Many scientists believe that MSG stimulates glutamate receptors in the tongue to augment meat-like flavors.

Asians originally used a seaweed broth to obtain the flavor-enhancing effects of MSG, but today MSG is made by a fermenting process using starch, sugar beets, sugar cane, or molasses.

Glutamate itself is in many living things: It is found naturally in our bodies and in protein-containing foods, such as cheese, milk, meat, peas, and mushrooms.

Some glutamate is in foods in a "free" form. It is only in this free form that glutamate can enhance a food's flavor. Part of the flavor-enhancing effect of tomatoes, certain cheeses, and fermented or hydrolyzed protein products (such as soy sauce) is due to the presence of free glutamate.

Hydrolyzed proteins, or protein hydrolysates, are acid-treated or enzymatically treated proteins from certain foods. They contain salts of free amino acids, such as glutamate, at levels of 5 to 20 percent. Hydrolyzed proteins are used in the same manner as MSG in many foods, such as canned vegetables, soups, and processed meats.

Scientific Review

In 1959, FDA classified MSG as a "generally recognized as safe," or GRAS, substance, along with many other common food ingredients, such as salt, vinegar, and baking powder. This action stemmed from the 1958 Food Additives Amendment to the Federal Food, Drug, and

Cosmetic Act, which required premarket approval for new food additives and led FDA to promulgate regulations listing substances, such as MSG, which have a history of safe use or are otherwise GRAS.

Since 1970, FDA has sponsored extensive reviews on the safety of MSG, other glutamates and hydrolyzed proteins, as part of an ongoing review of safety data on GRAS substances used in processed foods.

One such review was by the FASEB Select Committee on GRAS Substances. In 1980, the committee concluded that MSG was safe at current levels of use but recommended additional evaluation to determine MSG's safety at significantly higher levels of consumption. Additional reports attempted to look at this.

In 1986, FDA's Advisory Committee on Hypersensitivity to Food Constituents concluded that MSG poses no threat to the general public but that reactions of brief duration might occur in some people.

Other reports gave similar findings. A 1991 report by the European Communities' (EC) Scientific Committee for Foods reaffirmed MSG's safety and classified its "acceptable daily intake" as "not specified," the most favorable designation for a food ingredient. In addition, the EC Committee said, "Infants, including prematures, have been shown to metabolize glutamate as efficiently as adults and therefore do not display any special susceptibility to elevated oral intakes of glutamate."

A 1992 report from the Council on Scientific Affairs of the American Medical Association stated that glutamate in any form has not been shown to be a "significant health hazard."

Also, the 1987 Joint Expert Committee on Food Additives of the United Nations Food and Agriculture Organization and the World Health Organization have placed MSG in the safest category of food ingredients.

Scientific knowledge about how the body metabolizes glutamate developed rapidly during the 1980s. Studies showed that glutamate in the body plays an important role in normal functioning of the nervous system. Questions then arose on the role glutamate in food plays in these functions and whether or not glutamate in food contributes to certain neurological diseases.

Anecdotal Evidence

Many of these safety assessments were prompted by unconfirmed reports of MSG-related adverse reactions. Between 1980 and 1994, the Adverse Reaction Monitoring System in FDA's Center for Food Safety and Applied Nutrition received 622 reports of complaints about

MSG. Headache was the most frequently reported symptom. No severe reactions were documented, but some reports indicated that people with asthma got worse after they consumed MSG. In some of those cases, the asthma didn't get worse until many hours later.

Also, several books and a TV news show have reported widespread and sometimes life-threatening adverse reactions to MSG, claiming that even small amounts of manufactured glutamates may cause adverse reactions.

A problem with these unconfirmed reports is that it is difficult to link the reactions specifically to MSG. Most are cases in which people have had reactions after, but not necessarily because of, eating certain foods containing MSG.

While such reports are helpful in raising issues of concern, they do not provide the kind of information necessary to describe who is most likely to be affected, under what conditions they'll be affected, and with what amounts of MSG. They are not controlled studies done in a scientifically credible manner.

1995 FASEB Report

Prompted by continuing public interest and a flurry of glutamate-related studies in the late 1980s, FDA contracted with FASEB in 1992 to review the available scientific data. The agency asked FASEB to address 18 questions dealing with:

- the possible role of MSG in eliciting MSG symptom complex

- the possible role of dietary glutamates in forming brain lesions and damaging nerve cells in humans

- underlying conditions that may predispose a person to adverse effects from MSG

- the amount consumed and other factors that may affect a person's response to MSG

- the quality of scientific data and previous safety reviews.

FASEB held a two-day meeting and convened an expert panel that thoroughly reviewed all the available scientific literature on this issue.

FASEB completed the final report, over 350 pages long, and delivered it to FDA on July 31, 1995. While not a new study, the report offers a new safety assessment based on the most comprehensive existing evaluation to date of glutamate safety.

Among the report's key findings:

- An unknown percentage of the population may react to MSG and develop MSG symptom complex, a condition characterized by one or more of the following symptoms:

  - burning sensation in the back of the neck, forearms and chest

  - numbness in the back of the neck, radiating to the arms and back

  - tingling, warmth and weakness in the face, temples, upper back, neck and arms

  - facial pressure or tightness

  - chest pain

  - headache

  - nausea

  - rapid heartbeat

  - bronchospasm (difficulty breathing) in MSG-intolerant people with asthma

  - drowsiness

  - weakness.

- In otherwise healthy MSG-intolerant people, the MSG symptom complex tends to occur within one hour after eating 3 grams or more of MSG on an empty stomach or without other food. A typical serving of glutamate-treated food contains less than 0.5 grams of MSG. A reaction is most likely if the MSG is eaten in a large quantity or in a liquid, such as a clear soup.

- Severe, poorly controlled asthma may be a predisposing medical condition for MSG symptom complex.

- No evidence exists to suggest that dietary MSG or glutamate contributes to Alzheimer's disease, Huntington's chorea, amyotrophic lateral sclerosis, AIDS dementia complex, or any other long-term or chronic diseases.

- No evidence exists to suggest that dietary MSG causes brain lesions or damages nerve cells in humans.

- The level of vitamin B_6 in a person's body plays a role in glutamate metabolism, and the possible impact of marginal B_6 intake should be considered in future research

- There is no scientific evidence that the levels of glutamate in hydrolyzed proteins causes adverse effects or that other manufactured glutamate has effects different from glutamate normally found in foods

Ingredient Listing

Under current FDA regulations, when MSG is added to a food, it must be identified as "monosodium glutamate" in the label's ingredient list. Each ingredient used to make a food must be declared by its name in this list.

While technically MSG is only one of several forms of free glutamate used in foods, consumers frequently use the term MSG to mean all free glutamate. For this reason, FDA considers foods whose labels say "No MSG" or "No Added MSG" to be misleading if the food contains ingredients that are sources of free glutamates, such as hydrolyzed protein.

In 1993, FDA proposed adding the phrase "(contains glutamate)" to the common or usual names of certain protein hydrolysates that contain substantial amounts of glutamate. For example, if the proposal were adopted, hydrolyzed soy protein would have to be declared on food labels as "hydrolyzed soy protein (contains glutamate)." However, if FDA issues a new proposal, it would probably supersede this 1993 one.

In 1994, FDA received a citizen's petition requesting changes in labeling requirements for foods that contain MSG or related substances. The petition asks for mandatory listing of MSG as an ingredient on labels of manufactured and processed foods that contain manufactured free glutamic acid. It further asks that the amount of free glutamic acid or MSG in such products be stated on the label, along with a warning that MSG may be harmful to certain groups of people. FDA has not yet taken action on the petition.

Copies of the 1995 FASEB report are available for $50 each by writing to FASEB at 9650 Rockville Pike, Bethesda, MD 20814.

Chapter 32

Red Wine, Histamine, and Headache

Foods containing histamine, especially red wine, can induce headaches and other symptoms in individuals who are intolerant to histamine. This review article describes the biochemical basis for histamine intolerance, lists foods and beverages which are rich in histamine, and provides practical information on the treatment of this cause of chronic headaches.

Histamine intolerance occurs in people who have an impaired ability to degrade histamine because of reduced activity or a complete lack of the enzyme diamine oxidase. This enzyme, which is located in the jejunal mucosa, plays a clinical role in the normal metabolism of histamine.

In experimental models, headaches have been induced by infusion of histamine as well as by ingestion of red wine. Histamine-induced headache is a vascular headache, and nitric oxide probably plays a role in its causation.

Histamine is found in all types of wine, beer, certain fish such as sardines and anchovies, ripened cheeses, hard cured sausages, and a few vegetable products, including pickled cabbage, spinach, and tomato ketchup. Concentrations in red wine are generally higher than those in other foods and beverages. Red wine contains 20- to 200-fold more histamine than white wine.

"Red Wine, Histamine, and Headache," in *Nutrition Research Newsletter*, June 1996, vol. 15, no. 6, p. 72(1) Copyright 1999, *Nutrition Research Newsletter*. Reprinted with permission of John Wiley & Sons, Inc.

The recommended treatment for histamine intolerance is a histamine-free diet. Such diets are relatively simple to follow, inexpensive, and nutritionally adequate (provided that milk is consumed as a calcium source in place of cheese). Vitamin B_6 supplementation is also helpful in patients with histamine intolerance, presumably because it is crucial for diamine oxidase activity. Antihistamine drugs are also of value at the beginning of treatment and in case of dietary errors.

The authors recommend that histamine containing foods and beverages should be labeled for the benefit of individuals following a histamine-free diet. They also recommend that when physicians evaluate patients with chronic headaches, they should consider histamine intolerance early in their diagnostic investigations, since both the diagnosis and treatment of this condition are relatively simple.

Resource

Reinhart Jarisch and Felix Wantke, "Wine and Headache," *International Archives Allergy and Immunology* 110(1): 7-12 (May 1996).

Chapter 33

Beer-Related Anaphylaxis

Tingling in the face, trouble breathing, and hives—all from one glass of beer? Although it sounds extreme, those with allergy to barley can experience these and other symptoms after only a small amount of the brewed beverage.

Three case studies in the *Journal of Allergy and Clinical Immunology* (May 1999) illustrate the severity of allergy to beer and the need for physicians and affected consumers to take this condition seriously.

Researchers in Madrid, Spain studied three patients who suffered anaphylactic reactions after consuming beer. The patients experienced a range of symptoms including a tingling sensation in the face, lip or tongue angioedema, chest tightness, coughing, fainting, and generalized urticaria.

The research team prepared an extract from barley-made beer and performed skin prick testing. The three patients had positive skin prick test results, while 20 control patients had negative test responses. The study indicates that barley-made beer is a potential culprit of severe anaphylaxis and barley-sensitive patients should be questioned about beer tolerance.

Anaphylaxis is a severe allergic reaction that affects multiple systems in the body. Symptoms can include severe headache, nausea and

From "Researchers Say Beer Anaphylaxis Under-Recognized," in *Doctor's Guide to the Internet*, May 14, 1999; © 1999 P\S\L Consulting Group Inc. Reprinted by permission. *Doctor's Guide to the Internet* is at http://www.docguide.com.

vomiting, sneezing and coughing, abdominal cramps, diarrhea, hives, swelling of the lips, tongue and throat, itching all over the body, and anxiety. The most dangerous symptoms include breathing difficulties, a drop in blood pressure and shock—all of which can be fatal.

Part Four

Allergy Triggers

Chapter 34

Allergens and Irritants in the Home

Chapter Contents

Section 34.1

Common Household Irritants

From "Allergy Action," by Diane Kittower, in *Today's Homeowner*, April 1997, vol. 93, no. 814, p18(1). Copyright © 1997 Times Mirror Magazines Inc.. Reprinted with permission.

If the first signs of spring make you itch to begin painting, remodeling or even simply cleaning house, make sure your itch does not become literal. Many home-related products must be used with extra care by anyone who suffers from asthma, allergies, or chemical sensitivities.

Painting. Use water-based (latex) paint with low levels of or no volatile organic compounds (VOCs). Besides reducing the irritation that comes with VOCs, these paints are easier to work with and clean up than oil-based paints are; what's more, they're just as durable.

Remodeling. Along with keeping dust down as much as possible, try to avoid plywood or paneling made with adhesives that contain formaldehyde, a suspected carcinogen that causes upper respiratory irritation. Interior paneling, cabinets, and countertops made with particleboard probably contain urea-formaldehyde, which is the most irritating. Construction-grade, "exterior glue" plywood is made with a phenolic-resin-based adhesive and emits much less formaldehyde.

Cleaning the air. Very dry air is a problem for asthmatics. On the other hand, too much moisture encourages the growth of mold and mildew, both common allergens. The American Lung Association recommends aiming for a household humidity level of 30 to 50 percent. You can measure the relative humidity in your house with an inexpensive (and low-tech) hygrometer or with a $25 electronic version.

Kitchen and bathroom exhaust fans, air-conditioning, and a dehumidifier can help reduce humidity. If you want to add moisture with a portable or built-in humidifier, look for a molecular model, which evaporates water with a fan. Keep humidifiers and dehumidifiers clean to discourage mold and mildew.

When humidity rises above 50 percent, dust mites are more likely to be a problem. These microscopic critters can set off an allergic reaction. They love carpeting, so consider installing hardwood, linoleum, or ceramic-tile flooring instead.

Housecleaning. Even a house that's white-glove clean can harbor dust mites, but that's no reason to avoid spring cleaning. In fact, banishing dirt from the 12 typical trouble spots is crucial (see "The Dirty Dozen"). Just be sure people with asthma and those with allergies don't vacuum. And whoever does should use a machine with a high-efficiency filter to trap particulates.

The average household stocks some 50 chemicals for cleaning and other purposes. As they evaporate, they send irritating vapors into the air. Store them in a garage or, better yet, consider some good old-fashioned alternatives. A combination of baking soda and a little water makes an effective scouring powder, and a solution of equal parts lemon juice and water makes a good grease cutter.

The Dirty Dozen

Minute as they are, mold, dust mites, pollen, viruses, and bacteria spark allergic reactions ranging from mild discomfort to severe asthma. These 12 trouble spots require extra attention and cleaning:

- Dirty air conditioners, humidifiers, and dehumidifiers
- Bathrooms without vents or windows
- Kitchens without vents or windows
- Dirty refrigerator drip pans
- Laundry rooms with unvented dryers
- Unventilated attics
- Bedding
- Carpeting
- Closets on outside walls
- Dirty heating and air-conditioning filters and ducts
- Water damage around windows, the roof of the basement
- Cats and dogs

Section 34.2

The Home Environment and Chemically Sensitive People

From "Environmental Allergies," by Ken Scharabok, in *Countryside & Small Stock Journal*, September/October 1997, vol. 81, no. 5, p. 63(2). © 1997 *Countryside & Small Stock Journal*; reprinted with permission.

If you suffer from severe allergies, after having yourself tested, also test your house.

In addition to harboring dust and dirt, it has been found that carpeting can contain more than 350 chemicals. Manufactured woods, such as particle board, can have a high formaldehyde content, which is toxic (Plywood used on the exterior and roofing is considered to be safe.)

Some insulation can contain up to twelve percent formaldehyde by volume. Heating and air conditioning ducts can harbor and recycle dust and plant spores. Paints, sealers, glues, and stains can contain organic or inorganic compounds.

Construction of airtight houses has only compounded the problem because of the limited air exchange between interior and exterior.

For homes with a central heating and air conditioning system, a filtration system can be installed to reduce airborne organic particles, such as pollens, but it may not reduce chemical or inorganic fumes or particles. However, much beyond filtration systems, it may not be cost effective to try to retrofit a house to reduce or eliminate allergy problems. Thus, some extremely sensitive families have had to build a new house to be as dust- and chemical-free as possible.

This can include no wall-to-wall carpeting; no manufactured wood products inside the house (which includes some cheaper grades of furniture); use of only pure fiberglass insulation; installation of a water filtration system; using radiant electric heat; installation of a high-quality ventilation and air filtration system; and using only paints, sealers, glues, and stains which have either no or a very low level of volatile inorganic or organic compounds.

In some cases trace elements or minerals in the water supply have been identified as the cause of allergies. Some occur naturally from the source of the water, others may be added by the water distribution company. While chlorine, to prevent disease, and fluoride, to protect teeth, are commonly known water additives, others include phosphates, sodium hydroxide, caustic sodas, silicates, aluminum sulfate, ferric chloride, potassium permanganate, and polymers. Some are added to control taste and odors. Others are added to protect water pipes from rusting or from leaching lead or copper into the water flow. All are considered to be safe, but the water comes with no warning label on its contents.

Some people have been found to be extremely reactive to some of these compounds and they may not be removed, or even effectively reduced, by using a reverse-osmosis water filtration system. This sometimes requires a separate water supply or even the purchase of large quantities of bottled or spring water. However, even the pipes from a private well may contain some compounds which leach into the water flow.

If severe allergies occur after moving to a new location or suddenly, suspect it is from an environmental source. The cause may require extensive research. For example, one of your children graduates to a new school and then suffers an allergic reaction. It may be from a different water supply, construction material used, or the site itself may have previously been a landfill or factory site. Then again it may be a daughter using lipstick for the first time and she is allergic to a compound in it.

Section 34.3

Environmental Control of Dust Mites

House dust sensitivity, documented by dermal sensitivity to dust mite allergen, is found in 10 percent of the general population and 90 percent of asthmatic patients.[1] Dust mites, the most common of which is *Dermatophagoides pteronyssinus*, are the cause of dust allergy.[2] We have learned the importance of these minute arthropods, measuring 0.33 mm, from data gathered in Papua, New Guinea, and elsewhere. Asthma was extremely rare in the Papua, New Guinea, highlands before the introduction of cheap cotton blankets. These blankets, rarely washed, have been shown to harbor large numbers of dust mites. The widespread use of these mite-infested blankets raised the incidence of asthma in adults in that area from 0.15 percent to 7.3 percent. The New Guinea data strongly suggest that mites cause allergic airway disease. That area now has one of the highest incidences of asthma in the world.[2]

Exposure to dust mites can cause chronic allergic diseases in atopic persons. Dust mite allergens are an important environmental cause of asthma. In many patients, asthma symptoms could be markedly decreased or, perhaps, prevented by reduction of exposure.[3]

Measuring Mite Allergens

Most of the information about house dust mite allergens has been determined for the *D. pteronyssinus* allergen, *Der p I*,[3] which is derived from mite feces and is the major dust mite allergen.[4] Allergen levels are generally described as levels of *Der p I*. The First International Workshop on house dust mite allergens proposed two threshold levels for risk. Exposure to levels greater than 2 μg per g [micrograms per gram] of *Der p I* in house dust is associated with an increased risk of sensitization, and levels greater than 10 μg per g are associated with a risk of acute asthma symptoms.

Mites flourish in the same environment in which humans are comfortable. They require warmth and humidity for survival. In very cold or dry climates, dust mite allergen levels are generally less than 2 μg per g. In more humid areas, levels usually range between 2 μg per g and 15 μg per g. Regions where the climate is favorable for mite growth for much of the year (coastal tropical and subtropical areas) have mean levels in the range of 10 to 40 μg per g.[4] Mites grow well in houses with about 60 percent relative humidity[5]; levels below 50 percent inhibit growth. Mites are also temperature sensitive. They are killed by washing in hot water (above 55°C [130°F]).[3] Dust mites grow from egg to adult in a month and then live for about another month.

Primary Prevention of Asthma

In an attempt to identify opportunities for the primary prevention of asthma, British investigators prospectively followed 67 children with one allergic parent for 10 years.[6] The homes of these children were found to have significant dust loads, especially in the mattresses. Levels were 2.4 μg per g of *Der p I* dust on living room floors, 4.3 μg per g on bedroom floors, and 18.4 μg per g in the mattresses. All of the 16 atopic children who had asthma at age 11 were skin-test sensitive to the house dust mite. (One nonatopic child had clinical asthma symptoms.) All but one of the children with asthma at age 11 had been exposed to more than 10 μg per g of *Der p I* antigen at age one.

In this study, the only areas of the home found to have this average antigen load were the mattresses. Use of a simple, zippered mattress cover could reduce such exposure significantly and possibly prevent some cases of asthma. The study also showed a dose response to the allergens. The age of first episode of wheezing was inversely related to the level of exposure to dust mite antigen at age one. An allergic predisposition is inherited; the expression of allergic disease is dependent on exposure.

Secondary Prevention of Asthma

In a rigorously controlled bedroom environment, investigators studied 20 mite-allergic asthmatic children.[7] They recommended a rigorous regimen to remove dust mites from the bedroom, by far the most important room for atopic patients.

The bedroom changes produced dramatic improvement. The patients with dust-free bedrooms had wheezing on only 2 percent of the days of the study, compared with 27 percent in the control group. Medications were needed in only 2 percent of study patient days, as opposed to 60 percent of control patient days. Also, tolerance (bronchial reactivity) to histamine challenge was eight times that of control patients by the end of the study. Marked improvement in function and symptoms was noted after only one month in the rigorously controlled bedroom.

Mite Control in the Home

Various measures have been recommended for mite control in the home. Some are useful in reducing exposure to dust mite antigen; others appear to be useless.

Bedroom Modification

Mattresses provide dust mites with humidity, warmth, and exfoliated human skin for nutrition. Encasement of mattresses is the most important control measure. Inexpensive plastic mattress covers are readily available, but the slightly more expensive polyurethane covers are somewhat more comfortable.

The bedroom should be as easy to clean as possible. Hardwood, tile, or linoleum floors can be cleaned much more easily than carpet. A vacuumed flat floor of this type has a negligible level of allergens. Carpet that is laid on concrete is always humid and therefore mite-friendly, whereas hardwood on concrete is essentially mite-free.[8]

Humidity Control

Some investigators stress humidity reduction for primary control of mite allergens. One study[9] found that if the mite population were reduced during the winter, when central heating can result in humidity levels below 50 percent, it would remain low in those homes even when the summer brought more humid conditions. Air conditioning can provide effective humidity control to reduce mite population during the summer.[10]

Furniture Modification

Overstuffed furniture can harbor large numbers of mites and mite nests, because it provides a hospitable microclimate for mites. In periods of reduced humidity, they can withdraw deep into the furniture, where a more favorable humidity can be maintained for some time.[3] Sparsely stuffed furniture can reduce the mite population, as can custom furniture made with a polyurethane membrane enclosing the matting of the furniture.

Vacuum Cleaning

Weekly vacuum cleaning of carpets and upholstery is considered useful. An in-house vacuum system that moves dust outside the living space is most efficient. More frequent vacuum cleaning does not give greater benefit than a weekly schedule.[4] Although vacuuming helps remove fecal mite pellets, most mites remain after vacuum cleaning.

Filtration

Fecal mite pellets containing antigens become airborne only with household activity and settle rapidly (within 30 to 45 minutes). Air filtration therefore has little effect on airborne levels of *Der p I*. Although some investigators believe that filtration can be useful, research has shown that a specialized HEPA bedroom filter designed to wash filtered air over the atopic person's head does not reduce allergic symptoms or bronchial responsiveness.[11] Electronic air filters are not routinely recommended for allergen control.

Forced Air Heating

Forced air heating had in the past been suspected of disseminating allergens in the home. However, in a randomized, controlled study,[12] forced air heating did not worsen asthma symptoms or peak expiratory flow rates in patients with severe asthma.

Acaricides

Some clinicians recommend the use of acaricides to control mite allergens. Tannic acid is available as a 3 percent solution. Although it does not kill mites, it denatures and thus inactivates mite allergens in carpets. Good antigen reduction results, but the solution must be reapplied every two months.[13] Tannic acid is used much more commonly than miticidal compounds, such as benzyl benzoate, in treating bedroom carpets. Benzyl benzoate and tannic acid similarly reduce the allergen content of dust.[14]

Clinical Recommendations

Mite control in the home is an important aspect of secondary prevention for asthmatic patients. Circumstantial data suggest that primary prevention of asthma may be possible in children of atopic parents. These children might avoid asthma if the parents can provide a sleeping environment with a low dust mite concentration.[6] Similar measures are needed much less frequently in nonsleeping areas of the house A survey of the house can disclose particular "hot spots" that produce large amounts of mite growth, such as carpet on concrete.

Like other patients who require lifestyle modifications for chronic diseases, atopic patients can frequently accept a little change at a time, rather than attempting all changes at once.

References

1. Montanaro A. House dust, animal proteins, pollutants, and environmental controls. *J Allergy Clin Immunol* 1989;84(6 Pt 2):1125-8.

2. Dowse GK, Turner KJ, Stewart GA, Alpers MP, Woolcock AJ. The association between *Dermatophagoides* mites and the increasing prevalence of asthma in village communities within the Papua New Guinea highlands. *J Allergy Clin Immunol* 1985;75(1 Pt 1):75-83.

3. Tovey ER. Allergy exposure and control. *Exp Appl Acarol* 1992;16:181-202.

4. Dust mite allergens and asthma—a worldwide problem. *J Allergy Clin Immunol* 1989;83(2 Pt 1):416-27.

5. Platts-Mills TA, Chapman MD. Dust mites: immunology, allergic disease, and environmental control. *J Allergy Clin Immunol* 1987;80:755-75 [Published erratum appears in *J Allergy Clin Immunol* 1988;82(5 Pt 1):841].

6. Sporik R, Holgate ST, Platts-Mills TA, Cogswell N. Exposure to house-dust mite allergens (*Der p I*) and the development of asthma in childhood. A prospective study. *N Engl J Med* 1990;323:502-7.

7. Murray AB, Ferguson AC. Dust-free bedrooms in the treatment of asthmatic children with house dust or house dust mite allergy: a controlled trial. *Pediatrics* 1983;71:418,22.

8. Rose G, Woodfolk JA, Hayden ML, Plads-Mills TA. Testing of methods to control mite allergen in carpets fitted to concrete slabs [Abstract]. *J Allergy Clin Immunol* 1992;89:315.

9. Korsgaard J. House dust mites and absolute indoor humidity. *Allergy* 1983;38:85-92.

10. Lintner TJ, Schou C, Mulfinger LM, Guralnick MW, Brame KA. The effects of air conditioning on the prevalence of house dust mite allergens [Abstract]. *J Allergy Clin Immunol* 1991;87:320.

11. Antonicelli L, Bilo MB, Pucci S, Schou C, Bonifazi E Efficacy of an air-cleaning device equipped with a high efficiency particulate air filter in house dust mite respiratory allergy. *Allergy* 1991;46:594-600.

12. Dales RE, Fyfe M, Schweitzer J. Does forced air heating exacerbate asthma? *J Allergy Clin Immunol* 1992;90:803-7.

13. Miller JD, Miller A, Luczynska C, et al. Effect of tannic acid spray on dust-mite antigen levels in carpets [Abstract]. *J Allergy Clin Immunol* 1989; 83:262.

14. Woodfolk JA, Hayden ML, Couture N, Platts-Mills TA. Chemical treatment of carpets to reduce allergen: comparison of the effects of tannic acid and other treatments on protein derived from dust mites and cats. *J Allergy Clin Immunol* 1995;96:325-33.

—this section by Thomas A. Johnson Jr.

About the Author of This Section

The author, Thomas A. Johnson, Jr., M.D. is chairman of the Department of Family Medicine at St. John's Mercy Medical Center, St. Louis. After graduating from St. Louis University School of Medicine, Dr. Johnson completed a residency in family medicine at the University of Nebraska College of Medicine, Omaha.

Section 34.4

How to Croato a Dust-Free Bedroom

From "How to Create a Dust-Free Bedroom," a fact sheet prepared by the Office of Communications and Public Liaison, National Institute of Allergy and Infectious Diseases (NIAID), National Institutes of Health, Bethesda, MD 20892, June 1997.

Dust-sensitive individuals, especially those with allergies and asthma, can reduce some of their misery by creating a "dust-free" bedroom. Dust may contain molds, fibers, and dander from dogs, cats, and other animals, as well as tiny dust mites. These mites, which live in bedding, upholstered furniture, and carpets, thrive in the summer and die in the winter. The particles seen floating in a shaft of sunlight include dead mites and their waste products; the waste products actually provoke the allergic reaction.

The routine cleaning necessary to maintain a dust-free bedroom also can help reduce exposure to cockroaches, another important cause of asthma in some allergic people.

Most people cannot control dust conditions under which they work or spend their daylight hours. But everyone can, to a large extent, eliminate dust from the bedroom. To create a dust-free bedroom, it is necessary to reduce the number of surfaces on which dust can collect. The National Institute of Allergy and Infectious Diseases (NIAID) suggests the following guidelines, arranged from most important to least important:

- Carpeting makes dust control impossible. Although shag carpets are the worst type for the dust-sensitive person, all carpets trap dust. Therefore, hardwood, tile, or linoleum floors are preferred. Treating carpets with tannic acid eliminates some dust mite allergen, but tannic acid is not as effective as removing the carpet, is irritating to some people, and must be repeatedly applied.

- Keep only one bed in the bedroom. Most important, encase box springs and mattress in a dust-proof or allergen-proof cover (zippered plastic). Scrub bed springs outside the room. If a second bed must be in the room, prepare it in the same manner.

- Keep all animals with fur or feathers out of the room. People allergic to dust mites often are allergic to cats, dogs, or other animals.

- Use only washable materials on the bed. Sheets, blankets, and other bedclothes should be washed frequently in water that is at least 130°F. Lower temperatures will not kill dust mites. If you set your hot water temperature to a lower value (which is commonly done to prevent children from scalding themselves), wash items at a commercial establishment that uses high wash temperatures.

- Keep furniture and furnishings to a minimum. Avoid upholstered furniture and venetian blinds. A wooden or metal chair that can be scrubbed may be used in the bedroom. If desired, hang plain, lightweight curtains on the windows. Wash the curtains once a week at 130°F.

- To prepare the room for a dust-sensitive person, clean the room thoroughly and completely once a week; clean the floors, furniture, tops of doors, window frames, sills, etc., with a damp cloth or oil mop; air the room thoroughly; then close the doors and windows until the dust-sensitive person is ready to occupy the room.

- Air filters—either added to a furnace or a room unit—can be useful in reducing the levels of allergens. Electrostatic and high-energy particulate absorption (HEPA) filters can effectively remove many allergens from the air. If functioning improperly, however, electrostatic filters may emit ozone, which adversely affects the lungs of people with asthma.

- A dehumidifier may be helpful because house mites require high humidity to live and grow. Care should be taken to clean the unit frequently to prevent mold growth. However, while low humidity may reduce dust mite levels, it also may irritate the nose and lungs of some people.

- If the dust-sensitive person is a child, keep toys out of the bedroom that will accumulate dust. Avoid stuffed toys; use only washable toys of wood, rubber, metal, or plastic, and store them in a closed toy box or chest.

- Use a dacron mattress pad and pillow. Avoid fuzzy wool blankets or feather- or wool-stuffed comforters.

- To prepare the room for a dust-sensitive person, completely empty the room, just as if one were moving. Empty and clean all closets and, if possible, store contents elsewhere and seal closets. If this is not possible, keep clothing in zippered plastic bags and shoes in boxes off the floor. Give the woodwork and floors a thorough cleaning and scrubbing to remove all traces of dust. Wipe wood, tile, or linoleum floors with water, wax, or oil. If linoleum is used, cement it to the floor.

Although these steps may seem difficult at first, experience plus habit will make them easier. The results—better breathing, fewer medications, and greater freedom from allergy and asthma attacks—will be well worth the effort.

Chapter 35

Allergies to Animals

Chapter Contents

Section 35.1

Animal Allergies

Excerpted from "Something in the Air: Airborne Allergens,"
National Institute of Allergies and Infectious Diseases (NIAID),
February 1998.

Household pets are the most common source of allergic reactions to animals. Many people think that pet allergy is provoked by the fur of cats and dogs. But researchers have found that the major allergens are proteins secreted by oil glands in the animals' skin and shed in dander as well as proteins in the saliva, which sticks to the fur when the animal licks itself. Urine is also a source of allergy-causing proteins. When the substance carrying the proteins dries, the proteins can then float into the air. Cats may be more likely than dogs to cause allergic reactions because they lick themselves more and may be held more and spend more time in the house, close to humans.

Some rodents, such as guinea pigs and gerbils, have become increasingly popular as household pets. They, too, can cause allergic reactions in some people, as can mice and rats. Urine is the major source of allergens from these animals.

Allergies to animals can take two years or more to develop and may not subside until six months or more after ending contact with the animal. Carpet and furniture are a reservoir for pet allergens, and the allergens can remain in them for four to six weeks. In addition, these allergens can stay in household air for months after the animal has been removed. Therefore, it is wise for people with an animal allergy to check with the landlord or previous owner to find out if furry pets had lived previously on the premises.

Section 35.2

Coping with Allergic Reactions to Pets

From "Pet Column for the Week," by Kimberly Meenen, Information Specialist, University of Illinois, College of Veterinary Medicine, September 12, 1994; © 1994 University of Illinios; reprinted with permission.

For people who experience allergic reactions to their pets, understanding why the body's immune system causes the sneezing, watery eyes, and itching provide tips that may lessen or even avoid the discomfort many pet owners feel.

According to Dr. Karen Campbell, a small animal veterinarian at the University of Illinois College of Veterinary Medicine at Urbana, the bad news is that some people are genetically predisposed to develop allergies.

Familial atopy, says Dr. Campbell, is the tendency to develop allergies inherited from one's parents. With this condition, antibodies are made that bind to mast cells in the person's airway. When the right stimulus comes along (what scientists call an antigen, or more specifically, an allergen), it binds to the antibody, telling the mast cell to dump its contents, causing the asthmatic attack. A similar process occurs in the skin of some individuals, producing redness and itching.

The reason why people can acquire a new pet and not experience any of these symptoms until much later is due to the time required to produce these antibodies. Dr. Campbell says it can take anywhere from three weeks to three years for the body to build up enough of the exact same antibody so that an allergen can cross-link two identical antigens. This cross-linkage is the signal to mast cells to spill their contents.

While all this may seem discouraging, the good news is that some people can develop a lack of reactivity to the allergen following continued exposure, or through allergen immunotherapy (desensitization).

People are not allergic to their pet per se, but to products of their pet. These include dander, hair or skin proteins, fur, saliva, blood, and even urine from rodents. In order to determine what exactly a person is allergic to, Dr. Campbell advises pet owners to see an allergy

301

specialist. These allergists will perform prick, scratch, or intradermal skin tests that examine reactivity to as many as 70-80 possible allergens. Once the person knows what he or she is allergic to, a specific plan of action can prevent the need to get rid of a pet, if the pet is indeed the cause of the reaction.

"For people allergic to fur, get a breed of dog that doesn't shed," recommends Dr. Campbell. She lists poodles and Bedlington and Kerry blue terriers as dogs that fit into this category. Minimal shed ders include schnauzers and most other types of terriers.

Dander is a common culprit in allergies to dogs. The dogs can be bathed up to twice weekly to try to alleviate the excessive dander production. Be sure to use a medicated pet shampoo prescribed by a veterinarian, she advises, and not an inexpensive alternative which can dry out your pet's skin and worsen the problem. A non-allergic member of the family should brush the dog often, preferably outside. If these activities are impossible because of allergic discomfort, hire a professional to do the tasks for you.

Creme rinses can be used if the dog's skin dries out. Fatty acid supplements added to the pet's food may also be helpful in correcting a dry skin problem. Consult your veterinarian about possible fatty acid supplements for your pet. You may find that it is already getting ample amounts of fat in the diet and supplying more can be as harmful to your pet as it is to you.

For dogs who seem to have a problem with hair loss, excessive dander production, or oozing areas of the skin (exposing the dog's blood, another potential allergen), owners need to get the condition checked out before any program to decrease allergens in the environment could have a chance to work.

Cats present a unique situation. Being the conscientious groomers that they are, their fur is often covered with saliva, and this can produce allergic symptoms in people as well. Other potential sources of allergic stimuli are feathers, scales, molds, pollens, tobacco smoke, perfumes, carpet fibers, and house dust mites. Many people are allergic to more than one item.

Find out from a physician what your particular allergen is, and if it turns out to be pet- related, try some of Dr. Campbell's suggestions to reduce the allergens in the environment. Using air cleaners or filters is not a bad idea, either.

"If you are allergic to six things, get rid of three of them," Dr. Campbell advises, "and you may drop below your allergic threshold, and become symptom-free." Your physician may also be able to prescribe medications to lessen the symptoms associated with allergies.

Section 35.3

Don't Get Rid of That Cat Yet

"Don't Get Rid of That Cat Yet, Say Asthma Researchers," Press Release
From: Jeffrey Minerd, Office of Communications and Public Liaison, NIAID,
March 8, 2001.

Parents who worry that their household cat might trigger asthma in their children shouldn't be too quick to get rid of the pet, according to a study that appears in the March 10, 2001 issue of *The Lancet*. The study shows that high levels of cat allergen in the home decrease the risk of asthma, apparently by altering the immune response to cats.

The study, funded in part by the National Institute of Allergy and Infectious Diseases (NIAID), begins to uncover the immune system processes behind this phenomenon. This work was also supported by the National Institute of Environmental Health Sciences (NIEHS).

For many allergens, such as the house dust mite, the higher the level of exposure, the higher the likelihood of a person producing "allergic" antibodies (called immunoglobulin E or IgE antibodies). High allergen levels also increase a person's risk of becoming allergic and developing asthma.

Thomas A. Platts-Mills, M.D., Ph.D., and colleagues at the University of Virginia's Asthma and Allergic Diseases Center have shown that cat exposure is different. The researchers measured the levels of antibodies to cat allergen in 226 children, aged 12 to 14 years, and tested the children for asthma. They also measured the amount of cat allergens in the children's homes and discovered that low-to-moderate amounts of cat allergen seemed to trigger allergy, but high amounts reduced both IgE antibodies and the likelihood of asthma.

"This result alters the advice we give patients," says Dr. Platts-Mills. "I would not recommend that parents get rid of their cat because they are concerned their child might develop asthma. However, high exposure to cat allergen appears to be protective for some children and a risk factor for others. If the child is wheezing and has a positive skin test to cat allergen, then you should get rid of your cat."

The high levels of cat allergen prompted the children's immune systems to predominantly make immunoglobulin G (IgG) and IgG4 antibodies rather than IgE, explains Marshall Plaut, M.D., chief of the allergic mechanisms section at NIAID. "This research sheds more light on the relationship between allergen exposure and asthma. When investigators further understand this process, it might lead to new treatments for asthma."

Reference

T Platts-Mills et al. Sensitisation, asthma, and a modified Th2 response in children exposed to cat allergen: a populations-based cross-sectional study. *The Lancet* 357:752-56 (2001).

Chapter 36

Cockroach Antigens

Cockroach antigens are proteins found in the insects' feces, saliva, eggs, and shed cuticles that can trigger allergic reactions (and the corresponding formation of antibodies) when they become airborne and are inhaled by humans. Cockroach antigens produce allergic effects particularly in children, including respiratory symptoms and especially asthma. A recent study concluded that exposure to cockroach antigens may play an important role in asthma-related health problems among inner-city children. Skin tests to detect reactions to cockroach antigens produce positive results at rates second only to house dust mites.

Researchers at the United States Department of Agriculture's Agricultural Research Service (ARS), the Arkansas Children's Hospital Research Institute in Little Rock, Arkansas, and the U.S. Food and Drug Administration (FDA) have teamed up to identify cockroach antigens associated with triggering asthma. Their goal is to reduce asthma symptoms by finding and removing cockroach antigens from dwellings. A key milestone of their work is the development of a home test kit that uses polyclonal antibodies to detect cockroach antigens, which can then be eliminated with common household cleaners.

Controlling cockroach-induced asthma is difficult. Immunotherapy with injections of cockroach extracts brings little relief. And killing

From "Working the Bugs Out of Asthma," by Carol Potera, in *Environmental Health Perspectives*, Volume 105, Number 11, November 1997. *Environmental Health Perspectives* is published by the National Institute of Environmental Health Science (NIEHS).

cockroaches by fumigating homes with pesticides fails to significantly reduce allergic symptoms. During their search for better ways to prevent cockroach-induced asthma, the ARS researchers and their colleagues discovered that cockroach antigens persist in buildings for at least five years, even in the absence of cockroaches.

Tracking Cockroaches

Richard Brenner, a medical entomologist and research leader in the imported fire ants and household insects research unit of the ARS in Gainesville, Florida, set out to demonstrate the tenacity of cockroach antigens. In August 1990, Brenner and his colleagues infested a 1,040-square-foot building with 600 German cockroaches (*Blattella germanica*) captured at a Miami housing project. The facility was furnished with wall cabinets, countertops, a sink, refrigerator, electric stove, waste basket, and table. The activity of the cockroaches and their antigen distribution was monitored for five months while moving food and water sources.

Because insect pests redistribute themselves to optimize their survival in any environment, "all infestations are spatial in nature," says Brenner. However, research procedures and statistics traditionally used by entomologists fail to address these spatial relationships fully. So Brenner adapted spatial analysis, a statistical method developed by mining engineers to precisely target the subsurface distribution of minerals, to study the cockroaches.

Unlike traditional statistical methods that assume random sampling and independent observations, spatial analysis recognizes "spatial continuity," which is the phenomenon that samples taken close to each other will appear similar. This parallels ecological systems—trees tend to grow together in groves, grass occurs in continuous patches, and German cockroaches aggregate.

Spatial analysis is modeled by computer programs that generate a contour map showing areas of varying density, similar to topographic maps. Within a data set, sample locations are defined by X and Y spatial coordinates. Spatial analysis pairs each observation with each of the other observations, calculates the distance between the members of each pair, then determines how similar the values are in each pair. The information is then used to estimate values at unsampled locations within the study site.

In Brenner's German cockroach experiment, about 100 live traps, baited with bread soaked in beer, were placed overnight in a grid that covered the scope of ecological diversity in the test building. The next morning, trapped cockroaches were counted. Using these counts and spatial analysis, the researchers estimated the number of cockroaches at one-foot intervals, which added up to 1,040 locations within the facility.

Through spatial analysis Brenner learned that the cockroaches, which are very adaptable creatures, redistributed themselves rapidly after their food and water were relocated. This meant that allergens associated with them were probably broadly distributed as well. The next step was to devise a detection system that could determine the allergen distribution and how long the allergens persisted.

After five months of monitoring the cockroaches, Brenner's crew removed all the insects, closed the building without cleaning it, and set out to build a detection system. In December 1996, they returned with a prototype of the cockroach antigen test kit to determine whether these potential cockroach allergens persisted years later in the absence of cockroaches, and, if so, where they were distributed. Because German cockroaches only live where there are people, Brenner was certain no new ones had taken up residence in the closed building.

A 16-square-inch surface was swabbed at 110 locations, and the swabs were shipped to the laboratory of standards and testing at the FDA's Center for Biologics Evaluation and Research in Bethesda, Maryland, where they were analyzed with an enzyme-linked immuno-adsorbent assay (ELISA) using polyclonal antibodies to detect cockroach antigens. When the results were returned to Brenner and plugged into the spatial analysis computer program, the distribution of cockroach antigens matched to a remarkable degree the cumulative distribution of cockroaches found five years earlier. The researchers concluded that the allergen load, expressed by a newly created index called "cockroach hour equivalents," measured as high as 4,100 units five years after all cockroaches were removed. "The allergen load was still enormous. You can see why even when cockroaches are removed, asthma does not get better," says Brenner.

Next, the ARS researchers cleaned the facility with a common household cleaner. They took test swabs of the surfaces after cleaning and sent the samples to the FDA for ELISA testing. Spatial analysis showed that cleaning removed 90% of the cockroach antigens and highlighted where the rest remained. The researchers cleaned again, swabbed again, and tested with ELISA. This second cleaning reduced the allergen load to zero cockroach hour equivalents, and confirmed that common cleaners adequately eliminate cockroach antigens.

Perfecting a Home Test Kit

Testing for potential cockroach allergens in homes requires a detection probe that is both highly specific and environmentally sensitive. A monoclonal antibody to a single cockroach antigen fails to detect many others, because 15-20 proteins from several types of cockroaches, including German, American, and Asian varieties, are suspected of causing human allergic reactions, says microbiologist Chris Anderson, chief of the FDA's laboratory of standards and testing. To be environmentally sensitive to cockroach allergens in homes, a probe must be polyclonal, or capable of detecting all major cockroach antigens.

Perfecting the laboratory-based ELISA devised by Anderson's team into a simple, home-based test kit is the next challenge facing the cockroach researchers. The polyclonal ELISA includes two major cockroach antigens characterized and cloned by immunologist Ricki Helm, an associate professor of pediatrics at the Arkansas Children's Hospital Research Institute. Using physicochemical methods such as isoelectric focusing and gel electrophoresis, Helm identified a 36-kilodalton (kd) and a 90-kd antigen, both of which recognize IgE antibodies in serum from people with known cockroach allergies. The 90-kd allergen bound IgE in 77% (17 of 22) of patient sera tested. By definition, a major allergen produces an IgE response in more than 50% of allergic patients.

Other known cockroach antigens range in size from 6 to 100 kd. "Some people react to only one, others to 15 allergens," says Anderson. At this point, the researchers do not know the final combination of cockroach antigens that will be included in a home test kit, but the final mixture has to cover a practical, broad base, says Anderson.

In addition, the team needs to verify that cockroach antigens recovered from swabbed floors that test positive in the ELISA are allergens that trigger asthma. Work is underway to correlate the relationship between these antigens and asthma allergens. "This needs to be done before a test kit can be successful," says Anderson.

Preventing Cockroach-Induced Asthma

A study published in the May 8, 1997 issue of the *New England Journal of Medicine* highlighted the need to detect cockroach allergens in homes. Dust samples from the bedrooms of 476 inner-city asthmatic children were analyzed for dust mite, cat, and cockroach allergens. Multivariate analysis revealed that cockroaches were the most common cause of the children's asthma. In the children's bedrooms, 50.2% had cockroach allergen levels that exceeded the disease-induction threshold, compared with 9.7% for dust mite allergen levels and 12.6% for cat allergen levels. The rate of hospitalization for asthma was 3.4 times higher among children whose skin tested positive to cockroach allergens and whose bedrooms had high cockroach-allergen levels. The same group also had 78% more visits to health care providers, experienced significantly more wheezing, and missed more school because of asthma.

Brenner proposes that a cockroach allergen home test kit can help relieve asthmatic symptoms by precisely targeting the allergens and directing cleaning efforts. "We can have a positive impact on human health by eliminating the pests and their attendant allergens," he says. By analogy, he compares cockroach allergen contamination to having a nuclear waste spill in a home. Both are extremely dangerous even in small quantities—a picogram of cockroach allergen can kill a sensitive asthmatic—and both require clean-up procedures that find and remove all of the contamination. For example, he says, in the case of allergens, removing 95% clearly is good. But the remaining 5% could conceivably be entirely concentrated in one small location—for example, the corner of a child's playroom. Consequently, the remaining 5% is potentially a concentration that could be life-threatening to a severely cockroach-sensitive asthmatic. Brenner says, "That is the essence of our spatial analysis. It tells you exactly where the problem is, not just the magnitude."

Brenner foresees the test kit including many probes to check many sites in a home before and after cleaning with household cleansers. The cockroach allergen test kit could also be adapted by the pest control industry to assess, target, clean, resample, and verify that all cockroach allergens are eliminated. The technology is also helping to develop and test new cockroach repellents that are environmentally friendly.

The exact design of a commercial home test kit will be determined once partners from private industry are selected and patents are obtained. This novel approach of combining polyclonal antibodies for cockroach antigens with spatial analysis "allows us to take a holistic view of indoor environmental quality by examining surface contaminants," says Brenner, "and goes beyond simply testing indoor air quality."

Additional Reading

Brenner RJ. Preparing for the 21st century: research methods in developing management strategies for arthropods and allergens in the structural environment. In: *Proceedings of the 1st International Conference on Insect Pests in the Urban Environment* (Wildey KB, Robinson WH, eds.), Exeter: BPCC Wheatons Ltd ,1993;57-69

Rosenstreich DL, Eggleston P, Kattan M, et al. The role of cockroach allergy and exposure to cockroach allergen in causing morbidity among inner-city children with asthma. *N Engl J Med* 336:1356-1363 (1997)

Helm R, Cockrell G, Stanley JS, et al. Isolation and characterization of a clone encoding a major allergen (Bla g Bd90K) involved in IgE-mediated cockroach hypersensitivity. *J Allergy Clin Immunol* 98:172-180 (1996).

Chapter 37

Exposure to Pollens

Chapter Contents

Section 37.1

When Allergies Are in Season

From *Consumers' Research Magazine*, May 1995, vol. 78, no. 5, p26(5). ©1995 Consumers' Research Inc.; reprinted with permission.

The scene is a familiar one: Over a field of ragweed floats an invisible cloud of pollen grains as the plants try to reproduce. The trouble is the pollen lacks self-direction and is at the mercy of the wind and weather. As a result, the grains are soon carried by the wind into a nearby town. The pollen is inhaled by a child who has never been exposed to this substance before.

Once the pollen settles in the lining of the child's nose and throat (which closely resembles the sticky, moist plant stigma the pollen is seeking), the child's immune system overreacts because of some defect or predisposing genetic factor. It produces large numbers of antibodies, all designed to respond to ragweed pollen. Several of the antibodies attach themselves to cells in the child's nasal passages and upper respiratory tract. These cells, known as mast cells, contain strong chemicals called mediators, the best-known of which is histamine.

When the child inhales ragweed pollen again, proteins from the pollen bind to the specifically designed antibodies on the surface of the mast cells. This causes the mediators to burst from inside the mast cells, causing blood vessels in the nasal passages to swell and begin leaking fluid.

The child has begun a lifetime of suffering from "hay fever" —which involves neither hay nor a fever (the clinical term is allergic rhinitis). The hallmarks of this condition—which are familiar to some 35 million Americans—are sneezing, sniffling, a stuffy head, and red, watery eyes.

A bewildering array of over-the-counter products provide temporary relief for the hay fever sufferer. But allergy experts agree that the most effective antidote to hay fever is to avoid exposure as much as possible to symptom-causing pollen.

Table 37.1 will help you identify the high season for a variety of pollens in your area. You might be allergic to only one type of pollen, or you might be allergic to several. By identifying the pollens you're sensitive to and when they're in season, you can take steps to avoid contact with them while they're in the atmosphere.

The following advice from the American Academy of Allergy and Immunology will also help you minimize the effects of hay fever during pollen season:

- Keep windows closed at night; use air conditioning, which cleans, cools, and dries the air.

- Minimize early morning activity when pollen is most usually emitted (between 5:00 a.m. and 10:00 a.m.).

- Keep your car windows closed when you're out driving.

- Stay indoors when the pollen count or humidity is high and on windy days when dust and pollen are whipped up.

- Consider taking a vacation during the height of pollen season for your area to a place more pollen-free (such as the beach and seashore).

- Don't mow lawns or spend time around freshly cut grass; mowing stirs up pollen.

- Don't hang sheets or clothing out to dry, as pollen may collect in these items.

- Don't grow too many indoor plants.

[Table 37.1, listing the high pollen season for a variety of allergy-producing pollens, begins on page 314 and continues through p. 324.]

Table 37.1. High Pollen Seasons (Note: The climate, growing seasons, and vegetation vary drastically on the Hawaiian Islands, so the islands' pollen season has not been included in this chart.)

State/Region	Plant: Pollen Season

Alabama

Montgomery — Trees: mid January until early June
Grass: late April/early May until late September/early October
Ragweed: late August/early September until early October

Alaska — Trees: late March/early April until late June/early July
Grass: late May/early June until late August/early September
Dock-Plantain and Sage: late June/early July until late August/early September

Arizona

Kingman — Russian Thistle and Saltbush: mid June until late September
Ragweed: late July/early August until late October

Phoenix — Trees: late January until late April
Grass: late March until late October/early November
Amaranth-Chenopod: mid May until early December
Ragweed: mid September until late October/early November

Tucson — Trees: mid February until late May
Ragweed: mid February until late May and mid August until early to mid November
Grass: late February/early March until late May and late July until late October/early November
Amaranth-Chenopod: late July until late October/early November
Russian Thistle: late August until mid October

Arkansas

Little Rock/ Fort Smith — Trees: late January until mid May and late November until late December
Grass: early May until late September
Ragweed: mid August until mid October

314

California

Northwestern
Trees: late January until mid June
Grass: late March/early April until early September
Amaranth-Chenopod and Saltbush: late March/early April until mid September
Ragweed and Dock Plantain: early July until late November

San Francisco Bay
Trees: early January until late May and late August until late September
Grass: late March/early April until late June
Sage and Amaranth-Chenopod: late August until late September

Southern
Trees: mid January until late February/early March
Grass: late February/early March until late November
Russian Thistle: late June until late August
Ragweed and Sage: early July until late October

Colorado

Colorado Springs
Trees: late February/early March until late June
Grass: late March until early October
Amaranth-Chenopod: mid to late April until early November
Sage: late April until late November
Dock-Plantain: late May/early June until late August
Ragweed: late June until early November

Denver:
Trees: mid March until mid May
Grass: mid to late May until mid July
Amaranth-Chenopod: late May/early June until late September
Ragweed: late July until mid September

Connecticut
Trees: mid March until mid to late May
Grass: early May until early August
Ragweed: mid August until mid October

Delaware
Trees: early March until mid May
Grass: early May until early July
Ragweed: early August until late September

315

District of   Trees: early to mid March until mid May
Columbia   Grass: early May until mid July
    Ragweed: early August until late September

Florida

Miami   Trees: late January until late March
    Grass: late March until mid to late May and late July until late December
    Ragweed: mid to late May until late September

Tampa   Trees: early January until late May, mid to late September until early to mid October, and mid December until late December
    Grass: year round
    Ragweed: early August until late November/early December

Georgia

Atlanta   Trees: mid January until mid June
    Grass: late March/early April until late September
    Dock-Plantain: mid May until mid October
    Amaranth-Chenopod: late July until late October/early November
    Ragweed: late July until mid December

Augusta   Trees: mid January until mid to late May
    Grass: late April/early May until mid September
    Dock-Plantain: mid May until late September/early October
    Amaranth-Chenopod and Ragweed: mid to late August until early December

Idaho

Southern   Trees: mid March until late May/early June
    Grass: late April/early May until late July/early August
    Russian Thistle and Saltbush: early July until late September
    Dock-Plantain: mid to late July until early October

Illinois

Chicago   Trees: mid March until early June
    Grass: late May until early July
    Ragweed: mid August until late September

Indiana

Indianapolis   Trees: late February/early March until early to mid June
Grass: mid to late May until early July
Ragweed: mid August until late September/early October

Iowa

Ames   Trees: mid March until mid May
Grass: mid May until late August
Ragweed: mid August until late September

Kansas

Wichita   Trees: late February until late May
Grass: late April until late June
Russian Thistle and Amaranth-Chenopod: late July until late September
Ragweed: late August until early October

Kentucky

Lexington   Trees: late January/early February until late October
Grass: late March until late October
Dock-Plantain: late March until late May
Ragweed: late April until late November
Amaranth-Chenopod: late June until late October
Sage: late July/early August until late October

Louisville   Trees: late February/early March until mid June
Grass: mid April until late June
Ragweed: early August until early October

Lousiana

New Orleans/   Trees: early January until late March
LaFayette   Grass: late March until late November
Ragweed: mid July until mid October

Maine   Trees: late March until late May
Grass: mid to late May until early July
Ragweed: early to mid August until mid to late September

Maryland

Baltimore

Trees: mid March until late May
Grass: early April until mid September
Dock-Plantain: late April until late August/early September
Sage: mid May until mid June
Ragweed: late August until mid October

Massachusetts

Boston

Trees: mid March until late May
Grass: mid May until mid August
Ragweed: early to mid August until early October

Michigan

Detroit

Trees: mid to late March until early June
Grass: mid May until mid to late June
Ragweed: mid to late August until mid to late September

Kalamazoo

Trees: late March/early April until late May
Dock-Plantain: mid May until mid June
Grass: late May until mid July
Amaranth-Chenopod and Ragweed: mid August until mid September

Minnesota

Minneapolis/
Rochester

Trees: late March/early April until late May
Grass: mid May until mid July
Amaranth-Chenopod: mid July until early September
Ragweed: late July until late September

Mississippi

Vicksburg

Trees: late January/early February until late April/early May
Grass: early May until late September
Ragweed: late August/early September until early October

Missouri

St. Louis/
Kansas City

Trees: late February/early March until late May/early June
Grass: mid May until early July
Amaranth-Chenopod: late July until late September
Ragweed: early August until late September

318

Montana

Miles City   Trees: late March/early April until late May
Grass: late April/early May until late August/early September
Russian Thistle: mid July until early September
Ragweed and Sage: late July/early August until early October

Nebraska

Omaha   Trees: late February until mid June
Dock-Plantain: mid April until late July
Grass: mid May until late September
Amaranth-Chenopod: late June until early to mid October
Ragweed: mid August until early October
Sage: mid August until mid October

Nevada

Reno   Trees: late March/early April until late May/early June
Grass: late May/early June until late July
Russian Thistle and Dock-Plantain: late June/early July until late September
Sage: early August until early October
Ragweed: early September until late September

New Hampshire   Trees: late March/early April until late May/early June
Grass: mid May until late July
Ragweed: mid August until late September

New Jersey   Trees: late January until late June
Grass: late April/early May until late September
Dock-Plantain: mid May until mid September
Amaranth-Chenopod: late July/early August until early October
Ragweed: early August until late September

New Mexico

Albuquerque   Trees: late January until late June
Grass: late March until late May and late July/early August until late September
Amaranth-Chenopod: late May until late October
Sage: late July/early August until late September
Ragweed: late August until late September

New Mexico (continued)

Roswell   Trees: late January until late April
Grass: mid May until mid October
Amaranth-Chenopod and Saltbush: early June until late September
Ragweed and Sage: late August until late October

New York

NY City/   Trees: mid March until late May
Westchester   Grass: mid May until early July
County   Ragweed: early August until late September

Olean   Trees: mid March until late May
Grass: late May until late June
Ragweed: mid August until late September

Rochester   Trees: mid April until late May/early June
Grass: mid May until mid July
Dock-Plantain: late May/early June until late July
Amaranth-Chenopod and Ragweed: early August until late September

Watertown   Trees: late March/early April until mid July
Grass: late April/early May until late August
Dock-Plantain: late April/early May until late September
Ragweed: late June until late October
Amaranth-Chenopod and Russian Thistle: late July/early August until late October

North Carolina

Raleigh   Trees: mid January until late May
Grass: mid May until early July
Ragweed: early August until late September

North Dakota

Fargo   Trees: late March/early April until late May/early June
Grass: late May/early June until late July
Russian Thistle: late June until mid September
Ragweed: early July until mid September
Sage: early August until late September

Ohio

Cleveland   Trees: late March until early June
Grass: late May/early June until late July
Ragweed: early August until late September

Oklahoma

Oklahoma City   Trees: early January until early June
Dock-Plantain: early January until late April/early May
Grass: late February/early March until late October
Ragweed: mid to late August until late October

Tulsa   Trees: mid February until early June
Grass: late April/early May until late September
Amaranth-Chenopod: late June until early October
Ragweed: mid August until mid November

Oregon

East of   Trees: mid February until late August
Cascades   Grass: late April/early May until mid August
Amaranth-Chenopod: mid July until late September
Russian Thistle: mid July until late September
Sage: mid July until late September
Saltbush: mid July until late September

Portland   Trees: mid January until late May
Grass: late March/early April until mid July
Dock-Plantain: mid May until mid September
Amaranth-Chenopod: early April until mid August
Sage: late July/early August until early to mid October

Pennsylvania

Philadelphia   Trees: late February/early March until late June
Grass: late March until late July/early August
Amaranth-Chenopod: late June until early October
Dock-Plantain: mid June until late October/early November
Sage: mid July until late October/early November
Ragweed: early August until late October/early November

321

Pennsylvania (continued)

Pittsburgh   Trees: late February/early March until late June
Grass: late April/early May until late August/early September
Dock-Plantain: late April/early May until late September
Amaranth-Chenopod: late June until late September
Ragweed: late July/early August until late October/early November

Rhode Island   Trees: mid March until late May
Grass: late May until late July/early August
Ragweed: mid August until late September

South Carolina

Charleston   Trees: early February until late May
Grass: late May until early August
Ragweed: late August until early November

South Dakota   Trees: late February until late April
Grass: mid May until early July
Russian Thistle: late June until late September
Ragweed: mid to late July until late September
Sage: late August until late September

Tennessee

Knoxville   Trees: late January/early February until late May
Grass: late March until late September
Ragweed: late August until late October

Nashville   Trees: mid to late February until mid to late May
Grass: late March until mid August
Ragweed: early to mid August until mid to late October
Sage: early September until early October

Texas

Brownsville   Grass: mid January until late December
Tress: early February until late April
Ragweed: early May until mid September
Amaranth-Chenopod: mid May until mid September

Texas (continued)

Corpus Christi Trees: early January until late June, late August until
late September, and late October until late December
Grass: late February until late July and late August un-
til late November
Dock-Plantain: late February until late April/early May
Amaranth-Chenopod: late May until late June and late
July until late October
Ragweed: late August until late November

Dallas Trees: early January until late April, late August until
late September, and late November until late December
Grass: late March until late September
Ragweed: late August until late October

Utah

Salt Lake City Trees: late February/early March until early May
Grass: mid April until mid July
Russian Thistle: early July until early November
Ragweed: mid August until late October
Sage: late August until early November

Vermont

Trees: late March until late May
Grass: late May until late July
Ragweed: early August until mid to late September

Virginia

Richmond Trees: late January/early February until early June
Grass: mid May until early August
Ragweed: late August until late September

Washington

Eastern Trees: mid March until late April
Grass: late April until early July and late August until
late September
Russian Thistle and Saltbush: mid July until late Sep-
tember
Ragweed: early August until mid to late September

Seattle Trees: mid to late February until late April
Grass: mid to late April until late September/early Oc-
tober
Sage: late April/early May until late September/early
October

Washington (continued)

Vancouver Trees: late January/early February until late May/early June

Amaranth-Chenopod: mid April until mid August

Grass: mid to late April until early August

Sage: late May/early June until late September

West Virginia

Trees: mid March until early June

Grass: mid to late May until early to mid July

Ragweed: early August until late September

Wisconsin

La Crosse Trees: late March/early April until late May/early June

Grass: mid to late May until late July

Ragweed: early August until mid to late September

Marshfield Trees: late March/early April until mid June

Dock-Plantain: mid May until late August

Grass: mid to late May until late July/early August

Ragweed: early August until late September

Wyoming

Trees: mid to late March until late April

Grass: early June until late July

Ragweed and Russian Thistle: late June until early September

Sage: late July/early August until early October

Section 37.2

People with Allergies Can Enjoy Gardening

"The Hay Fever Harvest," by Bruce A. Berlow, in *Flower & Garden Magazine*, August-September 1995, vol. 39, no. 4, p. 20(2). © 1995 Bruce A. Berlow; reprinted with permission.

Most gardeners are well-prepared to cope with a variety of pests, from aphids to earwigs. But many aren't prepared to cope with one of the most stubborn garden pests of all—allergies. The problem is that a garden's bounty includes more than beans and begonias. There's also a rich harvest of pollens and molds, potent allergens for the 20 percent of gardeners who unfortunately suffer from hay fever or asthma. But with a little planning and preparation, most allergy sufferers can enjoy tending their flowers and vegetables without sneezing or wheezing.

An allergy—basically a misguided immune response—is an inflammatory reaction to foreign substances such as molds, dust, animals, or pollens. If this inflammation takes place in the membranes lining the eye and nose, we call it hay fever; if it occurs in the bronchial tubes, we call it asthma.

Pollens

Pollens, the tiny structures housing plant sperm, are the most common allergy triggers. Fortunately for gardeners, most flowers and vegetables don't produce the kind of pollen that causes allergy symptoms.

Plants generally rely on one of two methods for dispersing pollen: wind or insects. Wind-pollinated plants such as grasses, weeds, and trees rely on chance for their pollen to reach other plants in order to reproduce. Consequently, they produce massive quantities of powdery pollen—the kind that's easily inhaled into the respiratory tract.

Most flowers and vegetables, though, are insect-pollinated. In fact, the vast majority of terrestrial plants are insect-pollinated rather than wind-pollinated. Only about one-tenth of the approximately 300 flowering plant families rely on the inefficient airborne method of pollen dispersal. But these wind-pollinated plants make up for their relative scarcity by producing prodigious quantities of pollen. In a single growing season, one acre of grass can release nearly 40 pounds of pollen. And these pollens can travel for miles; significant amounts of grass and tree pollen have been detected even in the middle of the ocean.

In contrast to the random dispersal method of wind pollinators, insect pollinated plants have developed an efficient and cooperative arrangement with their pollinating partners. It's not just bees that do the work; other creatures such as butterflies, thrips, beetles, flies, ants, wasps, moths, and even birds (especially hummingbirds), bats, and sometimes small mammals help out. The flower's part of the bargain is to provide an appealing nectar, scent, or edible pollen to lure the pollinators.

Some flowering plants, notably orchids, have devised peculiar ways of attracting insect pollinators. One type of orchid has flower parts that resemble a female wasp. When the male attempts to mate with the flower, pollen is transferred. Another type of orchid resembles an enemy intruder, which invites attack by bees, thereby dispensing its pollen.

In order to stick to insects, these pollens are large and sticky, not easily inhaled, so they pose little risk for allergic gardeners. But by just working outdoors in your garden or flower bed, you're exposed to the small, airborne pollens that readily trigger allergies. These pollens are seasonal, tree pollens starting in early spring, grasses in the summer, and weeds extending into autumn.

Molds

The second culprit for allergic gardeners is mold, or fungi. Wherever you have an abundance of moisture and organic material, you have ideal conditions for growth of these primitive organisms, which release their allergenic spores into the atmosphere. And release they do—it's not unusual for mold spore counts to be a thousand times higher than the pollen count. In fact, molds represent the greatest proportion of airborne biomass. Furthermore, in some areas there are occasional "fungal showers," which lead to epidemics of severe asthma. A fungal shower occurs when a massive concentration of spores is released into the air. In New Orleans, for instance, the unloading of soybeans in the port area at harvest time unleashes a high concentration of fungal spores, causing epidemic asthma.

For years, allergists have warned mold-allergic patients to get rid of their houseplants. But there's some good news—a recent study shows that houseplants produce relatively little mold. On the other hand, a greenhouse represents a rich source of mold spores.

Molds can be found in other locations, too. They thrive in dark, undisturbed places, such as garages and sheds where gardening equipment is stored. But the most intense mold exposure of all is rotting vegetation—compost and piles of leaves. Not only can these fungal clusters trigger allergies, but they also harbor the fungus aspergillis, which can colonize asthmatic bronchial tubes, leading to a serious chronic respiratory disorder called aspergillosis.

Coping with Allergies

If you're one of the 35 million Americans with allergic respiratory disease, you have three options for coping with your symptoms. The first step is to minimize exposure to allergens. Fortunately, that doesn't mean giving up gardening, except in the most serious cases.

In order to reduce pollen exposure, it's important to know that there are bad pollen times. The highest pollen counts are encountered in the early morning and late afternoon. Furthermore, wind-pollinated plants tend to release their pollen during hot, windy conditions when the chances of dispersal are greatest. The other strategies for reducing pollen exposure are mostly common sense. For example, delegate to someone else the activities that are most likely to stir up allergens— mowing, raking, and turning the compost, for example. If no one else is available to help with these chores, an inexpensive pollen mask is a good second choice.

The medications used to treat allergies have come a long way in the past several years. They're not only more effective, but also freer of side effects. For red, itchy eyes, several new prescription allergy eye drops can be highly effective. There are also several newer antihistamines that control both eye and nasal symptoms without the drowsiness caused by earlier drugs. For itchy, sneezy noses, several types of nasal sprays are helpful, especially the cortisone-based sprays that are the most effective allergy treatments of all.

For gardeners with asthma, the menu of newer options is just as complete, from long-acting inhaled bronchodilators to inhaled anti-inflammatory and allergy-blocking sprays.

The final treatment option is immunotherapy, or desensitizing allergy shots. These work by inducing a gradual tolerance to inhaled allergens through injections of increasing doses of allergen extracts. Although a more cumbersome process than medications alone, shots may have an advantage because they treat the cause and not just the symptoms.

By being prudent about your exposures, and consulting with your physician or allergy specialist when necessary, there's no reason your sneezing or wheezing has to spoil your desire to garden.

About the Author of This Section

Dr. Bruce Berlow is a physician at the Sansum Medical Clinic in Santa Barbara, California. He is a veteran medical writer and an avid gardener.

Section 37.3

Additional Advice for Gardeners with Allergies

Excerpted from "Springtime Allergies," by Carol A. Prebich, in *Flower & Garden Magazine*, March-April 1998, vol. 42, no. 2, p. 12(1). © 1998 Carol A. Prebich; reprinted with permission.

When spring is just around the corner, most of us are simply itching to get out in the garden. Unfortunately, for some, the word "itching" has an altogether different meaning than a longing to have our hands in the soil.

I sought advice from Donald V. Belsito, Professor of Medicine and Director of the Division of Dermatology at Kansas University Medical Center. I want to share, in my lay-person manner, some of his insights on garden-related allergy and dermatology concerns.

Pollen and Mold

All of us who are hay fever sufferers know the symptoms of a day outdoors—red, itchy eyes, runny or stuffy noses. Another type of garden-related outbreak is eczema, or a red, itchy, scaly rash on the skin. These two types of allergies are caused by different mechanisms, and both can develop among gardeners.

Pollens can be a powerful source of irritation and are the most common of the allergy triggers for hay fever. Pollen is scattered by two methods—insects and wind. Fortunately, most vegetables and ornamental plants don't produce the kinds of pollen than can cause our allergy symptoms. Most vegetables and ornamentals are insect-pollinated, and these pollens are not easily inhaled. The wind-pollinated plants, such as trees, weeds, and grasses, do result in phenomenal amounts of pollen being dispersed. Just by being outdoors in the garden, a certain vulnerability occurs that will enhance the possibility of allergies.

Molds are an additional source of hay-fever allergens that can cause runny-nose symptoms. If you have a known allergy to molds, stay away from moist compost piles. If you must have one, have someone else care for it. And stay away from greenhouses. With the heat and humidity, greenhouses are a prime breeding place for mold, especially under wood surfaces.

When raking, mowing, or weeding, hay-fever-type molds and pollens can be stirred up. Again, if you are particularly sensitive and can have someone do these for you, all the better. Mold spore counts typically are many times greater than pollen counts. Check your local weather for the daily count.

Skin Conditions

Garden-related eczema can be caused by some of your garden products. Dr. Belsito recommends not using any type of latex garden gloves; use cloth or leather instead. If these are not readily available, opt for cotton glove liners. Be aware of the possibility that fungus in the soil can cause fungus in your nails. If you are generally susceptible, you can develop frictional dermatitis or psoriasis in areas of trauma when coming in contact with handles on mowers or rakes. And be sure your gardening tools are not rusty—this can release nickel, a common eczema-type allergen, especially in people sensitive to costume jewelry.

Also unpleasant to the gardener is poison ivy, especially during spring and early summer. Dr. Belsito reminds us of the age-old saying, "Leaves of three, let it be." Regrettably, there are many plants with leaves of three, so it's best to become familiar with the poison ivy variety, especially if you know you have a sensitivity to it. Be conscious of the fact that your outdoor pets can transfer the ivy resin to you—animals are not allergic to poison ivy, but if they happen upon it and some resin attaches to their fur, it can be transmitted to you by your petting them. Also, check rake handles or your garden gloves that have been inadvertently dropped for any ivy resin. An interesting fact that Dr. Belsito shared was winter-time reactions from poison ivy. The culprit? Firewood. If any ivy resins are on the logs, the smoke from a fire will throw them off, creating a situation that can be hazardous to any poison ivy-sensitive person in your home.

Time of Day and Weather

As for the time of day best for gardening with relation to allergies, Dr. Belsito recommends early morning or late in the day. But if another time of day works for you, by all means continue to garden then. Remember to use sunscreen, and be sure to check for offensive ingredients. (Check with your doctor if you are using any medications that would prevent you from being in the direct sun.) Be especially careful on hot, windy days, when large amounts of pollen are dispersed. A cloudy, cool day may be your best bet.

There is no one season of the year more offensive than another—it all depends on what you're allergic to. If it's trees and flowers, then spring is the time for caution; if it's ragweed, weeds, or grasses, then the fall would be your worst time.

A Final Word

If you suspect allergies, be evaluated by your doctor. There are a vast majority of irritants that can be ruled out, and by narrowing these down, it can make a world of difference in your life. Seeing a doctor early in the season and taking precautions before you're exposed to an allergen is much better than trying to treat the symptoms after they occur. Use common sense, read labels, be aware of your surroundings, and you can be one of the 60.5 million Americans who enjoy the number one leisure-time, stress-reducing, fun outdoor activity—gardening.

Chapter 38

Mold Allergies

Along with pollens from trees, grasses, and weeds, molds are an important cause of seasonal allergic rhinitis. People allergic to molds may have symptoms from spring to late fall. The mold season often peaks from July to late summer. Unlike pollens, molds may persist after the first killing frost. Some can grow at subfreezing temperatures, but most become dormant. Snow cover lowers the outdoor mold count dramatically but does not kill molds. After the spring thaw, molds thrive on the vegetation that has been killed by the winter cold.

In the warmest areas of the United States, however, molds thrive all year and can cause year-round (perennial) allergic problems. In addition, molds growing indoors can cause perennial allergic rhinitis even in the coldest climates.

What is mold?

There are thousands of types of molds and yeast, the two groups of plants in the fungus family. Yeasts are single cells that divide to form clusters. Molds consist of many cells that grow as branching threads called hyphae. Although both groups can probably cause allergic reactions, only a small number of molds are widely recognized offenders.

Excerpted from "Something in the Air: Airborne Allergens," National Institute of Allergy and Infectious Diseases (NIAID), February 1998.

The seeds or reproductive particles of fungi are called spores. They differ in size, shape, and color among species. Each spore that germinates can give rise to new mold growth, which in turn can produce millions of spores.

What is mold allergy?

When inhaled, microscopic fungal spores or, sometimes, fragments of fungi may cause allergic rhinitis. Because they are so small, mold spores may evade the protective mechanisms of the nose and upper respiratory tract to reach the lungs.

In a small number of people, symptoms of mold allergy may be brought on or worsened by eating certain foods, such as cheeses, processed with fungi. Occasionally, mushrooms, dried fruits, and foods containing yeast, soy sauce, or vinegar will produce allergic symptoms. There is no known relationship, however, between a respiratory allergy to the mold *Penicillium* and an allergy to the drug penicillin, made from the mold.

Where do molds grow?

Molds can be found wherever there is moisture, oxygen, and a source of the few other chemicals they need. In the fall they grow on rotting logs and fallen leaves, especially in moist, shady areas. In gardens, they can be found in compost piles and on certain grasses and weeds. Some molds attach to grains such as wheat, oats, barley, and corn, making farms, grain bins, and silos likely places to find mold.

Hot spots of mold growth in the home include damp basements and closets, bathrooms (especially shower stalls), places where fresh food is stored, refrigerator drip trays, house plants, air conditioners, humidifiers, garbage pails, mattresses, upholstered furniture, and old foam rubber pillows.

Bakeries, breweries, barns, dairies, and greenhouses are favorite places for molds to grow. Loggers, mill workers, carpenters, furniture repairers, and upholsterers often work in moldy environments.

Which molds are allergenic?

Like pollens, mold spores are important airborne allergens only if they are abundant, easily carried by air currents, and allergenic in their chemical makeup. Found almost everywhere, mold spores in some areas are so numerous they often outnumber the pollens in the air. Fortunately, however, only a few dozen different types are significant allergens.

In general, *Alternaria* and *Cladosporium* (*Hormodendrum*) are the molds most commonly found both indoors and outdoors throughout the United States. *Aspergillus, Penicillium, Helminthosporium, Epicoccum, Fusarium, Mucor, Rhizopus*, and *Aureobasidium* (*Pullularia*) are also common.

Are mold counts helpful?

Similar to pollen counts, mold counts may suggest the types and relative quantities of fungi present at a certain time and place. For several reasons, however, these counts probably cannot be used as a constant guide for daily activities. One reason is that the number and types of spores actually present in the mold count may have changed considerably in 24 hours because weather and spore dispersal are directly related. Many of the common allergenic molds are of the dry spore type—they release their spores during dry, windy weather. Other fungi need high humidity, fog, or dew to release their spores. Although rain washes many larger spores out of the air, it also causes some smaller spores to be shot into the air.

In addition to the effect of day-to-day weather changes on mold counts, spore populations may also differ between day and night. Day favors dispersal by dry spore types and night favors wet spore types.

Are there other mold-related disorders?

Fungi or microorganisms related to them may cause other health problems similar to allergic diseases. Some kinds of *Aspergillus* may cause several different illnesses, including both infections and allergy. These fungi may lodge in the airways or a distant part of the lung and grow until they form a compact sphere known as a "fungus ball." In people with lung damage or serious underlying illnesses, *Aspergillus* may grasp the opportunity to invade the lungs or the whole body.

In some individuals, exposure to these fungi also can lead to asthma or to a lung disease resembling severe inflammatory asthma called allergic bronchopulmonary aspergillosis. This latter condition, which occurs only in a minority of people with asthma, is characterized by wheezing, low-grade fever, and coughing up of brown-flecked masses or mucus plugs. Skin testing, blood tests, X-rays, and examination of the sputum for fungi can help establish the diagnosis. Corticosteroid drugs are usually effective in treating this reaction; immunotherapy (allergy shots) is not helpful.

Chapter 39

Insect Venom Allergies

Bees and ants are usually looking for food, not trouble. But cross their paths, or rather their nests, and you could feel the sting of their fury. About 100 people a year die from allergic reactions to bee stings. Fire ant bites can also be life-threatening.

After you have been stung once, you can become allergic to that insect's venom. The major offenders include members of the order *hymenoptera*— bees, wasps, hornets, yellow jackets, and fire ants. Biting flies, ticks, mosquitoes, and spiders can also cause allergic reactions, though they tend to be milder. A sting is never pleasant. The normal reaction is burning pain, redness, irritation, and itching. But an allergic reaction is worse: The area around the bite may swell and you may develop hives, breathing problems, a dry cough, nausea, abdominal pain, and vomiting.

Up to 2 million Americans have had allergic reactions to insect stings. Reactions can include a life-threatening anaphylactic reaction, a wild reaction of the immune system with a combination of symptoms, such as swelling of your lips, larynx, ears, eyelids, palms and the soles of your feet; hives; dizziness; wheezing or shortness of breath; and a sudden drop in blood pressure.

Recognizing Trouble

Most insect-sting allergies are to bees, hornets, wasps and yellow jackets. Fire ants cause problems mostly in the southeast.

From JohnsHopkins Health, online at http://www.intelihealth.com. ©1996-2000 InteliHealth Inc. Reprinted with permission of InteliHealth.

Honeybees, the most common of these stinging insects, aren't aggressive unless provoked. You can easily recognize them by their hairy bodies and bright yellow or black markings. They typically are found around flowers or clover. Once they sting, they die. They often leave their stinger behind.

Yellow jackets are the most aggressive of the stinging insects. Less "chunky" than bees, bright yellow with black markings, they hover around garbage cans, at picnics and wherever there are exposed foods, particularly those containing sugar. They will sting repeatedly, and they nest in the ground.

Hornets have short black bodies with yellow or white markings. They nest in trees or bushes and will sting repeatedly.

Wasps are hairless with narrow "waists" that separate their chests from their long, slim, lower bodies. They can be black, brown, or red. Wasps build nests in the caves of buildings and under rafters. They sting repeatedly.

Fire ants, native to the southeastern United States, are another common troublemaker in their home turf. Their stings cause intense burning. They often sting multiple times in a circle.

Prevention and Treatment

Of course, the best way to avoid getting an allergic reaction to insect venom is to avoid getting stung. Here's how:

- **Keep your distance.** Stay away from areas where insects congregate—namely in gardens and hedges, around fruit trees, and near garbage cans, picnic grounds, and other areas that attract insects. When dining outdoors, keep food covered until you're ready to eat, and clean up afterward. Garage and patio areas should be kept clean and free of debris, and garbage cans should be tightly sealed. If you encounter the insects, slowly back away. Don't swat at them, flail your arms, or make sudden movements that could trigger an attack.

- **Dress for success.** Bees, hornets and other flying insects are attracted to bright colors and floral patterns. So during picnic season, dress down—in white, khaki and other light solids, covering as much of your body as possible during late summer and early fall, when insects are at their peak. And avoid loose-fitting clothing; insects can become trapped in filmy garments.

Insects are also attracted to smells, so avoid wearing perfume, colognes or other fragrances—including suntan lotion, cosmetics, hair spray, and even deodorant—when around these bugs. And wear shoes rather than sandals outdoors to avoid face-to-foot contact with fire ants or low-flying bees, hornets or yellow jackets.

- **Check your car before you drive.** If you leave your car's windows open, check before getting in to make sure there are no flying insects are inside. Running the air conditioner while driving can keep you cool and help prevent on-the-road stings. Also, keep a can of insecticide in the car with you.

- **Advertise if you're allergic.** If you are allergic to insect venom, wear a Medic-Alert identification stating so. To order Medic-Alert identification, call 800-ID-ALERT. Many people with insect venom or food allergies carry a small kit containing a syringe of adrenaline (epinephrine) to use should they begin to develop signs of an anaphylactic reaction. If you are at risk for an anaphylactic reaction, it's also a good idea to wear a Medic Alert bracelet or necklace so that medical personnel will know what's wrong and how to treat you.

- **Scrape out the stinger.** If you get stung by a honeybee, the best way to avoid additional pain is to scrape out the stinger with a credit card or a long fingernail. If you try to pull it out, you'll squeeze the venom sac and accidentally release more venom. But scraping it out leaves the venom sac undisturbed.

  To ease the pain of a sting, take a pain reliever such as acetaminophen; ibuprofen or aspirin is even more effective. Young children should not be given aspirin because of the risk of Reye's syndrome. You could also make a paste by mixing water and meat tenderizer and applying it directly to the sting. Because insect venom is protein-based, meat tenderizer breaks down the protein and stops the pain. However, you must use a brand that contains papain, the active venom-busting ingredient.

- **Get your shots.** Once you've had a severe reaction to a stinging insect, you have about a 60 percent chance of having another anaphylactic reaction if stung again. But you can reduce your risk with venom therapy, which consists of getting injections

337

of minute amounts of venom from the same insect that causes your allergic reaction. The venom stimulates your immune system to become resistant to a future allergic reaction. Venom therapy is about 97 percent effective.

You will probably need about 6 to 20 injections, which will increase in dose. The injections will start on a weekly basis and then drop to bi-weekly. After this, you will be on a maintenance dosage, and need the injections about every 3 to 8 weeks. Venom therapy is recommended for adults, but not for children who have had only skin reactions (hives, itching).

Chapter 40

Poison Ivy, Poison Oak, and Poison Sumac

Chapter Contents

Section 40.1

Protect Yourself from Urushiol-Containing Plants

From "Protect Yourself from Poison Ivy," by Isadora B. Stehlin in *Consumers' Research Magazine*, August 1997 vol. 80, no. 8, p. 29(2). © 1997 Consumers' Research Inc.; reprinted with permission.

The poison ivy plant—along with its cousins poison oak and poison sumac—is the bane of millions of campers, hikers, gardeners, and others who enjoy the outdoors.

Approximately 85% of the population will develop an allergic reaction if exposed to poison ivy, oak, or sumac, according to the American Academy of Dermatology. Nearly one-third of forestry workers and firefighters who battle forest fires in California, Oregon, and Washington develop rashes or lung irritations from contact with poison oak, which is the most common of the three in those states.

Usually, people develop a sensitivity to poison ivy, oak, or sumac only after several encounters with the plants, sometimes over many years. However, sensitivity may occur after only one exposure.

The cause of the rash, blisters, and infamous itch is urushiol (pronounced "oo-roo-shee-ohl"), a chemical in the sap of poison ivy, oak, and sumac plants. Because urushiol is inside the plant, brushing against an intact plant will not cause a reaction. But undamaged plants are rare.

"Poison oak, ivy, and sumac are very fragile plants," says William L. Epstein, M.D., professor of dermatology, University of California, San Francisco. Stems or leaves broken by the wind or animals, and even the tiny holes made by chewing insects, can release urushiol.

Reactions, treatments, and preventive measures are the same for all three poison plants. Avoiding direct contact with the plants reduces the risk but doesn't guarantee against a reaction. Urushiol can stick to pets, garden tools, balls, or anything it comes in contact with. If the urushiol isn't washed off those objects or animals, just touching them—for example, picking up a ball or petting a dog—could cause a reaction in a susceptible person. (Animals, except for a few higher primates, are not sensitive to urushiol.)

Urushiol that's rubbed off the plants onto other things can remain potent for years, depending on the environment. If the contaminated object is in a dry environment, the potency of the urushiol can last for decades, says Epstein. Even if the environment is warm and moist, the urushiol could still cause a reaction a year later.

"One of the stories I tell people is of the hunter who gets poison oak on his hunting coat," says Epstein. "He puts it on a year later to go hunting and gets a rash."

Almost all parts of the body are vulnerable to the sticky urushiol, producing the characteristic linear (in a line) rash. Because the urushiol must penetrate the skin to cause a reaction, places where the skin is thick, such as the soles of the feet and the palms of the hands, are less sensitive to the sap than areas where the skin is thinner. The severity of the reaction may also depend on how big a dose of urushiol the person got.

Quick Action Needed

Because urushiol can penetrate the skin within minutes, there's no time to waste if you know you've been exposed. "The earlier you cleanse the skin, the greater the chance that you can remove the urushiol before it gets attached to the skin," says Hon-Sum Ko, M.D., an allergist and immunologist with the Food and Drug Administration's Center for Drug Evaluation and Research. Cleansing may not stop the initial outbreak of the rash if more than 10 minutes has elapsed, but it can help prevent further spread.

If you've been exposed to poison ivy, oak, or sumac, if possible, stay outdoors until you complete the first two steps:

- First, Epstein says, cleanse exposed skin with generous amounts of isopropyl (rubbing) alcohol. (Don't return to the woods or yard the same day. Alcohol removes your skin's protection along with the urushiol and any new contact will allow the urushiol to penetrate twice as fast.)

- Second, wash skin with water. (Water temperature does not matter.)

- Third, take a regular shower with soap and warm water. Do not use soap before this point because "soap will tend to pick up some of the urushiol from the surface of the skin and move it around," says Epstein.

- Clothes, shoes, tools, and anything else that may have been in contact with the urushiol should be wiped off with alcohol and water. Be sure to wear gloves or otherwise cover your hands while doing this and then discard the hand covering.

Dealing with the Rash

If you don't cleanse quickly enough, or if your skin is so sensitive that cleansing didn't help, redness and swelling will appear in about 12 to 48 hours. Blisters and itching will follow. For those rare people who react after their very first exposure, the rash appears after seven to 10 days.

Because they don't contain urushiol, the oozing blisters are not contagious nor can the fluid cause further spread on the affected person's body. Nevertheless, Epstein advises against scratching the blisters because fingernails may carry germs that could cause an infection.

The rash will occur only where urushiol has touched the skin; it doesn't spread throughout the body. However, the rash may seem to spread if it appears over time instead of all at once. This is either because the urushiol is absorbed at different rates in different parts of the body or because of repeated exposure to contaminated objects or urushiol trapped under the fingernails.

The rash, blisters, and itch normally disappear in 14 to 20 days without any treatment. But few can handle the itch without some relief. For mild cases, wet compresses or soaking in cool water may be effective. Oral antihistamines can also relieve itching.

The FDA also considers over-the-counter (OTC) topical corticosteroids (commonly called hydrocortisones under brand names such as Cortaid and Lanacort) safe and effective for temporary relief of itching associated with poison ivy.

For severe cases, prescription topical corticosteroid drugs can halt the reaction, but only if treatment begins within a few hours of exposure. "After the blisters form, the [topical] steroid isn't going to do much," says Epstein. The American Academy of Dermatology recommends that people who have had severe reactions in the past should contact a dermatologist as soon as possible after a new exposure.

Severe reactions can be treated with prescription oral corticosteroids. Phillip M. Williford, M.D., assistant professor of dermatology, Wake Forest University, prescribes oral corticosteroids if the rash is on the face, genitals, or covers more than 30% of the body. The drug must be taken for at least 14 days, and preferably over a three-week period, says the FDA's Ko. Shorter courses of treatment, he warns, will cause a rebound with an even more severe rash.

There are a number of OTC products to help dry up the oozing blisters, including:

- aluminum acetate (Burrows solution)
- baking soda
- Aveeno (oatmeal bath)
- aluminum hydroxide gel
- calamine
- kaolin
- zinc acetate
- zinc carbonate
- zinc oxide

Although desensitization, vaccines, and barrier creams have been studied over the past several decades for their potential to protect against poison ivy reactions, none have been approved by the FDA for this purpose.

Poisonous Plants

The famous rule "leaves of three, let it be" is good to follow, except that some of the plants don't always play by the rules and have leaves in groups of five to nine. To avoid these plants and their itchy consequences, here's what to look for.

Poison Ivy

- grows around lakes and streams in the Midwest and the East
- woody, ropelike vine, a trailing shrub on the ground, or a free-standing shrub
- normally three leaflets (groups of leaves all on the same small stem coming off the larger main stem), but may vary from groups of three to nine
- leaves are green in the summer and red in the fall
- yellow or green flowers and white berries

Poison Oak

- eastern (from New Jersey to Texas) grows as a low shrub; western (along the Pacific coast), grows to six-foot-tall clumps or vines up to 30 feet long
- oak-like leaves, usually in clusters of three
- clusters of yellow berries

Poison Sumac

- grows in boggy areas, especially in the Southeast
- rangy shrub up to 15 feet tall
- seven to 13 smooth-edged leaflets
- glossy pate yellow or cream-colored berries

Section 40.2

Poison Ivy Pointers for Parents

"Poison Ivy Pointers," in *Pediatrics for Parents*, December 1998, p. 3(1). Copyright © 1998 Pediatrics for Parents Inc.. Reprinted with permission.

The most common cause of allergic skin reactions is exposure to poison ivy and its "first cousins" poison oak and poison sumac. There are many misconceptions about these plants, all species of the plant genus *Rhus*, and the problems they can cause. Unless noted otherwise, whatever is said about poison ivy also applies to poison oak and poison sumac.

What Do These Plants Look Like?

That's a deceptively simple question. Poison ivy, poison oak, and the less common poison sumac have different appearances in different parts of the country. It's best to check with your local health department or a local college's botany department for pictures and descriptions of each of these plants.

Where Is Poison Ivy Found?

None of these weeds are found in Hawaii or Alaska, but they are in every other state. They don't grow very well above 4,000 feet altitude. Poison ivy is found east of the Rockies, poison oak west of the Rockies. The rarer poison sumac is found in the Northeast, swampy areas such as central Florida, and occasionally in the Midwest.

How Is Poison Ivy Spread?

All three of these plants contain a colorless to slightly yellow oil called urushiol. It's in the canals in the plant's leaves. When the fragile leaves are damaged, the oil leaks out and onto what touches the leaf. The oil may remain on clothing, boots, dog fur, or whatever rubs against the damaged leave. Even the ashes from a fire of burning poison ivy may have urushiol on them and, if they contact a child's skin, can cause a rash.

Some people who don't go into the woods or fields still get poison ivy. How? One way is their pets roam in fields or woods, brush against poison ivy, pick up the oil of their fur, come in the house, and transmit the oil to their owners.

How Does a Child Become Sensitized to Poison Ivy?

First there has to be an exposure to poison ivy, poison oak, or poison sumac. It usually takes 1 to 2 days for the rash to first appear. Accompanying the rash is redness, itching, and blisters. The blisters will usually heal in 10-14 days. In about 10% of people the first signs of a reaction appear within 4 to 8 hours.

Remember that if your child is sensitive to any one of the three plants, then he is sensitive to all them. That's because all three have the same type of oil in their leaves, and that's what causes the reaction.

What Should I Do If My Child Has Been Exposed to Poison Ivy?

Washing the exposed skin with water often removes all the urushiol. However, decontamination is better. One of the best ways to do this is to pour large amounts of rubbing (isopropyl) alcohol on the exposed area followed by a good washing with water. One advantage of rubbing alcohol is that it can actually extract some of the oil that has partially penetrated into the skin. Don't use premoistened towelettes or alcohol pads — they just spread the oils to other areas of the body.

The downside to using rubbing alcohol is that it removes the natural protective oils of the skin. If your child is exposed again to poison ivy after a decontamination with rubbing alcohol, his natural skin barriers are weakened and more of the urushiols will penetrate into his skin.

All clothing, canvas shoes, linens, etc. that have been exposed to poison ivy should be washed. It's a myth that the fluid in the blisters can spread the poison ivy.

How Can I Protect My Child?

There are two preparations that dermatologists generally agree work: StokoGard outdoor cream and Ivy Block. StokoGard provides 4-8 hours of protection. Initially your child will smell like a dead fish, but this odor disappears. Once the outdoor activity is finished, the substance must be washed off. Ivy Block is made from an organoclay from Arizona. It works by binding with the urushiol so it can't penetrate the skin. It doesn't need to be washed off.

What about Treatment?

The treatment depends on the severity of the reaction. A few children develop a severe reaction that requires treatment in a hospital emergency department with potent steroids.

For less severe reactions but still serious reactions, oral steroids are often needed. This potent drug will help lessen the swelling and itching. The drug should be taken for two to three weeks with the dose being slowly decreased. It should not be stop suddenly.

If your child only has a localized skin reaction with some itching, blister, and swelling, then a steroid cream may be all that's necessary. Most of the over-the-counter steroids are not strong enough to help much with the symptoms. It generally takes 7-10 days for the rash to go away no matter what treatment is used.

Calamine lotion will help with the itching and crust formation. Cool water also helps as does oatmeal soaks, bicarbonate of soda and acetic acid/vinegar in water. Antihistamines help only if the itching is severe or if your child is having trouble sleeping.

Remember no matter what you do, it will take time for the rash to go away and nothing speeds that up.

What about Desensitization?

This used to be done, but about 10 years ago the FDA found that this didn't work. Although it's possible to get some of the preparations used for desensitization, it's illegal.

Chapter 41

Hypersensitivity and Allergic Reactions to Drugs

Chapter Contents

Section 41.1

Drug Allergies

Causes and Risks

Drug allergies occur when there is an allergic reaction to a medication. This is caused by hypersensitivity of the immune system, leading to a misdirected response against a substance that does not cause a response in most people. The body becomes sensitized (the immune system is triggered) by the first exposure to the medication. The second or subsequent exposure causes an immune response.

Reactions to drugs are uncommon, but almost any drug can cause an adverse reaction. Reactions range from irritating or mild side effects (such as nausea and vomiting), to allergic response including life-threatening anaphylaxis. Some drug reactions are idiosyncratic (unusual effects of the medication). For example, aspirin can cause nonallergic hives (no antibodies formed), or it may trigger asthma.

"True" drug allergies involve the production of antibodies and the release of histamine and other chemicals. Most drug allergies cause minor skin rashes and hives. However, other symptoms occasionally develop and life-threatening acute allergic reaction involving the whole body (anaphylaxis) can occur. Serum sickness is a delayed type of drug allergy that occurs a week or more after exposure to a medication or vaccine.

Penicillin and related antibiotics are the most common cause of drug allergies. Other common allergy-causing drugs include sulfa drugs, barbiturates, anticonvulsants, insulin preparations (particularly animal sources of insulin), local anesthetics such as Novocain, and iodine (found in many X-ray contrast dyes).

Prevention

There is no known way to prevent development of a drug allergy. In people who have a drug allergy, avoiding the medication is the best means to prevent an allergic reaction. In some cases, the medication may be given safely after pre-treatment with corticosteroids (such as prednisone), antihistamines (such as diphenhydramine), and/or epinephrine.

Symptoms

- hives (common)
- skin rash (common)
- itching of the skin or eyes (common)
- wheezing
- swelling of the lips

Symptoms of anaphylaxis include:

- nasal congestion
- difficulty breathing
- cough
- blueness of the skin (cyanosis), including the lips or nail beds
- fainting, lightheadedness
- dizziness
- anxiety
- confusion
- slurred speech
- rapid pulse
- sensation of feeling the heart beat (palpitations)
- nausea, vomiting
- diarrhea
- abdominal pain or cramping

Signs and Tests

An examination of the skin may show hives, skin rash, or angioedema. Difficulty breathing, wheezing, and other symptoms may indicate anaphylactic reaction.

Skin testing may confirm allergy to penicillin-type medications. Testing may be ineffective (or in some cases, dangerous) for other medications. A history of allergic-type reaction after use of a medication is often considered adequately diagnostic for drug allergy. (No further testing is required to demonstrate the allergy.)

Treatment

The treatment goal is relief of symptoms.

Antihistamines usually relieve common symptoms (rash, hives, itching). Prednisone or topical (applied to a localized area of the skin) corticosteroids may also be recommended. Adrenergic bronchodilators may be prescribed to reduce asthma-like symptoms (moderate wheezing, cough, and so on.) Epinephrine— inhalation or injectable—is used to treat anaphylaxis.

The offending medication should be avoided. Health care providers (including dentists, hospital personnel, etc.) should be advised of drug allergies before treating the allergic patient. Identifying jewelry or cards (such as Medic-Alert or others) may be advised.

Occasionally a penicillin allergy responds to desensitization (immunotherapy) in which increasing doses (each dose of the drug is slightly larger than the previous dose) are given to improve tolerance of the drug.

Prognosis

Most drug allergies respond readily to treatment. A few cases cause severe asthma or anaphylaxis.

Complications

- discomfort
- asthma
- anaphylaxis (life threatening)

Call your health care provider if you are taking a medication and develop symptoms indicating drug allergy. Go to the emergency room or call the local emergency number (such as 911) if you have difficulty breathing or develop other symptoms of severe asthma or anaphylaxis; these are emergency conditions.

Section 41.2

Serum Sickness

Definition

Scrum sickness is a group of symptoms caused by a delayed immune response to certain medications or antiserum (passive immunization with antibodies from an animal or another person).

Causes and Risks

Serum is the clear fluid portion of blood. It does not contain blood cells but does contain many proteins, including antibodies, which are formed as part of the immune response to protect against infection.

Antiserum is a preparation of serum that has been removed from a person or animal that has already developed immunity to a particular microorganism. It contains antibodies against that microorganism. An injection of antiserum (passive immunization) may be used when a person has been exposed to a dangerous microorganism against which the person has not been immunized. It provides immediate (but temporary) protection while the person develops a personal immune response against the toxin or microorganism. Examples include antiserum for tetanus and rabies exposure.

Serum sickness is a hypersensitivity reaction similar to allergy. The immune system misidentifies a protein in antiserum as a potentially harmful substance (antigen) and develops an immune response against the antiserum. Antibodies bind with the antiserum protein to create larger particles (immune complexes). The immune complexes are deposited in various tissues, causing inflammation and various other symptoms. Because it takes time for the body to produce antibodies to a new antigen, symptoms do not develop until 7 to 14 days after exposure to the antiserum.

Exposure to certain medications (particularly penicillin) can cause a similar process. Unlike other drug allergies, which occur very soon after receiving the medication for the second (or subsequent) time, serum sickness can develop 7 to 14 days after the first exposure to a medication. The drug molecules probably combine with a protein in the blood before being misidentified as an antigen.

Serum sickness is different from anaphylactic shock, which is an immediate reaction with more severe symptoms.

Prevention

There is no known way to prevent the development of serum sickness. People who have experienced serum sickness, anaphylactic shock, or drug allergy should avoid future use of the antiserum or drug.

Symptoms

- skin rash
- itching (pruritus)
- hives
- joint pain
- fever

Note: The symptoms develop 1 to 2 weeks after exposure to antiserum or medication.

Signs and Tests

The lymph nodes may be enlarged and tender to palpation. Occasionally, shock-like symptoms will develop (such as pale skin, low blood pressure, and light headedness).

Treatment

The goal of treatment is the relief of symptoms. Topical corticosteroids or other soothing topical (applied to a localized area of the skin) medications may relieve discomfort from itching and rash. Antihistamines may shorten the duration of illness and help to relieve rash and itching. Nonsteroidal anti-inflammatory medications may relieve joint pain. Corticosteroids such as prednisone may be prescribed for severe cases.

Causative medications should be stopped. Future use of the medication or antiserum should be avoided. Health care providers (such as dentists and hospital personnel) should be advised of drug allergies before treating the patient. Identifying jewelry or cards (such as Medic-Alert or others) may be advised.

Prognosis

The symptoms usually resolve within a few days. The antiserum or medication should be avoided in the future.

Complications

- discomfort
- shock (rare)
- increased risk of anaphylaxis for future exposures to the substance

Call your health care provider if medication or antiserum has been given within the last 2 weeks and symptoms of serum sickness appear.

Section 41.3

Allergic Reactions to Agents Used in Chemotherapy

From "Hypersensitivity reactions - a new addition to IL-2 toxicity,"
by Michelle Marble in *Cancer Biotechnology Weekly*, July 3, 1995 p8(3),
© Charles Henderson, Publisher 1995; reprinted with permission.

A University of Southern California chemoimmunotherapy clinical trial has produced a surprising addition to the interleukin-2 (IL-2) repertoire.

G.R. Heywood et al. published the first report which describes IL-2 induced hypersensitivity reactions to chemotherapy ("Hypersensitivity Reactions to Chemotherapy Agents in Patients Receiving Chemoimmunotherapy with High-Dose Interleukin 2," *Journal of the National Cancer Institute*, June 21, 1995;87(12):915-922).

Many previous studies of chemotherapy agents combined with IL-2 have been published with no mention of hypersensitivity to the chemotherapy agents.

"The data presented here suggest that allergic reactions to cisplatin and dacarbazine, generally regarded as an uncommon phenomena, are quite common in patients receiving high-dose IL-2 and interferon alfa," wrote Heywood et al.

The authors noticed the unexpected hypersensitivity reactions in the early stages of a clinical trial studying the efficacy of combination chemoimmunotherapy for the treatment of patients with metastatic melanoma. One section of patients received high-dose IL-2 and interferon alfa in addition to standard chemotherapy and the other section received standard chemotherapy (i.e., cisplatin, tamoxifen and dacarbazine).

Thirty-one metastatic melanoma patients were included in the study. None of the patients had received previous chemotherapy, but all had had previous surgery. Fifteen of the patients were treated with chemotherapy alone, and 16 were treated by combination chemoimmunotherapy. The patient groups were balanced in terms of sex, age, and stage of disease.

Three patients in each treatment arm had received previous immunotherapy; three chemotherapy patients had received prior IL-2 based regimens for metastatic disease. Two of the three in the chemoimmunotherapy arm had been treated with a cellular vaccine, and one with levamisole as adjuvant therapy.

Ten of the 16 patients in the chemoimmunotherapy arm of the study exhibited significant allergic reactions while receiving the chemotherapy regimens. None of the 15 patients in the chemotherapy arm demonstrated any allergic reaction symptoms.

The allergic manifestations generally arose at the end of the second course or during the third course of therapy in all 10 patients. Most of the reactions consisted of generalized edema, erythema, pruritis, urticaria, and tingling or burning that occurred within several hours of the IV chemotherapy agents. Four patients developed hypotension requiring fluid resuscitation. Two of the four required further assistance and were transferred to an intensive care unit for monitoring. Four of the ten patients had hypersensitivity reactions severe enough to limit further chemotherapy.

All patients in the chemotherapy group lost weight, and had decreased white blood cell counts and eosinophil counts that did not change significantly. All patients in the chemoimmunotherapy group gained statistically significant amounts of weight, and had elevated white blood cell counts and increased eosinophil counts. These effects were more prominent in the ten with hypersensitivity reactions.

The authors suggested that hypersensitivity reactions occurred in all of the 16 in the chemoimmunotherapy group as all of them exhibited weight gain, increased eosinophil counts and elevated white blood cell counts. The six without obvious hypersensitivity reactions had reactions, but they were considered subclinical.

"The mechanism by which IL-2 may induce hypersensitivity reactions to chemotherapy agents might be explained by amplification of IL-2R-bearing T helper cells," wrote Heywood et al.

In more detail, IL-2 could stimulate the proliferation of T helper cells that promote IgE production by B cells. In the case of the Th2 subset, it could stimulate secretion of IL-4 and IL-5, the authors said. Additionally, it has been demonstrated that eosinophils express the low-affinity IL-2R p55. High-dose IL-2 may directly increase signal transduction in those eosinophils, causing degranulation and histamine release.

"In this study, the suggestion that IL-2 induced the hypersensitivity reaction to cisplatin or dacarbazine is strengthened by the absence of any adverse reactions in a concurrently treated, randomly assigned control group that received an identical chemotherapy regimen alone," Heywood et al. said.

Hypersensitivity reactions to combination chemotherapy, interferon alfa and IL-2 regimens have not been reported previously. The authors noted that the differences between their study and the other studies was chemotherapy immediately followed by high-dose IL-2. They suggested that the IL-2-associated hypersensitivity reactions were dose and schedule dependent.

Hypersensitivity reactions occurred within several hours after chemotherapy administration in patients who had previously received one to two cycle of high-dose IL-2. This suggested to the authors that the prior IL-2 therapy sensitized the patients to subsequent cisplatin or dacarbazine. There were no toxicities noted with tamoxifen therapy.

The authors recommended caution when treating patients with multiple cycles of chemoimmunotherapy, especially when high-dose IL-2 is planned. They also recommended the prophylactic use of H1 and H2 histamine blockers.

"We recommend that investigators using regimens that combine IL-2 and chemotherapy agents prospectively monitor their patients for chemotherapy-related type I hypersensitivity reactions, a new addition to the toxic effects of IL-2," concluded Heywood et al.

Section 41.4

Hypersensitivity Reactions to Anticonvulsants and ACE Inhibitors

From "Hypersensitivity reactions to anticonvulsants, ACE inhibitors, and other drugs," by Marti Jill Rothe and Jane M. Grant-Kels, in *Consultant*, February 1998, vol. 38, issue 2, p. 301(6), © 1998 Cliggott Publishing Company; reprinted with permission.

Most cutaneous drug reactions do not have major sequelae. However, significant morbidity and even mortality may be associated with drug hypersensitivity syndromes, urticaria and angioedema, Stevens-Johnson syndrome (SJS), and toxic epidermal necrolysis (TEN).[1] In this article, we concentrate specifically on aromatic anticonvulsant hypersensitivity syndrome, severe reactions to minocycline, and angioedema induced by angiotensinconverting enzyme (ACE) inhibitors.

Anticonvulsant Hypersensitivity

Hypersensitivity reactions may develop in a small percentage of patients treated with phenytoin, carbamazepine, and phenobarbital. Approximately 80% of affected patients are allergic to all three of the aromatic anticonvulsants. The reaction is thought to be the result of abnormal detoxification of arene oxide metabolites of the anticonvulsants, although hypersensitivity may also develop in persons who manifest normal detoxification.

Signs and Symptoms

Unlike the common morbilliform drug reactions, which develop approximately 1 week after the causative medication is initiated and have minimal systemic involvement, anticonvulsant hypersensitivity is a multisystem reaction that may not be evident until several months after initiation of drug therapy. It may assume a variety of manifestations, including morbilliform eruptions, exfoliative erythroderma, generalized pustular exanthems, pseudolymphoma, and SJS/TEN.

TEN occurs most commonly with reexposure to an aromatic anticonvulsant after a prior episode of hypersensitivity or with continued exposure despite an ongoing hypersensitivity reaction.

Patients with anticonvulsant hypersensitivity appear to have a toxic condition and may manifest any of a number of signs and symptoms, including fever, malaise, facial edema, conjunctivitis, pharyngitis, leukocytosis with eosinophilia, lymphadenopathy, hepatosplenomegaly, elevated liver enzyme levels, nephritis, arthritis, and transient hypothyroidism.

Treatment

Management of anticonvulsant hypersensitivity includes discontinuation of the medication, supportive care, initiation of high-dose systemic corticosteroids, and substitution of an antigenically unrelated anticonvulsant, such as divalproex. Even when the causative medication is discontinued, signs and symptoms may wax and wane for several weeks to months—particularly as systemic corticosteroids are tapered. Deaths have been reported as a consequence of prominent hepatic impairment, rechallenge with an aromatic anticonvulsant, and continued use of the anticonvulsant resulting from a failure to recognize the hypersensitivity syndrome.

Similar hypersensitivity reactions have been observed in patients treated with allopurinol, dapsone, sulfonamides, gold, and minocycline.

Adverse Reactions to Minocycline

Recently, a number of centers have reported serious adverse reactions to minocycline in patients treated for acne. The first such report, by Gough and colleagues,[2] described minocycline-induced autoimmune hepatitis in 16 patients and a systemic lupus erythematosus (SLE)-like syndrome in 11 patients; notification of these adverse reactions was made to a drug safety committee.

In addition, Gough and colleagues[2] prospectively identified minocycline-induced polyarthritis and hepatitis in five patients, polyarthritis in one, and chronic active hepatitis in one. In six of the patients tested for antinuclear antibodies, results were positive.

The dose of minocycline ranged from 50 to 100 mg bid in 32 of the patients; 1 patient took an overdose of 6 g. The duration of minocycline therapy ranged from 9 days to 6 years. Two patients died, and 1 required a liver transplant.

Investigators from Canada subsequently described minocycline-induced reactions in six patients with hypersensitivity syndrome, six with serum sickness-like reactions, and one with drug-induced SLE.[3] Hepatic failure necessitated liver transplant in one patient. Hypersensitivity reactions develop after an average of approximately 24 days of minocycline therapy; serum sickness, after an average of approximately 16 days; and drug-reduced SLE, after an average of 2 years. A follow-up article reviewed the comparative safety of tetracycline, minocycline, and doxycycline.[4]

The FDA noted 1 report of minocycline-induced autoimmune hepatitis and 32 reports of minocycline-induced SLE-like syndrome from 1972 through February 1996.[5]

Signs and Symptoms

The features of minocycline hypersensitivity syndrome are similar to those of the anticonvulsant syndrome: rash (morbilliform, exfoliative erythroderma, SJS/TEN, pustular exanthems), fever, lymphadenopathy, hepatitis, pneumonitis, and leukocytosis. Features of minocycline-induced serum sickness include urticaria, fever, arthralgias, and lymphadenopathy. Deaths have occurred secondary to hepatic failure, pancytopenia, and myocarditis.

Treatment

Minocycline-induced reactions generally resolve with discontinuation of the medication and recur with rechallenge. Severe reactions warrant treatment with systemic corticosteroids such as prednisone, typically starting with a dosage of 1 mg/kg/d that is tapered slowly over 2 to 3 weeks.

Although one patient who had minocycline-induced pneumonitis subsequently took doxycycline without complication,[3] cross-reaction patterns are not known. Thus, no form of tetracycline should be prescribed for patients who experience severe reactions to minocycline. Shapiro and colleagues[4] recommend avoidance of tetracycline antibiotics by first-degree relatives of patients with hypersensitivity reactions to tetracyclines.

Despite the gravity of the minocycline-induced reactions described above, the vast majority of patients who take minocycline for acne do not experience significant adverse reactions, even with long-term use.[6] The value of monitoring antinuclear antibodies, hepatic and renal function, and complete blood cell count at baseline and periodically during therapy has not been established. Shapiro and colleagues[4] recommend laboratory evaluation only if symptoms develop while a patient is being treated with antibiotics. They also recommend avoiding minocycline in patients with a personal history of SLE or a history of SLE in a first-degree relative.

ACE Inhibitor Induced Angioedema

Signs and Symptoms

ACE inhibitors have been associated with a number of adverse cutaneous reactions, including pemphigus, exfoliative erythroderma, lichen planus-like reactions, pityriasis rosea-like reactions, and angioedema.[7,8] Angioedema develops in 0.1% to 0.7% of patients who are treated with ACE inhibitors. It often occurs in the absence of urticaria and preferentially affects the tongue and lips as well as periorbital, buccal, laryngeal, pharyngeal, and subglottic tissues.

ACE inhibitors increase local levels of bradykinin—a potent vasodilator—and reduce production of angiotensin II—potent vasoconstrictor. The vasodilatory effects, rather than immunologic mechanisms, are thought to mediate ACE inhibitor-induced angioedema.

Although most cases of angioedema associated with ACE inhibitors develop within the first week of therapy, onset may be delayed by months or years and episodes may be intermittent. Lack of awareness of delayed onset and intermittent reactions may account for failure to identify an ACE inhibitor as the cause of angioedema.

Patients with a history of acquired or hereditary angioedema may be at greater risk for ACE inhibitor-induced angioedema; these agents are therefore contraindicated in this group of patients. Black patients have also been reported to be at greater risk for ACE inhibitor-induced angioedema.

Treatment

General measures include discontinuation of the ACE inhibitor, initiation of intravenous antihistamines and corticosteroids, and subcutaneous administration of epinephrine. Surgical intervention may be necessary to maintain patent airways. Oral antihistamines and a tapering course of oral corticosteroids may be required after the patient has been stabilized. Substitution of another ACE inhibitor is contraindicated.

Clinical Highlights

- Significant morbidity and even mortality may be associated with hypersensitivity syndromes, although these reactions are relatively rare.

- Anticonvulsant hypersensitivity is a multisystem reaction that may not develop until several months after drug therapy initiation. It may manifest as morbilliform eruptions or more serious cutaneous disorders. Management includes discontinuation of the causative medication, initiation of an antigenically unrelated anticonvulsant, supportive therapy, and high-dose systemic corticosteroids.

- Minocycline hypersensitivity syndrome can produce rash, fever, lymphadenopathy, hepatitis, and other disorders. Minocycline-induced reactions generally resolve when the medication is discontinued and recur with rechallenge. No form of tetracycline should be prescribed for patients who react adversely to minocycline.

- Angiotensin-converting enzyme inhibitors may produce a variety of cutaneous disorders, including angioedema that preferentially affects the tongue and lips. Most cases develop soon after initiation of therapy, although onset may be delayed by months or years. Acute therapy includes intravenous antihistamines and corticosteroids as well as subcutaneous epinephrine.

References

1. Roujeau JC, Stern RS. Severe adverse cutaneous reactions to drugs. *N Engl J Med*. 1994;331:1272-1285.

2. Gough A, Chapman S, Wagstaff K, et al. Minocycline induced autoimmune hepatitis and systemic lupus erythematosus-like syndrome. *BMJ*. 1996; 312:169-172.

3. Knowles SR, Shapiro L, Shear NH. Serious adverse reactions induced by minocycline: report of 13 patients and review of the literature. *Arch Dermatol*. 1996; 132:934-939.

4. Shapiro LE, Knowles SR, Shear NH. Comparative safety of tetracycline, minocycline, and doxycycline. *Arch Dermatol*. 1997;133:1224-1230.

5. Singer SJ, Piazza-Hepp TD, Girardi LS, et al. Lupus-like re-
    action associated with minocycline. *JAMA*. 1997;277:295-296.

6. Gaulden V, Glass D, Cunliffe WJ. Safety of long-term high-
    dose minocycline in the treatment of ache. *Br J Dermatol*.
    1996;134:693-695.

7. Pillans PI, Coulter DM, Black P. Angioedema and urticaria
    with angiotensin converting enzyme inhibitors. *Eur J Clin
    Pharmacol*. 1996;51:123-126.

8. Sabroe RA, Kobza Black A. Angiotensin-converting enzyme
    (ACE) inhibitors and angio-oedema. *Br J Dermatol*.
    1997;136:153-158.

About the Authors of This Section

Dr. Rothe is associate professor of dermatology and director of
phototherapy and clinical services in the department of dermatology
at the University of Connecticut Health Center in Farmington. Dr.
Grant-Kels is professor and chair, department of dermatology, and
director of dermatopathology at the same institution.

Chapter 42

Latex Allergy

Chapter Contents

Section 42.1

Allergy to Latex Is Potentially Disabling

Excerpted from "Latex Allergy: Potentially Disabling," by Nancy Walsh D'Epiro, in *Patient Care,* Vol. 30, No. 3, February 15, 1996, pp.32-4. Copyright © 1996 Medical Economics Publishing Co. Reprinted with permission.

"Latex is the allergen of the '90s. We simply can't afford to sensitize and potentially lose a large segment of our highly trained, well-paid health care professionals," says Kevin J. Kelly, M.D., Director of Pediatric Allergy and Immunology at Children's Hospital of Wisconsin in Milwaukee. "I've seen physicians, surgeons, nurses, laboratory technicians, and researchers develop such severe occupational asthma that they become totally disabled professionally."

Latex allergy is an unexpected result of the adoption of universal precautions against infectious diseases in recent years. Because products manufactured from the milky sap of *Hevea brasiliensis* are impermeable to transmissible viruses—especially HIV and hepatitis—the demand for them has increased exponentially. Latex now is ubiquitous in the health care environment and is used in dressings, catheters, tapes, and, most notably, protective gloves. Before the adoption of universal precautions, an estimated 300 million gloves were used annually. This figure has grown to 9.6 billion per year.

The initial manifestation of latex allergy is an urticarial condition that develops on the hands, often after an initial contact dermatitis that may break down the skin barrier. In up to 50% of exposed persons, however, the condition also affects the respiratory tract. This occurs because high concentrations of powder on latex gloves become airborne and are inhaled by workers in hospitals and clinics. The result can be severe rhinoconjunctivitis, asthma, and anaphylaxis. Fatalities have occurred.

Approximately 15-17% of health care workers are now thought to be sensitized to latex, and many of them manifesting occupational asthma may have permanent respiratory sequelae that force them to leave their jobs. Anaphylaxis may occur in 5-10% of allergic persons.

Gloves causing asthma? Some unusual operating room events in the early 1990s helped researchers make the connection.

Wisconsin, 1991: Anaphylaxis during Surgery

The first report of contact urticaria involving rubber products appeared in 1979, and a scattering of further cases was seen throughout Europe in the 1980s. Then, in 1991, some unexpected events occurred. One was at Children's Hospital of Wisconsin, where an unexplained epidemic of anaphylactic reactions occurred during surgery.[1] Another took place at Henry Ford Hospital in Detroit, where a number of allergic reactions—including fatalities—were associated with barium enemas. Other children's hospitals were reporting similar unexplained incidents.

Dr. Kelly, who is also Associate Professor of Pediatrics at the Medical College of Wisconsin, Milwaukee, explains what happened at his hospital: "During a 6–7-month period in 1991, there were 12 episodes of anaphylaxis in our operating room. The likelihood of anaphylaxis during surgery ranges from 1 in 5,000 to 1 in 15,000. In a hospital such as ours, where we do about 7,500 operations each year, you might expect one case. In fact, the previous year, we had none."

Specialists from the Centers for Disease Control and Prevention (CDC) went to Milwaukee to help determine the cause of the epidemic. They reviewed the types of surgical procedures and the patient populations involved. This analysis revealed that 11 of the 12 reactions occurred in patients with spina bifida—yet only 152 operations out of the 7,500 involved this patient group. Because of the extremely high statistical connection between spina bifida and anaphylaxis during surgery, the CDC and FDA ordered a moratorium on elective surgery for children with spina bifida until the cause of the problem could be identified. It was a year before the latex connection was found.

Two years earlier there had been a report of two cases of latex allergy in children with spina bifida at Children's National Medical Center in Washington, D.C.[2] This prompted Dr. Kelly and his colleagues to consider the possibility of latex sensitization occurring during surgery. They found that 68% of all spina bifida patients in southeast Wisconsin were indeed sensitized to latex. "These children were being sensitized to latex very early in life, in numerous procedures exposing mucosal surfaces to the antigen," Dr. Kelly explains.

Young children with spina bifida typically undergo surgery at least twice a year because of the numerous genitourinary, neurologic, and orthopedic problems associated with the condition. Born with myelomeningocele [protrusion of the membranes of the brain or spinal cord through a defect in the skull or spinal column], most of these children undergo two surgical procedures during the first week of life, one to repair the spinal abnormality and the second to insert a shunt for hydrocephalus. This early and repeated exposure to latex during surgery resulted in an extremely high incidence of sensitization

Diagnosis: Clues and Hazards

Identifying the patient with latex allergy, particularly with symptoms of asthma, requires an awareness of the magnitude of the problem in the health care environment affecting both patients and workers. It's quite likely that patient groups other than children with spina bifida also are at risk if they undergo multiple procedures that allow contact with latex. Anyone who exhibits any allergic symptoms during surgery should be tested for latex hypersensitivity. So should any health care worker who complains of symptoms ranging from urticaria on the hands to severe and worsening asthma that appears to have a temporal relation to the workplace.

Serologic testing can be done easily in the primary care office, with results available in about a week. Several tests are available, and one has recently been approved by the FDA (Alastat Latex-Specific IgE Allergen Test Kit, Diagnostic Products Corp., Los Angeles). The sensitivity of these tests is limited, however—10-20% of positive results may be missed. More specific tests are available through reference laboratories, and a negative result in light of a strong history and clinical suspicion may warrant further investigation and referral to an allergist.

A standardized skin test extract has not yet been made commercially available, and improvised in-office challenge testing is highly undesirable. Because the antigen is water-soluble and easily washes out of the gloves, some clinicians have attempted skin testing with a saline solution into which a latex glove has been immersed. Others have tested by having the patient actually try on a wet glove. These practices are potentially dangerous and have led to systemic reactions. Any challenge testing for latex allergy should be done by specialists under carefully controlled conditions.

A curious but important diagnostic clue involves the phenomenon of cross-reactivity. Some persons with latex allergy also experience a positive response to several food substances, most notably bananas and other tropical fruits such as kiwi and passion fruit. Chestnuts and pitted fruits such as peaches and cherries also have been implicated. It is not yet known if some unidentified proteins in these foods that are similar to those present in latex are responsible.

Investigators have suggested that certain chemicals and enzymes sprayed on rubber trees to preserve the sap until it can be processed may be involved. Others also suggest that chemicals used as antioxidants and accelerants in rubber processing may contribute to the initial development of dermatitis.[3] In vitro reactivity doesn't necessarily translate into clinical reactivity, however, and immunologists are still investigating the nature and variability of the cross-reactivity seen with latex and certain foods. Until the connection is clarified, Dr. Kelly advises presuming a latex allergy in anyone who is exposed frequently to latex and exhibits an allergic reaction to one of these fruits, because true allergy to them is uncommon.

Looking for a Solution

Some have suggested that the burgeoning demand for latex gloves spurred by the AIDS epidemic was accompanied by changes in manufacturing practices intended to meet the increased demand but which inadvertently resulted in increased antigenicity. The manufacturers deny substantial changes in practice, however, according to Dr. Kelly. "And unfortunately," he says, "the question probably won't be solved in a scientific forum, but in a court of law." A number of individual and class-action product-liability suits have been filed against latex manufacturers, similar to those involving silicone breast implants.

While no one doubts the benefits of latex in protecting against infectious diseases, the magnitude of the latex allergy problem now is forcing some hard questions to be asked. Should the universal use of latex gloves be rethought? Dr. Kelly suggests that consideration be given to man-made alternatives with less antigenic potential, such as vinyl. He acknowledges that vinyl is more permeable than latex and is therefore a less effective barrier against HIV and hepatitis, but he points out that permeability does not necessarily translate into infection. Wearing gloves is imperfect protection: Latex won't stop needlesticks. "We have no proof that health care workers wearing other types of gloves would actually become infected at a greater rate than those wearing latex gloves," he observes.

Low-allergen gloves and alternatives for some other products are now available, and a Compendium of Non-Latex Gloves was published by the Medical Devices Bureau, Health Protection Branch, Health Canada, in July 1994. Until a broad solution to the problem is found, however, the American Academy of Allergy and Immunology recommends the following guidelines for preventing latex sensitization:[4]

- Patients in high-risk groups should be identified.

- All patients, regardless of risk group status, should be questioned about a history of latex allergy.

- All high-risk patients should be offered testing for latex allergy.

- Procedures on all patients with spina bifida should be performed in an environment free of latex—one in which no latex gloves are used by any personnel. In addition, there should be no latex accessories (catheters, adhesives, tourniquets, anesthesia equipment) that come into direct contact with the patient.

- Procedures on all patients with a positive history, regardless of risk group status, should be performed in an environment free of latex.

- Low-risk patients with no history of latex allergy are extremely unlikely to react to latex. At this time, routine testing is not recommended for such persons.

- Patients identified as latex-allergic by history or testing should be advised to obtain a Medic Alert bracelet and self-injectable epinephrine.

References for This Section

1. Kelly K, Sitlock M, Davis JP: Anaphylactic reactions during general anesthesia among pediatric patients—United States, January 1990-January 1991. *MMWR* 1991;40:437-443.

2. Slater JE: Rubber anaphylaxis. *N Engl J Med* 1989;320:1126-1130.

3. Sussman GL, Beezhold DH: Allergy to latex rubber. *Ann Intern Med* 1995;122:43-46.

4. Task Force on Allergic Reactions to Latex: Committee report. *J Allergy Clin Immunol* 1993;92:16-18.

Section 42.2

Latex Allergies Stretch beyond Rubber Gloves

Excerpted from "Latex Allergies Stretch beyond Rubber Gloves," in
Environmental Health Perspectives, Vol. 104, No. 9 [Online] September
1996. Available: http://ehpnet1.niehs.nih.gov/docs/1996/104-9/forum.html. Produced by the National Institute of Environmental Health Sciences (NIEHS),
National Institutes of Health (NIH).

Latex in the Air

With the number of latex allergies jumping from a single case report in 1979 to 6.5% of Americans in 1994, it would seem that latex
is dropping from the sky. A report in the January 1995 issue of the
Journal of Allergy and Clinical Immunology and a followup article
in the March 1996 issue of *Chest* find that urban air does contain latex particles, shed into the environment by normal tire wear.

Along a four-lane road in Denver, Colorado, a team from the Allergy
Respiratory Institute of Colorado led by immunologist Brock Williams
collected particulate air pollution. Their samples included black fragments containing latex proteins, which were recognized in tests by human antibodies to latex. More than half (58%) of the airborne debris was
small enough to be inhaled into the lungs. Airborne latex could partially
explain the rise in latex sensitization. "Until we know more about it,"
says Williams, "it's difficult to weigh the importance of airborne latex to
the overall problem. But it's probably in every city in the world with cars."

Because 57 latex proteins are known allergens, removing them is
impractical. So is avoiding rubber, which is found in 40,000 items,
including 300 medical products. To circumvent latex allergies, U.S.
Department of Agriculture (USDA) researchers at the Western Regional Research Center in Albany, California, have developed hypoallergenic rubber from guayule (*Parthenium argentatum*), a shrub
native to the southwestern United States. In clinical trials published
in the *Journal of Allergy and Immunology,* people allergic to *Hevea*
latex do not react to guayule.

The USDA team, headed by plant physiologist Katrina Cornish,
created processing methods to extract guayule and manufacture rubber

products with superior resilience, strength, and elasticity. The USDA granted an exclusive license for the patented technology to American Medical Products in Burlingame, California. The first guayule products will be medical supplies for latex-sensitive patients and medical workers. Cornish is continuing genetic studies to improve latex yields and adapt guayule for growth in diverse climates.

Section 42.3

Latex at Home and at Work

Excerpted from "NIOSH Alert: Preventing Allergic Reactions to Natural Rubber Latex in the Workplace," Publication No. 97-135 [Online] June 1997. Available: http://www.cdc.gov/niosh/latexalt.html. Produced by the U.S. Department of Health and Human Services (HHS).

A wide variety of products contain latex: medical supplies, personal protective equipment, and numerous household objects. Most people who encounter latex products only through their general use in society have no health problems from the use of these products. Workers who repeatedly use latex products are the focus of this text. The following are examples of products that may contain latex:

Emergency Equipment

Blood pressure cuffs

Stethoscopes

Disposable gloves

Oral and nasal airways

Endotracheal tubes

Tourniquets

Intravenous tubing

Syringes

Electrode pads

Personal Protective Equipment

Gloves

Surgical masks

Goggles

Respirators

Rubber aprons

Office Supplies

Rubber bands

Erasers

Hospital Supplies

Anesthesia masks

Catheters

Wound drains

Injection ports

Rubber tops of multidose vials

Dental dams

Household Objects

Automobile tires

Motorcycle and bicycle handgrips

Carpeting

Swimming goggles

Racquet handles

Shoe soles

Expandable fabric (waistbands)

Dishwashing gloves

Hot water bottles

Condoms

Diaphragms

Balloons

Pacifiers

Baby bottle nipples

Individuals who already have latex allergy should be aware of latex-containing products that may trigger an allergic reaction. Some of the listed products are available in latex-free forms.

Types of Reactions to Latex

Three types of reactions can occur in persons using latex products:

- Irritant contact dermatitis
- Allergic contact dermatitis (delayed hypersensitivity)
- Latex allergy

Irritant Contact Dermatitis

The most common reaction to latex products is irritant contact dermatitis—the development of dry, itchy, irritated areas on the skin, usually the hands. This reaction is caused by skin irritation from using gloves and possibly by exposure to other workplace products and chemicals. The reaction can also result from repeated hand washing and drying, incomplete hand drying, use of cleaners and sanitizers, and exposure to powders added to the gloves. Irritant contact dermatitis is not a true allergy.

Chemical Sensitivity Dermatitis

Allergic contact dermatitis (delayed hypersensitivity, also sometimes called chemical sensitivity dermatitis) results from exposure to chemicals added to latex during harvesting, processing, or manufacturing. These chemicals can cause skin reactions similar to those caused by poison ivy. As with poison ivy, the rash usually begins 24 to 48 hours after contact and may progress to oozing skin blisters or spread away from the area of skin touched by the latex.

Latex Allergy

Latex allergy (immediate hypersensitivity) can be a more serious reaction to latex than irritant contact dermatitis or allergic contact dermatitis. Certain proteins in latex may cause sensitization (positive blood or skin test, with or without symptoms). Although the amount of exposure needed to cause sensitization or symptoms is not known, exposures at even very low levels can trigger allergic reactions in some sensitized individuals.

Reactions usually begin within minutes of exposure to latex, but they can occur hours later and can produce various symptoms. Mild reactions to latex involve skin redness, hives, or itching. More severe reactions may involve respiratory symptoms such as runny nose, sneezing, itchy eyes, scratchy throat, and asthma (difficult breathing, coughing spells, and sneezing). Rarely, shock may occur; but a life-threatening reaction is seldom the first sign of latex allergy. Such reactions are similar to those seen in some allergic persons after a bee sting.

Who Is at Risk?

Workers with ongoing latex exposure are at risk for developing latex allergy. Such workers include health care workers (physicians, nurses, aids, dentists, dental hygienists, operating room employees, laboratory technicians, and hospital housekeeping personnel) who frequently use latex gloves and other latex-containing medical supplies. Workers who use latex gloves less frequently (law enforcement personnel, ambulance attendants, funeral-home workers, fire fighters, painters, gardeners, food service workers, and housekeeping personnel) may also develop latex allergy. Workers in factories where latex products are manufactured or used can also be affected.

Atopic individuals (persons with a tendency to have multiple allergic conditions) are at increased risk for developing latex allergy. Latex allergy is also associated with allergies to certain foods especially avocado, potato, banana, tomato, chestnuts, kiwi fruit, and papaya. People with spina bifida are also at increased risk for latex allergy.

Section 42.4

Preventing Latex Allergy

Scientists at Columbia University have developed a new topical hand cream that may prevent the two most common latex allergy reactions—sensitization to latex after prolonged exposure and contact dermatitis. Over 100,000 people in the United States are at risk for latex allergies, which cause itching and redness and in severe cases can lead to respiratory distress or even death.

Study author, Shanta Modak, Ph.D., associate research scientist at Columbia-Presbyterian Medical Center and lead researcher in the discovery of the cream, presented the findings today at the Interscience Conference on Antimicrobial Agents and Chemotherapy meeting in Toronto, Ontario.

Researchers investigated topical creams containing a new gel composition for their efficacy in preventing irritant dermatitis when used before wearing latex gloves. Scientists discovered that when the zinc gel composition was formulated in a special base, a gel matrix or protective coating structure is formed on the skin's surface. The matrix appears to react with and bind soluble latex proteins and other irritants known to produce allergies and may actually prevent the allergic response altogether.

Prevention of the initial onset of irritant dermatitis is critical, because these symptoms are prelude to more severe allergic reactions. And in the most severe cases, people left untreated with this condition—like those allergic to bee stings—risk respiratory distress or even death.

"This cream can prevent latex glove allergies for up to four hours when applied before putting on the gloves," Modak said. "Use of the cream may reduce health care workers' risk of becoming sensitized to latex after continued exposure and may help the tens of thousands of health care workers who suffer daily with chronic irritant dermatitis."

The cream was developed for health care workers who are or who may become allergic to natural latex rubber in gloves and other common irritants. It is estimated that between eight and 17 percent of all health care workers risk developing latex allergies, both from wearing the powdered latex gloves and/or from inhaling cornstarch particles, coated with latex allergen, that drift from the gloves into the air.

Preliminary clinical evaluation indicates the cream is safe for use by the general public and for those who are not allergic to latex. Columbia University licensed the anti-irritant cream called Allergy Guard™ to Virasept Pharmaceuticals Inc.

The study was funded by The Columbia-Presbyterian Medical Center surgery department and Virasept Pharmaceuticals.

Chapter 43

Clearing Up Cosmetic Confusion

Cosmetics run the gamut from eye shadow to deodorant sprays. And consumers' concerns and questions are just as varied as the products themselves.

"Consumers are so confused by the products out there because they all do so many different things," says Lynn Reniers, a licensed cosmetologist with Elizabeth Arden. "So it's important to send them away with a very clear understanding of product usage."

When FDA surveyed 1,687 consumers ages 14 and older in 1994 about their use of cosmetics, many of the responses pertained to consumer perceptions about cosmetic labeling claims. For example, many said they expect a product to prevent or slow the formation of wrinkles if it makes such a claim on its packaging. And nearly half of those surveyed felt that a product claiming to be "natural" should contain all natural ingredients. But do these products live up to their labeling claims?

Not necessarily. John Bailey, Ph.D., director of FDA's Office of Cosmetics and Colors, says, "Image is what the cosmetics industry sells through its products, and it's up to the consumer to believe the claims or not."

Behind the image, however, are real products, and consumers want to know what works and what doesn't.

"Clearing Up Cosmetic Confusion," by Carol Lewis. This article originally appeared in the May-June 1998 *FDA Consumer*. The version here is from a reprint of the original article (Publication No. FDA 98-5017) and contains revisions made in May 1998 and August 2000.

An understanding of FDA's cosmetic responsibilities can help consumers make wise, rational decisions about the cosmetics they buy.

Regulatory Authority

The regulatory requirements governing the sale of cosmetics are not as stringent as those that apply to other FDA-regulated products. Under the Federal Food, Drug, and Cosmetic (FD&C) Act, cosmetics and their ingredients are not required to undergo approval before they are sold to the public. Generally, FDA regulates these products after they have been released to the marketplace. This means that manufacturers may use any ingredient or raw material, except for color additives and a few prohibited substances, to market a product without a government review or approval.

But some regulations do apply to cosmetics. In addition to the FD&C Act, the Fair Packaging and Labeling Act requires an ingredient declaration on every cosmetic product offered for sale to consumers. In addition, these regulations require that ingredients be listed in descending order of quantity. Water, for example, accounts for the bulk of most skin-care products, which is why it usually appears first on these products.

Although companies are not required to substantiate performance claims or conduct safety testing, if safety has not been substantiated, the product's label must read "WARNING: The safety of this product has not been determined."

"Consumers believe that 'if it's on the market, it can't hurt me,'" says Bailey. "And this belief is sometimes wrong."

FDA's challenge comes in proving that a product is harmful under conditions of use or that it is improperly labeled. Only then can the agency take action to remove adulterated or misbranded products from the marketplace.

The Fine Line between Cosmetics and Drugs

The FD&C Act defines cosmetics as articles intended to be applied to the human body for cleansing, beautifying, promoting attractiveness, or altering the appearance without affecting the body's structure or functions. This definition includes skin-care creams, lotions, powders and sprays, perfumes, lipsticks, fingernail polishes, eye and facial makeup, permanent waves, hair colors, deodorants, baby products, bath oils, bubble baths, and mouthwashes, as well as any material intended for use as a component of a cosmetic product.

Products that intend to treat or prevent disease, or otherwise affect structure or function of the human body are considered drugs. Cosmetics that make therapeutic claims are regulated as drugs and cosmetics, and must meet the labeling requirements for both. A good way to tell if you're buying a cosmetic that is also regulated as a drug is to see if the first ingredient listed is an "active ingredient." The active ingredient is the chemical that makes the product effective, and the manufacturer must have proof that it's safe for its intended use. For products that are both drugs and cosmetics, the regulations require that active ingredients be listed first on these products, followed by the list of cosmetic ingredients in order of decreasing predominance.

Examples of products that are both cosmetics and drugs are dandruff shampoos, fluoride toothpastes, antiperspirant deodorants, and foundations and tanning preparations that contain sunscreen.

Before products with both a cosmetic and drug classification can be marketed, they must be scientifically proven safe and effective for their therapeutic claims. If they are not, FDA considers them to be misbranded and can take regulatory action.

Reading Is Believing

The ingredient list on a cosmetic container is the only place where a consumer can readily find out the truth about what he or she is buying. Consumers can check the listing to identify substances they wish to avoid. And becoming familiar with what cosmetics contain can help counter some of the alluring appeal showcased elsewhere on the product.

"Our best friend is the ingredient label," says beauty consultant and 14-year veteran consumer reporter Paula Begoun. "And spending the time to read it may be all that is needed to protect ourselves from hurting our skin."

But the ingredient list, although a mandatory requirement on cosmetics, is also the most difficult part of the label to understand. Bailey admits that most of us don't recognize the names of the ingredients listed because there are thousands available to chemists creating a wide variety of products. But there's no way to change that, he says, and still accurately identify the substances that are used.

Consumers can, however, obtain specific information about a cosmetic ingredient in various references, such as the *International Cosmetic Ingredient Dictionary and Handbook,* published by the Cosmetic, Toiletry, and Fragrance Association, available at many public libraries.

FDA recognizes the association as a reliable source of facts on substances that have been identified as cosmetic ingredients, as well as their definitions and trade names.

Cosmetic ingredient declaration regulations apply only to retail products intended for home use. Cosmetic samples and products used exclusively by beauticians in salons are not required to include the ingredient declaration. However, these products must state the distributor, list the content's quantity, and include all necessary warning statements.

They Can Be Irritating

Almost all cosmetics can cause allergic reactions in certain individuals. Often the first sign of a reaction is a mild redness and irritation. There is no list of ingredients that can be guaranteed not to cause allergic reactions, so consumers who are prone to allergies should pay careful attention to what they use on their skin.

Nearly one-quarter of the people questioned in FDA's 1994 cosmetics survey responded "yes" to having suffered an allergic reaction to personal care products, including moisturizers, foundations, and eye shadows.

"Because of the almost limitless combinations in all sorts of mixtures and formulations, it is virtually impossible to know if, when, or how anyone's skin will react to any cosmetic," Begoun says. She advises consumers to "buy with a healthy dose of skepticism," and to stop using an offending product and return it to the place of purchase. "Returning the product gives the cosmetics company essential information about how these formulas are working."

Beauty on the Safe Side

Serious injury from makeup is a rare occurrence, according to John Bailey, director of FDA's Office of Cosmetics and Colors. But it does happen. Good common sense and a few precautions can help consumers protect themselves against hazards associated with the misuse of cosmetics.

- Never drive and apply makeup. Not only does it make for dangerous driving, but hitting a bump in the road and scratching your eyeball can cause bacteria to contaminate the cut and could result in serious injury, including blindness.

- Never share makeup. Always use a new disposable applicator when sampling products at a cosmetics counter. Insist that salespersons clean container openings with alcohol before applying their contents to your skin.

- Never add liquid to a product to bring back its original consistency. Adding other liquids could introduce bacteria that can easily grow out of control.

- Stop using any product that causes an allergic reaction.

- Throw away makeup if the color changes or an odor develops. Preservatives degrade over time and may no longer be able to fight bacteria.

- Do not use eye makeup if you have an eye infection. Throw away all products you were using when you discovered the infection.

- Keep makeup out of sunlight. Light and heat can degrade preservatives.

- Keep makeup containers tightly closed when not in use.

- Never use aerosol beauty products near heat or while smoking because they can ignite. Hairsprays and powders may cause lung damage if inhaled regularly.

What Lies behind the Meaning

FDA has tried to establish official definitions for the use of certain terms such as "natural" and "hypoallergenic," but its regulations were overturned in court. So companies can use them on cosmetic labels to mean anything or nothing at all. Most of the terms have considerable market value in promoting cosmetic products to consumers, but dermatologists say they have very little medical meaning.

Some of the more common terms that consumers should be aware of include:

- **Natural:** implies that ingredients are extracted directly from plants or animal products as opposed to being produced synthetically. There is no basis in fact or scientific legitimacy to the notion that products containing natural ingredients are good for the skin.

- **Hypoallergenic:** implies that products making this claim are less likely to cause allergic reactions. There are no prescribed scientific studies required to substantiate this claim. Likewise, the terms "dermatologist-tested," "sensitivity tested," "allergy tested," or "nonirritating" carry no guarantee that they won't cause skin reactions.

- **Alcohol Free:** traditionally meant that certain cosmetic products do not contain ethyl alcohol (or grain alcohol). Cosmetic products, however, may contain other alcohols, such as cetyl, stearyl, cetearyl, or lanolin, which are known as fatty alcohols.

- **Fragrance Free:** implies that a cosmetic product so labeled has no perceptible odor. Fragrance ingredients may be added to a fragrance-free cosmetic to mask any offensive odor originating from the raw materials used, but in a smaller amount than is needed to impart a noticeable scent.

- **Noncomodogenic:** suggests that products do not contain common pore-clogging ingredients that could lead to acne.

- **Shelf Life (Expiration Date):** the amount of time for which a cosmetic product is good under normal conditions of storage and use, depending on the product's composition, packaging, preservation, etc. Expiration dates are, for practical purposes, a rule of thumb, and a product may expire long before that date if it has not been stored and handled properly.

- **Cruelty Free:** implies that products have not been tested on animals. Most ingredients used in cosmetics have at some point been tested on animals so consumers may want to look for "no new animal testing," to get a more accurate indication.

The list of ingredients, once again, can help consumers determine if there is any significant difference between products labeled similar to the above, and competing brands that don't make these claims.

Since the cosmetics industry often produces new, reworked versions of old ingredients, a wise consumer will take the time to read the labels to know what's in a product and how to use it safely. After all, consumers are likely to try other products with the same recognizable names. Once you have all the information, you can begin to make your own decisions about what products work best for you.

"There is really very little that's new under the sun," Bailey concludes, "and that certainly applies to cosmetics."

Prohibited Ingredients

The following ingredients, because of the dangers they impose, are either restricted or prohibited by regulation for use in cosmetics:

- bithionol
- mercury compounds
- vinyl chloride
- halogenated salicylanilides
- zirconium complexes in aerosol cosmetics
- chloroform
- methylene chloride
- chlorofluorocarbon propellants
- hexachlorophene
- methyl methacrylate monomer in nail products

Helping the Buyer Beware

Despite many questions about their safety, alpha hydroxy acids (AHAs) and beta hydroxy acids (BHAs) have become widely used in recent years. AHAs are derived from fruit and milk sugars, and are among the popular ingredients that attract customers with their claims to reduce wrinkles and age spots, and help repair sun-damaged skin.

FDA recommends that consumers take precautions with AHA and BHA products:

- Test any AHA/BHA-containing product on a small area of skin before applying to a larger area.
- Avoid the sun when possible.
- Use an effective sunscreen when using an AHA-containing product, even if you haven't used the product that day.
- Follow use instructions on the label.
- Do not exceed recommended applications.
- Do not use on infants and children.

Consumers should report cosmetic adverse reactions by calling their local FDA office, listed in the Blue Pages of the telephone book under U.S. Department of Health and Human Services. Call the Office of Cosmetics and Colors at 202-205-4706. More information on cosmetics is available by calling the Center for Food Safety and Applied Nutrition's outreach and information center at 1-888-723-3366 or by visiting the Cosmetics Page on the Center's Web site at www.fda.gov.

— by Carol Lewis

Carol Lewis is a staff writer for *FDA Consumer*.

Chapter 44

Fragrances and Health

Fragrance is ubiquitous in nature and plays a major role in both helping animals and humans locate food and enticing them to reproduce. Throughout history, humans have drawn fragrances from the natural environment for a variety of purposes, including use in religious and burial rituals, in aphrodisiacs, and to cover foul odors. In the late 1800s, the first fragrance containing synthesized ingredients was introduced. Since then, people have used chemicals extensively to mimic scents from nature.

Consumers' fascination with scent has increased with the manufacture of a multitude of scented "personal" products including cosmetics, lotions, soaps, oils, and perfumes. There are more than 1,000 body fragrances (including colognes, perfumes, and toilet waters) on the market today, according to The Fragrance Foundation, a non-profit educational arm of the fragrance industry. Furthermore, scents are now added to a slew of commercial products ranging from cleaning products to tissues, from candles to diapers.

While many people enjoy wearing perfumes and using scented products, there is a growing outcry from some people who claim that exposure to certain fragrances, including perfumes and scented products, adversely impacts their health. They report symptoms such as headaches, dizziness, nausea, fatigue, shortness of breath, difficulty with concentration, and allergy-like symptoms. It has been shown that many asthmatic patients have adverse reactions to perfumes and

"Scents and Sensitivity," by Brandy E. Fisher in *Environmental Health Perspectives*, Volume 106, December 12, 1998.

other fragrances, and some researchers hypothesize that exposure to fragrance may actually cause asthma. People who suffer from multiple chemical sensitivity (MCS), a health condition in which exposure to one chemical is thought to lead to adverse reactions to other chemicals, claim that exposure to fragrance triggers various symptoms, often to the point that sufferers are incapacitated or must forgo many of their usual activities to avoid exposure.

As information continues to surface on the issue of indoor air pollution, it appears that fragrances may represent part of the problem. Some researchers believe that exposure to the types of chemicals found in many scented products may contribute to the development and exacerbation of sick building syndrome, a health condition allegedly caused by indoor air pollution. The chemicals in perfumes, colognes, and deodorants worn by employees add to the chemical mixtures in indoor air, as do fragrances in cleaning products. In addition, some building owners pump certain fragrances—believed to evoke an emotional response that results in increased work productivity—through office ventilation systems.

Claudia Miller, an associate professor of environmental and occupational medicine at the University of Texas Health Sciences Center in San Antonio, says that several studies indicate that 15-30% of the general population report some sensitivity to chemicals, including fragrances, and 4-6% report that chemical intolerance has a major impact on their quality of life. Of these people, more than 80% report that exposure to fragrances is bothersome. Miller, who has conducted extensive research on MCS and coauthored the book *Chemical Exposures: Low Levels and High Stakes*, adds that many Gulf War veterans report new chemical intolerances since the war, including sensitivity to fragrances.

Gerald McEwen, vice president of science at the Cosmetic, Toiletry, and Fragrance Association, a Washington, DC–based trade association for the personal care products industry, says that fragrance materials in most products are at very low concentrations, and that people who claim to be adversely affected by scented products may actually be reacting to other chemicals in the products or in their environments. He says that affected people are more likely to identify fragrances as the offending agents because they are readily noticeable. McEwen further suggests that reactions to fragrance could be psychological. "This could be a conditioned response just as easily as an organic response," he says.

This theory has many proponents, including Sally Satel, a lecturer in psychiatry in Yale University School of Medicine's department of psychiatry. In her article, published in the May 1997 issue of *Psychiatric Times*, Satel refers to MCS, sick building syndrome, and other chemical sensitivity illnesses as having "elements of paranoia and hypervigilance (directed toward the physical environment), somatization (as well as stress-induced psychosomatic symptoms), hypochondriasis, hysteria, and suggestibility."

Components of Fragrances

The process of developing fragrances is a complex mixture of chemistry and art. Not only must the chemicals used be compatible, the combination must also be aesthetically pleasing to the nose. Synthetic ingredients are less expensive than natural ingredients, and can be created year-round, while the supply of natural ingredients depends on season and availability. Once synthetic ingredients were introduced to the marketplace, perfumes and fragrance materials became more widespread as the demand and supply increased. It is estimated that there are more than 3,000 chemicals used in the manufacture of fragrances. Synthetic organic chemicals constitute more than 80-90% (by weight and value) of the raw materials used in flavor and fragrance formulations. A single fragrance may contain as few as 10 chemicals or as many as several hundred. Like many other chemicals and chemical mixtures in widespread use today, little is known about the impact fragrances have on human health.

Because of the complex and competitive nature of fragrance development, manufacturers were given the right to protect their products through state trade secret laws, which allow them to not disclose the ingredients to anyone. Due to the secrecy surrounding fragrance ingredients, claims of adverse reactions to fragrances may be difficult or impossible to link to particular fragrance chemicals. Such secrecy also makes it difficult for researchers to study the health effects of fragrances. "Because of the number of chemicals and their different volatilities, polarities, and other properties, analysis is expensive and technically sophisticated," says Lance Wallace, an environmental scientist in the EPA's Office of Research and Development in Reston, Virginia.

As part of efforts to identify substances that contribute to indoor air pollution, Wallace and colleagues conducted a study to identify volatile organic compounds emitted by fragranced products. These compounds can be both toxic and carcinogenic and have been associated with the symptoms of sick building syndrome.

The study, published in the proceedings of the Air and Waste Management Association's 84th Annual Meeting and Exhibition, held June

16–21 1991, examined 31 selected scented products, including perfumes, soaps, and deodorants. The brand names were not revealed because only one semiquantitative analysis was made for each sample; therefore, the results could not be said to be indicative of that sample's typical composition. The researchers identified a total of 150 unique chemicals in the 31 products. Chemicals that appeared in more than half of the products included ethanol, limonene, linalool, ß-phenethyl alcohol, and ß-myrcene. The authors point out that few of these chemicals have been tested for carcinogenicity, but say that some, such as α-pinene, are known mutagens and others, such as camphor, have known toxic effects at high concentrations. Limonene has been tested for carcinogenicity and was observed to cause cancer in male rats, but not in mice or female rats. Wallace cautions that, while the chemicals have been identified as components of fragrances, health effects may occur at far higher doses than what may typically be found in fragrances.

Mary Lamielle, executive director of the National Center for Environmental Health Strategies, a national nonprofit organization dedicated to finding creative solutions for environmental health problems, points out that, even though the chemicals may be present at low levels in perfumes and products, people generally do not experience just a single exposure. "These same chemicals are cropping up in many different products," she says.

Self-Regulated Industry

Currently, the fragrance industry is essentially self-regulated in the United States. The FDA's Office of Cosmetics and Colors has jurisdiction over perfumes and fragrances used in cosmetics, but does not require an approval process or premarket clearance for perfumes or cosmetics containing fragrance, says John Bailey, Jr., director of the office. Therefore, the FDA does not technically have jurisdiction over products until they are on the market. "It is up to the manufacturer to market a safe product," Bailey says. "If there's an identifiable public health risk, then certainly the agency can step in and take action." However, he says, "People claim to be sensitive to fragrances, but in spite of efforts to try to characterize the risk, the issue has defied a concise identification of a public health risk [and has] defied a good solid scientific definition. Therefore, the agency is not in a position to propose a change in regulation."

Due to the trade secret rules, the FDA does not require manufacturers to reveal fragrance ingredients to the agency, nor does it require them to list the fragrance ingredients on the products themselves. The manufacturer is simply required to list the collective term "fragrance" in the ingredients, a term that is often representative of a complex mixture of chemicals, Bailey says. But Bailey also says the industry does regulate itself through a safety review process, and that the FDA has periodically monitored this process.

Many manufacturers of fragrance chemicals conduct their own safety tests. In addition, the fragrance industry developed the Research Institute for Fragrance Materials (RIFM, pronounced "RIFF-um") in 1996 to conduct research on fragrance ingredients in order to ensure the safety of perfumery materials. According to Glenn Roberts, a spokesperson for RIFM, fragrance ingredients undergo a multistep testing process. "We are committed to developing safe products," Roberts says.

RIFM tests raw perfumery materials that are selected by an independent expert panel made up largely of academics, Roberts says. The ingredients are most commonly tested for allergenicity, phototoxicity, and general toxicity by oral and dermal routes. Some of the tests are conducted on animals while others, such as skin patch tests, are conducted on humans. To date, RIFM has tested more than 1,300 fragrance materials, and publishes test results in scientific journals such as *Food and Chemical Toxicology*, says Roberts. The National Toxicology Program has also conducted tests on many of these chemicals.

The results of the fragrance screenings are then submitted by RIFM to the International Fragrance Association (IFRA), an international organization composed of more than 100 fragrance manufacturers from 15 countries. IFRA reviews the data and establishes guidelines for the safe use of the materials. If a fragrance material is found to have neurotoxic, carcinogenic, phototoxic, or other adverse health effects, IFRA categorizes the material as restricted, and recommends amounts of the material for use in fragrance formulas. While many companies voluntarily adhere to the IFRA safety guidelines, they are not required by law to follow any of the group's recommendations, or to limit the use of any fragrance materials. Roberts points out that, while RIFM tests only the raw materials, the manufacturers of the finished fragrance products also often conduct safety tests.

Research on Fragrances and the Sense of Smell

Extensive research has been conducted on the allergic effects of fragrances on skin, and many fragrance materials have been shown to cause dermal allergic reactions. RIFM conducts most of its research on the dermal effects of fragrances, rarely testing the effects of inhaling fragrance chemicals. Roberts says, "It has always been the scientific opinion of the industry that the skin is the primary route of exposure [for fragrances]." However, he says the industry "continues to think about and look at" the issue of respiratory testing.

Not only is it difficult for nonindustry researchers to identify and quantify the actual components of fragrances, it is also challenging to study how inhaling these chemicals impacts human health because very little is known about the olfactory system, and very little research has been conducted on the passage of fragrance molecules into the body via this system. There is a strong link between the sense of smell and emotion; many researchers believe this is due to the proximity of the olfactory bulb to the limbic system, which popular media have dubbed "emotion central." The nasal passage offers a unique route of exposure for chemicals, which can proceed directly into the brain because of the proximity of these systems. "The olfactory/limbic tract is the most direct connection between our brains and the air we breathe," says Miller. "There is no blood-brain barrier." Studies have shown that in rodents, chemical molecules can move through the nose directly into the brain, passing through only one or two synapses. Miller says research indicates that molecules follow this same route in humans.

Fragrances and Non-Olfactory Responses

Another problem in studying fragrances, according to Dennis Shusterman, an associate clinical professor in the division of occupational and environmental medicine and director of the Upper Airway Biology Lab at the University of California at San Francisco, is the assumption that the only property of a fragrance chemical is its ability to stimulate the olfactory nerve and produce the sensation of smell. "In fact, [such chemicals] can stimulate both the olfactory and the trigeminal nerve, which mediates irritation," Shusterman says. Stimulation of receptors in the trigeminal nerve results in the perception of irritancy or pungency, causing sensations such as stinging, burning, piquancy, prickling, freshness, and tingling. This process is referred to as sensory irritation and can result in a localized neurogenic inflammation.

Many researchers believe that exposure to fragrance and other chemicals can indeed cause irritation, which can mimic the symptoms of allergies. James Wells, a professor of medicine at the University of Oklahoma Health Sciences Center in Oklahoma City, recounts that in his private practice as an allergist, he has encountered many patients who complain of reactions to specific perfumes or fragrances. He has observed that in a vast majority of the cases, the reaction to the fragrances is one of irritation, not allergy. Wells says the reactions to irritants are less responsive to treatment than allergies, and that avoiding the offending chemicals appears to be the only effective solution. Wells stresses that he has not conducted research, but that in his clinical experience, he has found that these patients also react to other irritants, such as detergents, cleansers, and deodorizers that emit volatile chemicals into the air.

Despite the similarity of the symptoms, though, Shusterman says existing studies indicate that the process behind chemical-induced irritation is a different phenomenon from allergies altogether. Shusterman adds that many studies have indicated that people who have preexisting nasal allergies such as hay fever either perceive or react more strongly to irritant chemicals.

The Indoor Environment

William Cain, a professor of surgery, Enrique Cometto-Muniz, an associate research scientist, and colleagues at the Chemosensory Perception Laboratory at the University of California at San Diego are conducting extensive research on the sense of smell and sensory irritation from chemicals in the indoor environment. Cometto-Muniz says the goal of the research is to provide further insight into the sense of smell so that it can be as well understood as the visual and aural senses. "We know very well the electromagnetic spectrum to which the eye responds and the vibrational spectrum to which the ear responds, but we don't know the chemical spectrum to which the nose responds," he says.

Cain says an important issue to consider in investigating the effects of fragrance on the body is differentiating between psychological irritation from unpleasant chemical odors and actual sensory irritation from chemicals. Because of the strong tie between the sense of smell and emotion, researchers say foul odors emitted by certain chemicals can provoke people to believe their health is being impacted when, in fact, the offending substance may be benign.

Cain and Cometto-Muniz are working to establish the odor and irritant thresholds of chemicals—at what level a chemical first is an odorant and then becomes an irritant. Identifying such thresholds will aid in distinguishing the psychological response to odor from measurable nasal and eye irritation. The involvement of anosmics, or people who have no sense of smell, in the studies allows for the "perfect opportunity to differentiate what is a trigeminal response from an olfactory response," says Cometto-Muniz.

So far, the group has successfully established the threshold levels of physiological irritation for several chemical mixtures. Their research has indicated that the higher the number of chemicals being combined, the lower their individual levels need to be to cause sensory reactions. Areas they plan to further investigate include chemical mixtures, as well as the role of time in sensory irritation and sense of smell. Cometto-Muniz says that when a person is exposed to an odor, the sensation appears to diminish over time as the person seemingly adapts to the odor, while sensory irritation occurs in an opposite manner—as time passes, irritation increases. While there are still many questions about how long-term sensory irritation may affect health, Cometto-Muniz points out that "sensory irritation is there to warn us that continued exposure could potentially be dangerous."

Toxic Effects of Fragrance Products

One of the few studies that has looked at the effects of inhalation of specific fragrance chemicals and perfumes was conducted at the private Anderson Laboratory in West Hartford, Vermont, by Rosalind Anderson, founder and owner of the laboratory, and Julius Anderson, vice president. The goal of the study was to determine whether fragrance products can produce acute toxic effects in mammals. The Andersons exposed laboratory mice to five fragrance products—four colognes and one toilet water. The mice breathed the emissions of the products for 1 hour and then were tested using the ASTM-E-981 method to evaluate sensory irritation and pulmonary irritation, as well as a functional observational battery to look for changes in the nervous system function.

The study, published in the March-April 1998 issue of *Archives of Environmental Health*, showed that the emissions of the fragrances produced various combinations of sensory irritation, pulmonary irritation, decreases in expiratory airflow velocity, and alterations of the functional observational battery indicative of neurotoxicity. Neurotoxicity was more severe after mice were repeatedly exposed to the products.

The Andersons say the findings indicate that some fragrance products produce toxic effects in at least one mammalian species. In the study's conclusions, they wrote, "Collectively, the experimental data and chemistry predict that some humans exposed to these fragrance products might experience some combination of eye, nose, and/or throat irritation; respiratory difficulty; possibly bronchoconstriction or asthma-like reaction; and central nervous system reactions (for example, dizziness, incoordination, confusion, fatigue). The results of our study might help explain why some individuals report an intolerance to [fragrance products] and why some [fragrance products] can exacerbate airflow limitation in some asthmatics."

Fragrances and Chemical Sensitivity

Miller says it's important to recognize that many people who report sensitivities to fragrances also report sensitivities to other chemicals. Because fragrances are noticeable, they may be more commonly reported as causing symptoms than other chemicals. Miller conducted a study, published in the March-April 1995 issue of *Archives of Environmental Health*, that surveyed 112 people who reported onset of MCS following a well-documented exposure to either a pesticide exposure or remodeling of a building. Miller and colleagues hypothesize that MCS may be explained by what they call toxicant-induced loss of tolerance, a two-part process involving a single high-level chemical exposure followed by subsequent triggering of symptoms by everyday exposure to chemicals.

Respondents were asked to identify possible trigger exposures via inhalation and ingestion and report symptoms. About 90% of respondents reported that perfumes triggered their symptoms, but Miller stresses that many other exposures triggered symptoms as well, including insecticides, traffic exhaust, new carpet, paint, and various foods. The most frequently reported symptoms included lethargy, memory difficulties, feelings of depression, dizziness, "spaciness," and shortness of breath.

Fragrance and Children

One other issue to consider is that of the effect of fragrance exposure on children's health. Today, many children's products are scented, and there are many fragrances marketed specifically toward children. Betty Bridges, a registered nurse and founder of the Fragranced Products Information Network, a Web site containing information about chemicals used in scented products and their health effects, says that children may be more susceptible to the effects of such products because of their smaller size, their higher respiratory rate, and their thinner skin. However, little research has been done on this issue.

A Fragrance-Free Future?

Some patient groups claim that in the next decade, the issue of fragrance will be as controversial as today's tobacco smoke issue. They say the debate over people's right to smoke versus others' right to breathe clean air could also be applied to fragrance. McEwen calls the comparison between tobacco smoke and fragrances "absurd," saying "Fragrances are scents that are basically taken from nature. They have been around forever. There is no process of combustion involved and they are not addictive."

However, many organizations are taking the fragrance sensitivity issue seriously. At an American Chemical Society meeting held in August 1998 in Boston, Massachusetts, attendees were asked not to wear fragrances due to the number of chemically sensitive people attending the meeting. Miller says that requests for people to refrain from wearing scented products are appearing with more frequency on social invitations, as well as in public meeting notices. At the University of Minnesota School of Social Work in Minneapolis, signs are posted at entrances to the department, stating, "Some persons employed or studying in the School of Social Work report sensitivities to various chemical-based or scented products. We ask for everyone's cooperation in our efforts to accommodate their health concerns."

In recent years, perhaps in response to the abundance of fragrance encountered by people on a daily basis, the trend of scenting products has been somewhat reversed. Many manufacturers are now removing fragrance from products and touting "fragrance-free" and "unscented" versions of products such as laundry detergent and fabric softeners.

However, chemically sensitive patients warn that, even though a product is labeled unscented or fragrance-free, it doesn't necessarily mean that it contains no fragrance chemicals. As studies have documented, manufacturers will often add masking chemicals to cover the scent of other chemicals in the product, resulting in a product that does not produce a detectable scent.

As for manufacturers that label their products as fragrance-free or unscented, Bailey says the FDA requires them to list the term "fragrance" in the ingredients when any fragrance materials are used — even masking ingredients. If the manufacturer fails to list fragrance ingredients, the FDA has the power to take regulatory action.

Whether the fragrance issue can and will be regulated remains to be seen. The U.S. Postal Service passed a regulation in April 1990 stating that "a fragrance advertising sample is nonmailable unless the sample meets the following requirement: It must be sealed, wrapped, treated, or otherwise prepared in a manner reasonably designed to prevent individuals from being unknowingly or involuntarily exposed to the sample." The California state government expanded the concept of that rule in 1992 by passing a regulation stating that "Any fragrance advertising insert contained in a newspaper, magazine, mailing, or other periodically printed material shall contain only microencapsulated oils. Glue tabs or binders shall be used to prevent premature activation of the fragrance advertising insert." In addition, several magazines now offer a "scent-free" version at the subscriber's request.

Lamielle and others are working to raise awareness of the issue of fragrance sensitivity. "Unfortunately, a lot of people don't realize that this is a serious issue, because it sounds so trivial," she says. "There's a huge population who do get sick from these products." In order to help solve the problem, Lamielle says that people should use less-toxic, unscented products and be considerate of those who are affected by fragrance sensitivity.

The issue of the environmental health effects of fragrances is complex, controversial, and slowly garnering more public attention. While Lamielle and Bridges say the number of people claiming to be affected by fragrances seems to be growing, Roberts says the fragrance industry has not seen an increase in complaints from consumers. "Fragrance helps many people enjoy their lives, but if there is a problem, we hope that [consumers] will call the manufacturers and we'll work to resolve it. We are always open to new ideas," says Roberts.

McEwen says it is important not to forget the many benefits of fragrances. They are used in the identification of different products, for instance by distinguishing a cough syrup from an emetic. They can also mask objectionable odors in certain products. "Fragrance really is like beautiful colors, beautiful music—a sensory phenomenon. It makes life better," McEwen says.

In the end, however, the only indisputable fact is that there is a lack of research on the issue. Says Miller, "It's worrisome, and should be explored with good, careful scientific studies."

Chapter 45

Indoor Air Quality and Health

Chapter Contents

Section 45.1

Workplace Air Quality

"Sick Days at Work," by Kathryn S. Brown in *Environmental Health Perspectives*, Volume 104, Number 10, October 1996; produced by the National Institute of Environmental Health Sciences (NIEHS), available online at http://ehpnet1.niehs.nih.gov.

Early in her medical career, Rebecca Bascom became puzzled by a stream of patients complaining of respiratory problems. Bascom, a pulmonary specialist, ran standard lung tests on these patients, whose lungs, surprisingly, seemed to function normally. "With everybody I had seen before . . . I knew the tests to order, the way to treat them," recalls Bascom, now director of the University of Maryland School of Medicine's Environmental Research Facility. "With this group, there just wasn't any [test] that seemed to work." It turns out Bascom's patients were being made ill by substances in the air in their offices. These patients were among the first wave of office workers to complain of a set of symptoms that is now referred to as sick building syndrome (SBS).

According to the World Health Organization, up to 30% of new and remodeled buildings worldwide contain enough pollutants to make workers ill. Asbestos, radon, and environmental tobacco smoke can cause lung cancer or chronic pulmonary disease. And pollutants like volatile organic compounds (VOCs) and bioaerosols—airborne particles emitted by fungi and bacteria—may be causing equally hazardous, though less well-understood, illnesses. Scientists have identified more than 1,500 indoor air pollutants from sources such as carpets, photocopiers, and ventilation ducts.

Researchers suggest that symptoms of SBS result from a complex, hard-to-study blend of pollutants that affects individuals differently. In response, scientists are wielding a range of research tools—from epidemiology studies to air chamber studies—to solve the indoor air pollution problem.

A Growing Concern

The problem of indoor pollution has generated concern among the scientific community around the world. In the United States, up to

21 million employees are exposed to poor indoor air quality, according to the Occupational Safety and Health Administration. Several major office buildings have recently made headlines by being diagnosed as "sick." At a New York office used by Memorial Sloan-Kettering Cancer Center, environmental investigators found high levels of carbon monoxide that forced more than 700 workers into temporary quarters. At Boston's Suffolk County Courthouse, a fume-emitting waterproofing compound caused over 800 employees to move to makeshift offices elsewhere. And in Washington, DC, health investigators discovered toxic fungi and poor ventilation in the Department of Transportation's headquarters. Again, workers had to evacuate.

Jim Young, a spokesperson for the New York Committee for Occupational Safety and Health (NYCOSH), a nonprofit advocacy group for workers, says he receives about 300 telephone calls a month from workers worried about their health. The majority of these calls, he says, involve indoor pollutants. "Indoor air quality is probably the most prevalent occupational health problem that we hear about," Young says. "There have just been more and more calls over time."

Researchers trace a rise in indoor air pollution to the 1970s when the energy crisis dictated a cut in air-handling costs. In 1973, the American Society of Heating, Refrigerating, and Air-Conditioning Engineers (ASHRAE) reduced the professional standard for the minimum amount of outdoor air brought into buildings by 70%. In the past, office employees had received 20-30 cubic feet of outdoor air per minute per person (cfm/p). The 1973 recommendation called for heating, ventilation, and air-conditioning (HVAC) systems to provide a minimum of just 5 cfm/p of outdoor air.

This outdoor air cutback accompanied a gradual rise in the use of photocopiers, laser printers, personal computers, and other equipment that may release chemical fumes. What's more, architectural designs changed and sealed windows, wall-to-wall carpeting, and fiberglass or particle board materials that may also contribute to the problem were increasingly used in buildings.

Researchers say that lower ventilation rates combined with increased exposure to indoor pollutants might explain the rash of SBS-type illnesses. According to the EPA, most Americans spend up to 90% of their time indoors, whether at the office or home. The EPA also suggests many indoor pollutants are concentrated at levels 2-5 times higher than outdoor levels. Other researchers suggest that psychological factors associated with the work environment including monotonization, loss of privacy, electronic monitoring of productivity, a faster work pace, and bad management practices may also play a role by increasing worker stress and compounding awareness of symptoms.

Too Little Data

Still, despite the statistics and plausible explanations, studies of hazardous buildings suffer from a lack of data as well as disagreements over sampling techniques, exposure assessments, and nomenclature. "Think of it this way," says John Spengler, a professor of environmental science and physiology at Harvard University, "when you're doing classic epidemiology, you may have to control a lot of variables, but you're still just making observations about individuals or groups of individuals. When you talk about buildings, you expand the inherent variability. You have to consider stress, job dissatisfaction, vibration, noise, lighting. There are so many factors that it's much more difficult to study. So there has yet to be a 1,000-building study."

Understanding and fixing indoor air pollution problems hasn't been as easy as researchers hoped. "Ten years ago, as epidemiologists we anticipated that we would figure out the causes [of SBS] by studying the atmosphere in buildings and diagnosing the probability [of illness] by knowing what's in the air," remarks Michael Hodgson, an associate professor of occupational and environmental medicine at the University of Connecticut. "But that has not worked because of limitations in our study designs, sampling frames, and exposure assessment strategies." Simply increasing ventilation rates, for example, hasn't solved the problem in every instance, although studies show that symptoms do improve when rates are increased from the current professional design standard of 25 cfm/p of outdoor air to 50cfm/p. In 1990, ASHRAE modified its ventilation guidelines, recommending that building owners return outdoor air flow rates to around 20 cfm/p. Still, indoor air pollution complaints continue.

Ongoing uncertainty leaves builders and engineers without any indoor air regulatory standards to follow, notes Hillel Koren, director of the human studies division at the EPA's National Health and Environmental Effects Research Laboratory. "It would be very difficult, at this point, to create [regulatory standards]," Koren says. "In outdoor pollutants, like ozone, there are ambient national quality standards and a scientific database. In indoor air, we are at an early stage of establishing, characterizing, and developing good biomarkers and endpoints. Here, we are just getting started." Still, Hodgson argues that regulatory standards have always lagged behind good professional standards and that adoption of the ASHRAE standard would solve a lot of the health complaints.

A Volatile Situation

At first, Mary Ann Mazzella, an administrative aide at New York University, began suffering from headaches. Then she began to have sinus problems. Soon she noticed she was feeling lethargic. Eventually, on hot days, she got so nauseous at the office that she'd call it quits and head home early. "I never got to the point where I was seriously ill," says Mazzella, "but I felt terrible."

With help from her local union, Mazzella got her office building's blueprints and surmised the source of her misery: industrial fumes and poor ventilation. "I work in a renovated factory building," Mazzella says. "We're supposed to have fresh air ducts every few feet. We don't. We have no windows. And the air conditioning shuts down for days at a time."

In fact, the photocopying room in Mazzella's building lacked a filtering system to flush out air rich in VOCs, including formaldehyde and ozone, which are emitted by photocopiers. This is a common oversight, according to indoor air researchers. Reporting in the July 1995 issue of the *ASHRAE Journal*, Hodgson and colleagues noted that, "In our experience, complaints around photocopiers abound, presumably because of ventilation inadequate for the needs imposed by this particular source."

In addition to photocopiers, a variety of building equipment and materials including paint, cleaning compounds, glues, silicone caulking material, insecticides, laser printers, personal computers, photographic equipment, fiberglass, and carpeting can give off irritating chemicals. Like Mazzella, employees affected by this chemical soup report a number of allergy-like symptoms.

Researchers often classify VOC sources based on how fast their emissions decline. For example, solid, dry materials like carpet or particle board are "slow decay" sources, meaning they strike the air with an initial blast of chemicals, then emissions slowly fall. Wet products like paints, adhesives, or waxes are "fast decay" sources that release most of their chemicals within minutes to days, though VOCs may be emitted for months or even years.

One wet product to gain attention in recent years is the adhesive glue used to install some carpets. Such glue can infuse the air with VOCs such as formaldehyde. Because of these chemicals, manufacturers recommend that new carpet owners temporarily turn up their ventilation systems.

Some workers may be more susceptible to VOC emissions than others. A myriad of factors ranging from noise to harsh lighting can aggravate symptoms of illness, making employees more aware of their physiological reactions. Awareness of an unusual odor, such as one emanating from carpeting, for example, can even make employees suspicious of air quality that is actually acceptable. "Smell plays a role because people smell things they don't expect to and [believe] there must be something wrong," explains William Cain, a professor of surgery and head of the Chemosensory Perception Laboratory at the University of California at San Diego. "They think that if something smells bad, it may be bad for you. That really isn't a good toxicological rule."

Cain is conducting experiments to separate the psychological effects of odor from measurable nasal inflammation and eye irritation, which more accurately pinpoint building-induced health problems. Cain and colleagues administered mixtures of VOCs to two sets of people: those with a normal sense of smell, and anosmics, or those without a sense of smell. In both groups of people, the researchers established threshold levels of physiological irritation for mixtures of chemicals like ethyl acetate, butanol, and benzene. "Every organic compound has an odor threshold and an irritation threshold," says Cain. "At some point above these thresholds, people can sense irritation. Our work entails measuring the difference. We use people without a sense of smell to measure the point where things truly become irritating."

So far, Cain and colleagues have found that the more chemical compounds that are combined, the more likely they are to cause physiological reactions. "If you want to be rash, you might say we get increasing additivity [more reactions between chemicals] with increasing complexity. You may have nine components in a study, and the real environment has 100 components. By the time you get to 100, you really have a tremendously more potent stimulus than you would predict by just knowing the individual components involved."

The additivity of VOCs may have foiled many attempts to discern toxic levels of chemicals in a building. Traditionally, environmental investigators simply measured the levels of individual airborne chemicals. But this approach overlooks the interaction between those chemicals. "The whole theory since the 1930s has operated on a flawed philosophy that maximum allowable concentrations were the best way [to measure indoor pollutants]," says Hodgson. "That helps explain why people have symptoms even while [equipment] perceives low levels."

Unfortunately, Cain says, research into VOC interaction is technical and expensive. "The problem is that we've got hundreds of chemicals. If we're going to talk about health effects that we're interested in, we've got to begin building the database one chemical at a time. Looking at the task, it seems almost insurmountable. But it's the tried-and-true path."

Koren is one researcher willing to travel that path. He and his colleagues are conducting a number of chamber studies in which they expose subjects to controlled amounts of VOCs. Using nasal wash to measure a subject's reactions and ocular examinations, the scientists can look for objective biological changes that indicate inflammation. "Our procedures allow us to measure changes that would lead to irritation and congestion, which are some of the most prominent complaints of SBS," Koren says.

Rather than build a database one chemical at a time, Koren hopes to find a model or prototype of VOCs to represent whole families of compounds with similar structures. "Ideally, once we find some clinical endpoints, I'd like to work with epidemiologists who can identify sick buildings, engineers to monitor exposure, biologists of various disciplines that can analyze whatever we find," Koren says. "It's got to be the kind of research that can integrate studies."

Invisible Zoo

Abundant as they may be, VOCs are not the only hazards to inhabit office air. Fungi, bacteria, viruses, algae, and other microbes lurk inside air ducts, grow around ceiling tiles, and thrive on almost any warm, damp surface.

Microbes need only four basic ingredients to survive: organic nutrients on which to feed, moisture (whether from humid air or standing water), a surface on which to grow, and darkness. Fungi usually travel from outdoors into a building, so high concentrations of mold or fungi occur in buildings surrounded by trees or shrubs. Once the microbes get inside, they capitalize on the nourishing environment of indoor humidity, dust, and dirt.

While their living requirements are minimal, microbes' health effects are quite substantial. Bacteria and fungi can produce airborne particles called bioaerosols, such as spores or mycotoxins. These bioaerosols can leave employees with symptoms such as coughing, headaches, and other allergic reactions. Buildings left vacant or recently renovated are particularly susceptible to microbe invasions.

Researchers suggest that renovating a building may increase the concentration of indoor air contaminants 1,000-fold.

Like VOCs, microbial contamination can be difficult to assess and treat. Current microbiological techniques are very limited, says Mark Mendell, an epidemiologist with the Cincinnati office of the National Institute for Occupational Safety and Health. "For one thing," he says, "conventional measurements typically only measure organisms that will actually grow on culture, but it is not only the living organisms that can cause problems. Nonliving spores, or pieces of organisms, or substances released from organisms can all have health effects, either allergic or toxic. For example, there are substances called mycotoxins (released from fungi) and endotoxins (contained in gram-negative bacteria) that are known to have serious adverse health effects at high levels in agricultural environments. A variety of evidence now suggests that both of these may be causing health effects at high levels in some indoor environments as well, but these substances are not usually measured indoors."

Koren and others are trying to identify what makes a person susceptible to irritation from biological contaminants. Koren's microbe research includes buildings and homes, both of which can host high levels of fungi and other microbes. Koren is studying interactions between outdoor and indoor pollutants. "Our question is, does exposure to outdoor pollutants like ozone increase a person's sensitivity to [indoor pollutants] like dust mites," Koren says. "We hope to help other agencies come up with prevention policies that take into account how the indoor environment fits with the outdoor environment."

In one experiment, Koren and colleagues exposed asthmatic study participants sensitive to dust mites to ozone and later to allergens carried by dust mites found in homes. Results appear to show that the combined contaminants spur a much stronger asthmatic reaction than either does alone.

Filling in the Gaps

Because little data exists on VOCs, microbes, and other indoor pollutants, researchers are furiously working to fill in the gaps. For example, the EPA's Indoor Air Division is about halfway through a study of 100 randomly-chosen office buildings across the United States with the goal of creating basic pollution data on typical buildings.

"There isn't a lot of information about the quality of air in office buildings now," explains Susan Womble, an EPA environmental scientist and manager of the project, called Baseline Information on Indoor

Air Quality in Large Buildings, or BASE. "So when people investigate sick building syndrome, for example, they don't have anything to compare their measurements to."

With the help of 40 experts, the EPA developed a standardized protocol—including characterization of a building, environmental monitoring, and questionnaires on health symptoms—with which to inspect buildings. "We expect to use the data for trends and to help us spot indicators that we should be following up on," Womble says. "We're hoping that this will also give us some insight into other studies that we need to target."

Meanwhile, James Woods, an environmental design professor and director of the Center for Building Health, Safety, and Productivity at Virginia Polytechnic Institute and State University, is working on a different approach: communication between practitioners. Because indoor air pollution spans many fields, epidemiology, microbiology, occupational medicine, and engineering specialists often find themselves working at cross purposes. Woods explains, "A clinician is going to approach the problem from the patient's perspective. A public health person is going to look at preventive measures. Engineers look at specific buildings. Policy makers look at sets of buildings. We want to try to get that all together and be able to address problems."

Eventually, Woods hopes to establish standardized methods of defining, tracking, and treating buildings that, over time, experience varying rates of pollution. "I think awareness [of building pollution] is changing," Woods says. "So the social trend is greater demand for improved performance of buildings. That includes thermal conditions, lighting, acoustic, and ergonomic factors." Woods notes that such factors affect employee stress, which in turn aggravates most health symptoms. "If you address just one of these factors, the level of stress is not affected well enough. You've got to address all of them."

While these researchers attempt to refine existing approaches, others are examining often overlooked pollutants. At Cornell University, Alan Hedge, a professor of design and environmental analysis, blames some indoor health complaints on manmade mineral fibers dropped into the air by ceiling tiles, insulation, and ventilation systems. In a recent study, Hedge and colleagues discovered high rates of employee health complaints correlated with high numbers of manmade mineral fibers in settled dust. In another study, after installing filter systems that collected the fibers, Hedge says, the number of complaints plummeted.

Hedge stumbled across the mineral fiber phenomenon while investigating a building for VOC contamination. "We were inside the building when one employee said to me 'I'm sure there's something in this building. I've got an air filter on my desk. Would you take a look at it?'" Hedge recalls. "I shook the filter out and looked at some samples on [microscope] slides. I was absolutely astonished to find samples full of what looked like glass fibers."

Intrigued, Hedge began reading up on mineral fibers. He learned that in the 1960s—when homes were built using fiberglass in the linings of ductwork—residents complained of health problems similar to today's SBS. He also discovered a number of building practices introduced in the 1970s that might be implicated in illnesses, such as the use of fiberglass in broad ceiling spaces or insulation placed inside the ventilation system where mineral fibers can shred and rain down on employees. "Inhaling [fibers] is like swallowing a . . . javelin," Hedge says. "If you swallow them end-ways, they can get quite far. The fiber pieces are three to eight microns in diameter and up to 30 microns long. They can cause fiber damage to epithelial cells of your eyes, nose, and throat." Hedge also believes fibers cause skin irritation and other symptoms.

Hedge says many researchers, steeped in the study of microbes or VOCs, have yet to seriously pursue the mineral fiber-illness relationship. However, researchers in England are working on similar studies, and Hedge is planning further studies on fibers.

Regulation Unlikely

At least for the time being, enforced regulations on workplace air quality appear unlikely. The closest policy makers have come is a 1994 proposal by OSHA that addressed a wide range of pollutants, including tobacco smoke. The proposed legislation called for employers to implement and maintain controls for many known pollutants. The proposal also asked employers to develop indoor air quality compliance plans and do inspections to make sure those plans work. While many indoor air researchers and activists supported the OSHA proposal, even more building owners, managers, and employers opposed it. "In our period of public comment we received over 115,000 comments," says Debra Janes, a health scientist and project manager at OSHA. "It's hard to find anyone who wants to take responsibility [for indoor air pollution]. And nobody wants to be cited over something they have no control over. Say there's a wet photocopier with solvents that are leaking. The building manager will say, 'That's not related to the building design. Why should we be responsible?'" Given the blast of negative responses, Janes says, it will take OSHA "a while" to review the responses received during the comment period.

The EPA continues to emphasize voluntary building standards to prevent indoor air pollutants. "We think there are incentives for doing it voluntarily," says Elissa Feldman, deputy director of the EPA's indoor air division. "Some real estate markets have rentable office space that's overflowing. [Quality indoor air] is a niche that some building owners could use to their advantage. It's also true that indoor air costs increasingly are associated with liability. In a big lawsuit, [the victim] can go after everybody from the architect to the general contractor and everybody along the way. Plus, getting a reputation as a sick building is really death to a marketable property."

The only way to tighten indoor air regulation and improve patients' diagnoses is to amass a broad collection of studies on poorly understood pollutants, researchers say. However, says Koren, "We are experiencing dwindling funding for this important health issue. There is a great deal of research that has only begun and that needs to be pursued vigorously to improve our understanding of the risks associated with the indoor air environment. And that is our number one goal."

Section 45.2

Sick Building Syndrome

"Indoor Air Facts No. 4 (Revised)," U.S. Environmental Protection Agency (EPA), April 1991, modified November 9, 2000. Available at http:// www.epa.gov/iaq/pubs/sbs.html.

Introduction

The term "sick building syndrome" (SBS) is used to describe situations in which building occupants experience acute health and comfort effects that appear to be linked to time spent in a building, but no specific illness or cause can be identified. The complaints may be localized in a particular room or zone, or may be widespread throughout the building. In contrast, the term "building related illness" (BRI) is used when symptoms of diagnosable illness are identified and can be attributed directly to airborne building contaminants.

A 1984 World Health Organization Committee report suggested that up to 30 percent of new and remodeled buildings worldwide may be the subject of excessive complaints related to indoor air quality (IAQ). Often this condition is temporary, but some build ings have long-term problems. Frequently, problems result when a building is operated or maintained in a manner that is inconsistent with its original design or prescribed operating procedures. Sometimes indoor air problems are a result of poor building design or occupant activities.

Indicators of SBS include:

- Building occupants complain of symptoms associated with acute discomfort, for example, headache; eye, nose, or throat irritation; dry cough; dry or itchy skin; dizziness and nausea; difficulty in concentrating; fatigue; and sensitivity to odors.

- The cause of the symptoms is not known.

- Most of the complainants report relief soon after leaving the building.

Indicators of BRI include:

- Building occupants complain of symptoms such as cough; chest tightness; fever, chills; and muscle aches.

- The symptoms can be clinically defined and have clearly identifiable causes.

- Complainants may require prolonged recovery times after leaving the building.

It is important to note that complaints may result from other causes. These may include an illness contracted outside the building, acute sensitivity (for example, allergies), job related stress or dissatisfaction, and other psychosocial factors. Nevertheless, studies show that symptoms may be caused or exacerbated by indoor air quality problems.

Causes of Sick Building Syndrome

The following have been cited causes of or contributing factors to sick building syndrome:

Inadequate Ventilation

In the early and mid 1900's, building ventilation standards called for approximately 15 cubic feet per minute (cfm) of outside air for each building occupant, primarily to dilute and remove body odors. As a result of the 1973 oil embargo, however, national energy conservation measures called for a reduction in the amount of outdoor air provided for ventilation to 5 cfm per occupant. In many cases these reduced outdoor air ventilation rates were found to be inadequate to maintain the health and comfort of building occupants. Inadequate ventilation, which may also occur if heating, ventilating, and air conditioning (HVAC) systems do not effectively distribute air to people in the building, is thought to be an important factor in SBS. In an effort to achieve acceptable IAQ while minimizing energy consumption, the American Society of Heating, Refrigerating and Air-Conditioning Engineers (ASHRAE) recently revised its ventilation standard to provide a minimum of 15 cfm of outdoor air per person (20 cfm/person in office spaces). Up to 60 cfm/person may be required in some spaces (such as smoking lounges) depending on the activities that normally occur in that space (see ASHRAE Standard 62-1989).

Chemical Contaminants from Indoor Sources

Most indoor air pollution comes from sources inside the building. For example, adhesives, carpeting, upholstery, manufactured wood products, copy machines, pesticides, and cleaning agents may emit volatile organic compounds (VOCs), including formaldehyde. Environmental tobacco smoke contributes high levels of VOCs, other toxic compounds, and respirable particulate matter. Research shows that some VOCs can cause chronic and acute health effects at high concentrations, and some are known carcinogens. Low to moderate levels of multiple VOCs may also produce acute reactions. Combustion products such as carbon monoxide, nitrogen dioxide, as well as respirable particles, can come from unvented kerosene and gas space heaters, woodstoves, fireplaces and gas stoves.

Chemical Contaminants from Outdoor Sources

The outdoor air that enters a building can be a source of indoor air pollution. For example, pollutants from motor vehicle exhausts; plumbing vents, and building exhausts (for example, bathrooms and kitchens) can enter the building through poorly located air intake vents, windows, and other openings. In addition, combustion products can enter a building from a nearby garage.

Biological Contaminants

Bacteria, molds, pollen, and viruses are types of biological contaminants. These contaminants may breed in stagnant water that has accumulated in ducts, humidifiers and drain pans, or where water has collected on ceiling tiles, carpeting, or insulation. Sometimes insects or bird droppings can be a source of biological contaminants. Physical symptoms related to biological contamination include cough, chest tightness, fever, chills, muscle aches, and allergic responses such as mucous membrane irritation and upper respiratory congestion. One indoor bacterium, *Legionella*, has caused both Legionnaires disease and Pontiac fever.

These elements may act in combination, and may supplement other complaints such as inadequate temperature, humidity, or lighting. Even after a building investigation, however, the specific causes of the complaints may remain unknown.

A Word about Radon and Asbestos

SBS and BRI are associated with acute or immediate health problems; radon and asbestos cause long-term diseases which occur years after exposure, and are therefore not considered to be among the causes of sick buildings. This is not to say that the latter are not serious health risks; both should be included in any comprehensive evaluation of a building's IAQ.

Building Investigation Procedures

The goal of a building investigation is to identify and solve indoor air quality complaints in a way that prevents them from recurring and which avoids the creation of other problems. To achieve this goal, it is necessary for the investigator(s) to discover whether a complaint is actually related to indoor air quality, identify the cause of the complaint, and determine the most appropriate corrective actions.

An indoor air quality investigation procedure is best characterized as a cycle of information gathering, hypothesis formation, and hypothesis testing. It generally begins with a walkthrough inspection of the problem area to provide information about the four basic factors that influence indoor air quality:

- the occupants
- the HVAC system
- possible pollutant pathways
- possible contaminant sources.

Preparation for a walkthrough should include documenting easily obtainable information about the history of the building and of the complaints; identifying known HVAC zones and complaint areas; notifying occupants of the upcoming investigation; and, identifying key individuals needed for information and access. The walkthrough itself entails visual inspection of critical building areas and consultation with occupants and staff.

The initial walkthrough should allow the investigator to develop some possible explanations for the complaint. At this point, the investigator may have sufficient information to formulate a hypothesis, test the hypothesis, and see if the problem is solved. If it is, steps should be taken to ensure that it does not recur. However, if insufficient information is obtained from the walk through to construct a hypothesis, or if initial tests fail to reveal the problem, the investigator should move on to collect additional information to allow formulation of additional hypotheses. The process of formulating hypotheses, testing them, and evaluating them continues until the problem is solved.

Although air sampling for contaminants might seem to be the logical response to occupant complaints, it seldom provides information about possible causes. While certain basic measurements, for example, temperature, relative humidity, CO_2, and air movement, can provide a useful "snapshot" of current building conditions, sampling for specific pollutant concentrations is often not required to solve the problem and can even be misleading. Contaminant concentration levels rarely exceed existing standards and guidelines even when occupants continue to report health complaints. Air sampling should not be undertaken until considerable information on the factors listed above has been collected, and any sampling strategy should be based on a comprehensive understanding of how the building operates and the nature of the complaints.

Solutions to Sick Building Syndrome

Solutions to sick building syndrome usually include combinations of the following:

- **Pollutant source removal or modification** is an effective approach to resolving an IAQ problem when sources are known and control is feasible. Examples include routine maintenance of HVAC systems, for example, periodic cleaning or replacement of filters; replacement of water-stained ceiling tile and carpeting; institution of smoking restrictions; venting contaminant source emissions to the outdoors; storage and use of paints, adhesives, solvents, and pesticides in well ventilated areas, and use of these pollutant sources during periods of non-occupancy; and allowing time for building materials in new or remodeled areas to off-gas pollutants before occupancy. Several of these options may be exercised at one time.

- **Increasing ventilation rates** and air distribution often can be a cost effective means of reducing indoor pollutant levels. HVAC systems should be designed, at a minimum, to meet ventilation standards in local building codes; however, many systems are not operated or maintained to ensure that these design ventilation rates are provided. In many buildings, IAQ can be improved by operating the HVAC system to at least its design standard, and to ASHRAE Standard 62-1989 if possible. When there are strong pollutant sources, local exhaust ventilation may be appropriate to exhaust contaminated air directly from the building. Local exhaust ventilation is particularly recommended to remove pollutants that accumulate in specific areas such as rest rooms, copy rooms, and printing facilities.

- **Air cleaning** can be a useful adjunct to source control and ventilation but has certain limitations. Particle control devices such as the typical furnace filter are inexpensive but do not effectively capture small particles; high performance air filters capture the smaller, respirable particles but are relatively expensive to install and operate. Mechanical filters do not remove gaseous pollutants. Some specific gaseous pollutants may be removed by adsorbent beds, but these devices can be expensive and require frequent replacement of the adsorbent material. In sum, air cleaners can be useful, but have limited application.

- **Education and communication** are important elements in both remedial and preventive indoor air quality management programs. When building occupants, management, and maintenance personnel fully communicate and understand the causes

412

and consequences of IAQ problems, they can work more effectively together to prevent problems from occurring, or to solve them if they do.

Section 45.3

Does Carbonless Copy Paper Contribute to Indoor Air Quality Problems?

"Dangerous Duplicates," *Environmental Health Perspectives*, Volume 106, Number 6, June 1998. Produced by the National Institute of Environmental Health Sciences (NIEHS).

Brenda Smith's health problems, including headaches, high blood pressure, and sensitivity to perfumes, began in 1981 and have grown progressively worse during the past 17 years. Smith, 49, believes her health problems can be traced to her job as a service representative for Bell Atlantic in Virginia Beach, Virginia, where she frequently worked with carbonless copy paper (CCP). "Carbonless copy paper is the culprit," Smith says. "We handled CCP and breathed its fumes, but no one warned us about it."

Smith, who was fired from her job at Bell Atlantic in 1993, is one of several plaintiffs who have filed product liability lawsuits against the Mead Corporation, Appleton Papers, Inc., Moore Business Forms, Inc., and other CCP manufacturers. The plaintiffs, who claim they have developed formaldehyde sensitization and have suffered deterioration of their allergic, immunologic, and respiratory systems, are seeking $3 million in compensatory damages.

Introduced commercially in 1954, CCP is used to make multiple paper copies of an original document simultaneously. The paper is coated with microencapsulated droplets of colorless dyes and solvents that break when pressure is applied through writing or typing. The released dyes form an image on the backing sheet, copying the writing without the use of carbon paper.

"CCP is a pervasive presence in the workplace," says Charles Schmidt, an associate in engineering in the department of environmental engineering at the University of Florida at Gainesville, who has been studying CCP. "It's cheap and an easy way of copying mundane items like invoices, office forms, and credit card receipts."

"The number of environmental health complaints about CCP is both disappointing and frustrating," says Henricka Nagy, a toxicologist at the National Institute for Occupational Safety and Health (NIOSH). "At this point, we really can't do much about the issue because we don't have much science to explain it." Reports about adverse effects in workers exposed to CCP began appearing in the scientific literature in the late 1960s, and NIOSH has since reported symptoms anecdotally associated with its use. Symptoms attributed to exposure by touch include eczema, tingling, dryness, irritation, redness, and itchiness of the skin, while those attributed to inhalation exposure include asthma, headaches, fatigue, hoarseness, throat tickle, joint pain, nasal congestion, and respiratory tract irritation.

But despite numerous studies, CCP's environmental health effects still remain a controversial issue in the scientific literature. While several researchers have concluded that some people are affected by the chemicals released in using the paper, CCP manufacturers and other scientists say past studies, including a 1987 investigation by NIOSH, have failed to find a link between CCP and worker illnesses. According to a *Federal Register* notice posted February 12, 1997, "On June 12, 1987, NIOSH published a *Federal Register* notice (52 FR 22534) requesting comments and secondary data on the toxicity of carbonless copy paper. At that time, it was determined, based on the submitted information, that insufficient data were available to conclude that the relationship between the exposure to carbonless copy paper and suggested health effects was a causal one."

No standards for recommended exposure limits exist for CCP, although there are OSHA permissible exposure limits, NIOSH recommended exposure limits, or American Conference of Environmental Hygienists threshold limit values for most of the active ingredients contained in CCP. In the past three decades, the published scientific literature has identified numerous chemicals and other substances used in CCP's manufacture, including resin, kaolin, starch, styrene, mineral oil, sanatasol oil, butadiene latex, hydrogenated terphenyls, aluminum silicate, organic dyes, diaryl ethanes, alkyl benzenes, isoparaffins, diisopropyl naphthalenes, dibutyl phthalate, aliphatic compounds, and aromatic compounds such as alkyl substituted biphenyls, although polychlorinated biphenyls have not been used since the early 1970s.

"CCP is a complex issue because we can compile a list of 1,000-plus chemicals that can be used in its manufacture," explains Rick Niemeier, a senior scientist and toxicologist at NIOSH. "There is no magic formula [for the manufacture of CCP] and it's all proprietary." However, Robert Tardiff, president of the Bethesda, Maryland-based Sapphire Group, a scientific research firm that deals with risk management issues, asserts that "several dozen compounds, certainly less than 100, are used in the manufacture of CCP coatings used in the United States."

Schmidt says his CCP study revealed that potentially dangerous chemicals are being used to make CCP, and that these chemicals can escape into the air as well as penetrate the skin. Schmidt found that biphenyl oil, one of the substances found in the microcapsules, flows out when the tiny bubbles are broken, either when the paper is handled or when a person writes on the top sheet. Moreover, further tests indicated that the biphenyl oil can be absorbed through the skin and could possibly help further the penetration of other compounds, such as formaldehyde, dye cursors, and hydrocarbon solvents. Schmidt says, however, "I can't really say whether CCP is causing environmental health problems. . . . It would be up to a toxicologist to take my findings and make a determination."

In the summer of 1997, the Mead Corporation, a major CCP manufacturer, asked Tardiff to review the scientific literature on their product. Tardiff spent four months doing the study. "Mead asked me to provide a dispassionate third-party analysis," Tardiff explains. "All of the available data I examined indicate that CCP, as [it] currently is being used, is unlikely to have injurious consequences for humans."

The studies of both Tardiff and Schmidt now form part of more than 14,000 pages of scientific literature relating to CCP that are currently being studied by a task force headed by Niemeier. In February 1997, NIOSH posted a notice in the *Federal Register* requesting comments on the possible adverse health effects of working with CCP. The task force started the review in September 1997 and expected to take six months to complete its charge, but Niemeier reveals, "It's going to take longer because the docket has been flooded with information."

As for the health problems of Smith and the other plaintiffs who have filed CCP law suits, Niemeier says, "I suspect that they may be a little more sensitive than the general population, but the problem is that many of the symptoms said to be associated with exposure to CCP are very similar, if not identical, to indoor air quality problems. Is it an issue of CCP, indoor air quality, or multiple chemical sensitivity? I honestly can't say at this point."

Chapter 46

Exercise-Induced Severe Allergic Reaction

Of the various allergies that sports medicine professionals encounter, exercise-induced anaphylaxis and cholinergic urticaria are
among the most underappreciated. Though the conditions are rare,
it's important to become familiar with them because they can be
life threatening. This review of two cases of exercise-induced anaphylaxis and one case of cholinergic urticaria is intended to help
physicians diagnose and treat patients who have sports-related
allergies.

Case One

A 20-year-old male college soccer player presented after having
had three episodes of diffuse urticaria associated with a sensation
of throat thickening, audible wheezing, and mild shortness of
breath. Each episode occurred within 1 hour of completing strenu-
ous exercise. The first had occurred in the early evening at practice, starting with discrete hives on the extremities that quickly
spread over his entire body, and progressing to dysphagia [diffi-
culty in swallowing] and mild symptoms of stridor [vibrating sound
heard during respiration caused by obstruction of air passages]

From "Identifying Exercise Allergies: Exercise-Induced Anaphylaxis and
Cholinergic Urticaria," by Tom Terrell, M.D., M.Phil.; David O. Hough, M.D.;
and Raquelle Alexander, M.D., in *The Physician and Sportsmedicine,* Vol. 24,
No. 11, November 1996 [Online]. Available: http://www.physsportsmed.com.

within minutes. The episode resolved 30 minutes after he stopped exercising. The second episode occurred midday in hot, humid conditions while the patient was playing football on a beach during spring break.

His symptoms—facial and lip swelling and dysphagia—were treated with prednisone and diphenhydramine. Playing volleyball while on prednisone produced no symptoms. The most recent episode had occurred while he was playing soccer and involved perioral [around the mouth] and facial swelling, mild dysphagia, and scattered truncal hives measuring 10 to 20 mm in diameter.

The patient's medical history was negative for atopic disease, viral respiratory infection, or other medical problems. He denied any allergies. His family history was positive for allergic rhinitis. The physical exam revealed no significant skin lesions. The patient's nasal passages had mild bilateral edema [swelling] with mucus. The remaining physical exam was normal.

The diagnosis was exercise-induced anaphylaxis with an atypical form of urticaria [hives].

The patient was taught about the signs and symptoms of anaphylaxis and about when to self-administer epinephrine. He was prescribed loratadine 10 mg once a day to be taken 1 hour before exercise and diphenhydramine hydrochloride 25 to 50 mg as needed for hives.

The patient did well using this regimen, even while running in hot summer conditions. He stopped taking his medications 5 months after the first episode and did not have a relapse until 11 months later. After the relapse, allergy skin testing performed by another physician demonstrated atopy. While playing beach football he had a relapse that consisted of periorbital edema [swelling around the eyes], skin itching, and scratchy voice with a lump in the throat, followed after several minutes by diffuse, pruritic [itchy] hiving and anterior chest tightness with a cough. After a cool shower, his symptoms resolved in 1 hour without treatment.

After this episode, his physician discontinued treatment with prophylactic antihistamines because of the possibility of masking the early warning signs of anaphylaxis. (Most allergists would not discontinue antihistamines for this reason.) The patient was instructed to take loratadine for pruritus associated with hiving, after symptoms of early anaphylaxis have resolved. Instructions on when and how to administer epinephrine were reinforced. The patient was advised to wear a medical alert bracelet and to exercise with a partner during cool times of the day.

Case Two

An 18-year-old female college runner presented after having two episodes of severe lightheadedness, dyspnea [difficulty in breathing], chest tightness, scalp pruritus, chills, and tunnel vision 5 minutes into vigorous runs. Subsequently, she developed a feeling of warmth over her face and upper body but no urticaria. She had no cough, dysphagia, or wheals and was not sure if she had had throat tightness. Taking a hot shower made the condition worse. A third episode was similar, but without lower-respiratory-tract symptoms. The episodes had occurred within 3 hours after meals.

The patient's history was significant for possible mild exercise-induced bronchospasm. Her family history revealed cat-induced allergic rhinitis. The exam was otherwise normal. Prick skin testing demonstrated isolated 2+ reactions to soy and pecan. Spirometry and exercise bronchoprovocation studies were normal.

The diagnosis was exercise-induced anaphylaxis with very mild exercise-induced bronchospasm.

Because her exercise-induced anaphylaxis might have had a food allergy component, the patient was asked to keep a food diary with future episodes, to avoid soy products, and to avoid exercise within 4 hours after meals. She was prescribed injectable epinephrine for anaphylaxis episodes and diphenhydramine as needed for hiving. She was lost to further follow-up.

Case Three

A 32-year-old woman presented with hives of 2 months duration on her arms, legs, and jaw line. The patient said her hives were worse in the evening and were exacerbated by hot showers, but not by exercise or sweating. She reported lip swelling but no face swelling. She denied having shortness of breath, breathing problems, nasal symptoms, sneezing, and watery eyes.

The patient's medical history was noncontributory; she took no medicines and denied medicine allergies. Her family history was significant for allergies. Her social history revealed that she had been making stressful wedding plans. The physical exam revealed small, nonconfluent hives of about 5 mm diameter on her arms; there was no dermatographism. Physical exam was otherwise unremarkable. Allergy testing was negative for dust, mold, and pollens.

The diagnosis was chronic cholinergic urticaria with angioedema [swelling of throat tissues]. Treatment included 25 mg hydroxyzine hydrochloride three to four times daily and 10 mg loratadine each day. Her symptoms abated in about 2 weeks, and she takes hydroxyzine as needed for occasional hives with hot showers.

What Sparks a Reaction?

The three major differential diagnoses considered in the case presentations are the physical urticarias: classic exercise-induced anaphylaxis, exercise-induced anaphylaxis variant syndrome, and cholinergic (generalized heat) urticaria. A familial form of exercise-induced anaphylaxis also exists.[1]

Exercise-induced anaphylaxis was described first by Maulitz, et al., in 1979.[2] It is more common in young people (the mean age at onset was 25 years), and the condition is twice as common in women as in men.[3] Clinical features include a flushing sensation, pruritus, gastrointestinal complaints such as vomiting, and throat tightness or choking. Diffuse, large urticarial wheals, angioedema, bronchospasm, and hypotension may occur.[4-11] Exercise-induced anaphylaxis may also progress to angioedema or full-fledged anaphylaxis. Angioedema sometimes presents with painful swelling of the face, extremities, and oral cavity.

In exercise-induced anaphylaxis variant syndrome, the wheals are smaller (2 to 4 mm) punctate lesions, and patients more frequently progress to anaphylaxis.

As the name implies, exercise-induced anaphylaxis occurs only with exercise, but various environmental, physiologic, hormonal, drug, and food stimuli have been reported as contributing factors.[12] Humid, warm, and cold conditions are known precipitants. Some individuals are more likely to experience symptoms if they are exposed to pollens or grasses. Drugs such as aspirin, nonsteroidal anti-inflammatories, over-the-counter cold remedies, and antibiotics have been shown to increase the risk of symptoms in patients who have exercise-induced anaphylaxis.[3] Increased emotional responses and menses may be cofactors in exercise-induced anaphylaxis episodes. The patient in case 2 might have had food-related exercise-induced anaphylaxis. Celery has been associated with 13 reported cases of exercise-induced anaphylaxis,[3] and wheat, shellfish,[2,13] and hazelnuts have also been implicated; however, any food may interact with chemical neuropeptides released during exercise to trigger an exercise-induced anaphylaxis episode.

Cholinergic urticaria is an allergic response to passive warming or exercise and is characterized by small (2 to 4 mm) pruritic papules [small, solid, usually conical elevations of the skin]. It very rarely leads to shock or anaphylaxis.[12] Studies have shown that it is most common in young people. In a study[14] of high school and university students aged 15 to 35, the highest prevalence was observed in the 26-to-28 age-group.

The major precipitating factor for cholinergic urticaria is any process that raises the core body temperature by 0.5°C to 1.5°C (0.9°F to 2.7°F), such as hot showers, anxiety, and exercise. By contrast, exercise-induced anaphylaxis does not occur without exercise.

The physical urticarias are IgE-mediated allergic reactions. Physical urticarias are chronic urticarias in which wheals can be reproduced by a physical stimulus (for example, cold, heat, pressure, vibration, light, exercise, water). The final pathway for exercise-induced anaphylaxis and cholinergic urticaria is the same: Antigen exposure crosslinks the IgE antibodies on mast cells, which causes the release of histamine and other mediators. Mast cell degranulation and the release of histamine and other mediators lead to symptoms.[15] Food may coprecipitate exercise-induced anaphylaxis through an IgE-mediated response when IgE antibodies to a specific food are present, or through a non-IgE-mediated response when gastrin and other hormones react with other neuropeptides released during exercise.[16] Etiologic theories involving respiratory heat loss and water loss have also been proposed.[17] One study[16] suggests that a central perception of temperature change is followed by an efferent [conveying nervous impulses] reflex that leads to cholinergic urticaria.

History, Signs, and Symptoms

The patient history plays a key role in differentiating exercise-induced anaphylaxis and cholinergic urticaria.[18] Cues such as the onset of symptoms with exercise or certain precipitating factors may point to one or the other. Cholinergic urticaria is more reproducible with exercise. In addition, patients who have cholinergic urticaria are more likely to have bronchospasm, whereas patients who have exercise-induced anaphylaxis are more likely to have upper-airway obstruction.

The symptoms the patient is experiencing during current episodes are the most accurate predictors of progression to anaphylaxis. Patients who have a history of anaphylaxis are less likely to have cholinergic urticaria. Clinical history is not predictive for future oropharyngeal edema and impending airway obstruction.

Exercise-induced anaphylaxis. Classic exercise-induced anaphylaxis is characterized by giant (10 to 25 mm) urticarial wheals that may coalesce. Other symptoms include cutaneous flushing, gastrointestinal problems, pruritus, and headache. In severe cases, the patient may have angioedema of the oropharynx and hands with stridor from upper-airway obstruction. The signs and symptoms of full-blown anaphylaxis include hypotension [very low blood pressure], syncope [fainting], and vascular collapse.

Exercise-induced anaphylaxis occurs exclusively with exercise, but some symptoms may be reproducible in a controlled, closely supervised lab that is prepared to treat acute anaphylaxis.[10] However, allergists and primary care sports medicine physicians do not use exercise testing to make the diagnosis of exercise-induced anaphylaxis. Symptoms may begin within 5 minutes of starting exercise and typically abate within 30 minutes to 4 hours after exercise, though headache may persist longer. Wade, et al.,[3] described the experiences of 199 patients who had classic exercise-induced anaphylaxis. Symptoms were usually precipitated by moderate-to-hard exercise, most frequently while jogging. Not surprisingly, attacks typically occurred early in activity, and exercising in a warm or humid environment or after eating increased the likelihood of attacks.[3] The most common symptom early in an episode was pruritus (92%). Attacks averaged twice a week, though frequency varied widely.[3] Two thirds of patients who have exercise-induced anaphylaxis have a family history of atopy, and half are atopic, which is not true of the other physical urticarias.

Cholinergic urticaria. The hallmark of cholinergic urticaria is smaller (2 to 4 mm) pruritic papules that are surrounded by macular erythema [spotty redness].[12] The rash usually occurs in a follicular distribution and appears on the neck, upper trunk, and proximal limbs. In severe reactions, lesions may coalesce into giant hives, and angioedema may develop. Patients who have cholinergic urticaria may have headache, palpitations, abdominal cramps, diarrhea, sweating, flushing, bronchospasm, or angioedema. Shortness of breath and wheezing occur more than with exercise-induced anaphylaxis. Decreases in forced expiratory volume in 1 second (FEV_1) and wheezing have been demonstrated in both spontaneous and experimentally induced cholinergic urticaria attacks.[18]

An attack usually occurs 2 to 30 minutes after a precipitant, and it lasts from 20 to 90 minutes.[19] On average, patients have the condition 7.5 years.[10] One study[20] demonstrated only a 14% spontaneous remission rate.

Diagnostic Studies

When the diagnosis is unclear from clinical history alone, laboratory and diagnostic tests are rarely helpful for exercise-induced anaphylaxis and cholinergic urticaria. The lab tests are nonspecific and expensive.

Exercise-induced anaphylaxis. Serum histamine evaluation is not useful because the level usually peaks within 30 minutes after anaphylaxis onset. However, serum tryptase levels, as a referral lab study, peak within 60 to 90 minutes of the onset of anaphylaxis and may provide evidence of mast cell activation if drawn within 3 hours.[21] Other factors, such as systemic mastocytosis and drug effects (aspirin use), may also cause nonspecific histamine and tryptase elevations. Exercise challenge tests are risky and nonspecific.

Cholinergic urticaria. The most specific diagnostic test for cholinergic urticaria involves passively warming an extremity with a heating blanket or warm water immersion to raise patients' core temperature by 0.5°C to 1.5°C (0.9°F to 2.7°F). In those who have cholinergic urticaria, serum histamine will increase with or without urticaria symptoms. The methacholine challenge test involves injecting methacholine with saline subcutaneously [beneath the skin] and watching for a cholinergic urticaria reaction. The test is not routine because the sensitivity is only 50%.[22]

Treatment

The first step in acute treatment for patients who present with hives, pruritus, and flushing and who have not been previously diagnosed as having exercise-induced anaphylaxis or cholinergic urticaria involves having patients stop exercising, getting them to a cool place, and administering an injection of diphenhydramine. If symptoms progress to wheezing, throat tightness, or lightheadedness, patients should receive an injection of epinephrine. If patients' symptoms resolve, the physician prescribes 10 mg oral loratadine, monitors patients closely, then sends them home with injectable epinephrine.

Exercise-induced anaphylaxis. Some patients who have exercise-induced anaphylaxis progress to full-blown anaphylaxis. When more advanced symptoms occur, injectable epinephrine is indicated. A repeat dose may be given in 15 to 20 minutes if the symptoms progress or do not resolve. Patients who have very mild symptoms, however, may not require epinephrine. Their symptoms may resolve within 5 to 10 minutes with minimal treatment. A clinician's experience and comfort level with treating this condition will dictate when he or she feels epinephrine is indicated. Acute treatment of anaphylaxis follows the standard ABC (airway, breathing, circulation) protocol: Place an intravenous line; give oxygen, intravenous fluids, epinephrine, and diphenhydramine; and transport the patient to an emergency room.[19] Patients who have developed anaphylaxis should be referred to an allergist.

Long-term treatment for exercise-induced anaphylaxis mandates intensive education of the patient and sports medicine team about the nature of the disease and its precipitants. Wearing a medical alert bracelet is essential. Patients should always carry injectable epinephrine that can be administered by trainers, coaches, or teammates when needed. Patients who have exercise-induced anaphylaxis should exercise with a partner during cool times of the day. In food-dependent cases, patients should avoid exercise within 4 hours after meals, and avoid eating celery or shellfish. If pruritus, cutaneous flushing, or throat tightness develops, the athlete should cease exercise and seek a cool place. If symptoms do not resolve within 5 to 10 minutes of exercise cessation, injectable epinephrine should be administered. If symptoms progress to lightheadedness, hives, throat tightness, or increased wheezing, injectable epinephrine should be given immediately. If epinephrine is given, the patient should be taken to an urgent care facility.

Prophylactic [preventive] treatment for exercise-induced anaphylaxis has been largely unsuccessful, unproved, and controversial. However, the mainstream treatment approach is to prescribe antihistamines. The majority of studies[23] have failed to show symptom improvement with antihistamines; however, a few studies[7] have shown a reduction in symptoms associated with histamine release. One study[7] showed similar benefits with tricyclic antidepressants (doxepin hydrochloride) and inhaled cromolyn sodium, but these medications are not used. Though allergists routinely prescribe sedating or nonsedating antihistamines,[7] a minority feel that these medications may mask the early warning signs and symptoms of anaphylaxis, such as cutaneous itching and rash.

To our knowledge, no study has demonstrated the utility of pairing antihistamines with histamine$_2$ receptor blockers for patients who have exercise-induced anaphylaxis or cholinergic urticaria. H$_2$ blockers used alone have no impact on the condition because of the pathophysiology involved in histamine release.

Patients who have exercise-induced anaphylaxis should not be prescribed beta blockers because they reduce the response to epinephrine—a beta agonist.

Cholinergic urticaria. Treatment for patients who have established cholinergic urticaria involves a dose of diphenhydramine or hydroxyzine at the time of flare-up. They are usually also taking hydroxyzine chronically, so it is safe to give a dose of diphenhydramine or another antihistamine.

Prophylactic treatment with antihistamines is effective for patients who have cholinergic urticaria. In one study,[20] 63% of patients who had cholinergic urticaria reported improvement with antihistamines. Treatment typically includes oral hydroxyzine hydrochloride at a dosage up to 50 mg four times a day. A consistent exercise program with gradual increases in intensity may help patients avoid a cholinergic urticaria reaction.[11] Because of the small risk of anaphylaxis, injectable epinephrine may be prescribed with clear instructions on indications and method of use.

A Risk-Reduction Role

Exercise-induced anaphylaxis and cholinergic urticaria are two allergic syndromes that those who care for sports teams or treat athletes may encounter. Rapid recognition and initiation of treatment for these entities can result in early resolution of the allergic mast-cell-mediated response before anaphylactic symptoms develop. Proper treatment may enable individuals to continue intense exercise.

References

1. Grant JA, Farnam J, Lord RA, et al: Familial exercise-induced anaphylaxis. *Ann Allergy* 1985;54(1):35-38.

2. Maulitz RM, Pratt DS, Schocket AC: Exercise induced anaphylactic reaction to shellfish. *J Allergy Clin Immunol* 1979;63(6):433-434.

3. Wade JP, Liang MH, Sheffer AL: Biochemistry of acute allergic reactions, in Tauber AI, Wintroub BU, Simon AS, et al (eds): *International Symposium on the Biochemistry of Acute Allergic Reactions,* Fifth International Symposium. New York City, Alan Liss, Inc, 1989, pp 175-182.

4. Casale TB, Keahey TM, Kaliner M: Exercise-induced anaphylactic syndromes: insights into diagnostic and pathophysiologic features. *JAMA* 1986;255(15):2049-2053.

5. Kaplan AP, Natbony SF, Tawil AP, et al: Exercise-induced anaphylaxis as a manifestation of cholinergic urticaria. *J Allergy Clin Immunol* 1981;68(4):319-324.

0. Sheffer AL, Austen KF. Exercise-induced anaphylaxis. *J Allergy Clin Immunol* 1980;66(2):106-111.

7. Sheffer AL, Austen KF: Exercise-induced anaphylaxis. *J Allergy Clin Immunol* 1984;73(5 pt 2):699-703.

8. Sheffer AL, Soter NA, McFadden ER, et al: Exercise-induced anaphylaxis: a distinct form of physical allergy: *J Allergy Clin Immunol* 1983;71(3):311-316.

9. Songsiridej V, Busse WW: Exercise-induced anaphylaxis. *Clin Allergy* 1983;13(4):317-321.

10. Briner WW Jr, Sheffer A: Exercise-induced anaphylaxis. *Med Sci Sports Exerc* 1992;24(8):849-850.

11. Briner WW Jr: Physical allergies and exercise: clinical implications for those engaged in sports activities. *Sports Med* 1993;15(6):365-373.

12. Nichols AW: Exercise-induced anaphylaxis and urticaria. *Clin Sports Med* 1992;11(2):303-312.

13. Eisenstadt WS, Nicholas SS, Velick G, et al: Allergic reactions to exercise. *Phys Sportsmed* 1984;12(12):95-104.

14. Zuberbier T, Althaus C, Chantraine-Hess S, et al: Prevalence of cholinergic urticaria in young adults. *J Am Acad Dermatol* 1994;31(6):978-981.

15. Sheffer AL, Soter NA, McFadden ER Jr, et al: Exercise-induced anaphylaxis: a distinct form of physical allergy. *Monogr Allergy* 1983;18:138.

16. Fink JN: *Medical Knowledge Self Assessment Program in the Subspecialty of Allergy and Immunology,* ed 1. Philadelphia, American College of Physicians, 1993.

17. Hough D, Dec K: Exercise-induced asthma and anaphylaxis. *Sports Med* 1994;18(3):162-172.

18. Silvers WS: Exercise-induced allergies: the role of histamine release. *Ann Allergy* 1992;68(1):58-66.

19. Kaplan AP: Urticaria and angioedema, in Middleton E (ed): *Allergy: Principles and Practice,* ed 3. St Louis, CV Mosby Co, 1988, pp 1377-1401.

20. Hirschmann JV, Lawlor F, English JS, et al: Cholinergic urticaria: a clinical and histologic study. *Arch Dermatol* 1987;123(4):462-467.

21. Schwartz LB, Yunginger JW, Miller J, et al: Time course of appearance and disappearance of human mast cell tryptase in the circulation after anaphylaxis. *J Clin Invest* 1989;83(5):1551-1555.

22. Kaplan AP, Gray L, Shaff RE, et al: In vivo studies of mediator release in cold urticaria and cholinergic urticaria. *J Allergy Clin Immunol* 1975;55(6):394-402.

23. Sheffer AL, Austen KF: Exercise-induced hives. *J Allergy Clin Immunol* 1984;73:704-707.

— by Tom Terrell, M.D., M.Phil.;
David O. Hough, M.D.; and
Raquelle Alexander, M.D.

Dr. Terrell is a sports medicine physician at Resurgens Orthopaedics in Atlanta and a past primary care sports medicine fellow at Michigan State University in East Lansing, Michigan. Dr. Hough died September 26, 1996. He was director of sports medicine and of the primary care sports medicine fellowship program at Michigan State University Sports Medicine in the Department of Family Practice at Michigan State. He was a fellow of the American College of Sports Medicine and the American Medical Society for Sports Medicine. Dr. Alexander is an allergist in Asheville, North Carolina.

Part Five

Diagnosis, Treatments, and Aids to Wellness

Chapter 47

Allergy Tests

Identifying specific allergens is helpful when pharmacotherapy isn't working or when complications like chronic sinusitis, otitis, or asthma have developed. Testing is advised, too, if the patient has tired of the treatment regimen and is ready to try immunotherapy for relief.

About one person in six has some form of allergy.[1] The more common presentations include IgE-mediated reactions of seasonal and perennial rhinitis, asthma, acute urticaria, immediate reactions to drugs or food, otitis, conjunctivitis, and atopic eczema. These are classified as immediate (type I) hypersensitivity reactions. Examples of other hypersensitivities include transfusion reactions (type II; antibody reactions with antigens on cell surfaces), farmer's lung and bird fancier's disease (type III; immune complex-mediated reactions), and contact dermatitis and fixed drug eruptions like late reactions to antibiotics (type IV; delayed-type cell-mediated reactions).

When Allergy Testing Is Useful

When a patient has the typical symptoms of allergic rhinitis—rhinorrhea, nasal congestion, itchy nose and eyes, and sneezing—certain medications are worth trying empirically before a referral for allergy testing. Remember, however, that the first principle of allergy treatment is allergen avoidance, not pharmacotherapy. Elimination or reduction of offending allergens can cure the disease or reduce the need for treatment.

If the patient has tried medical means to relieve allergic rhinitis and still has bothersome symptoms, allergy testing is recommended to confirm the diagnosis, uncover allergens that may not have been previously suspected, and steer therapy. Testing is advised, too, if the patient is no longer willing to comply with the regimen required to produce results or when complications such as sinusitis, otitis media, or asthma have occurred. Turn also to testing when allergy symptoms require treatment for more than three or four months each year and both you and the patient want to identify the cause (see Table 47.1).

Ask yourself these questions when considering allergy testing: How severe are the symptoms, and how easily are they controlled? How long do the symptoms last? Are they perennial? Is the patient taking one medication to control symptoms or many? Is the treatment expensive? Is the patient willing to continue taking medication regularly? Finally, how old is the patient? IgE levels decline steadily and allergic symptoms tend to diminish in the fifth or sixth decade of life. A 16-year-old is likely to spend many more years taking medication than is a 60-year-old, who may eventually be able to do without drugs entirely.

Table 47.1. Criteria for Allergy Testing

Refer patients for allergy testing when

- They have bothersome, persistent rhinitis.

- The condition or its treatment is interfering with performance or causing significant absences from school or work.

- Quality of life is significantly affected.

- Complications such as sinusitis, otitis media, hearing loss, asthma, significant snoring, loss of sleep, or bronchitis arise.

- Medical treatments have not adequately resolved symptoms, or additional diagnostic approaches are required.

- Systemic corticosteroids are required to quell symptoms, or untoward reactions to other therapeutic approaches have occurred.[6]

Allergy testing is not always necessary to know that you are dealing with an allergy. Sometimes the history, symptoms, and physical exam are enough to make the diagnosis. If, for example, your patient lives on the east coast or in the midwest and coughs, sneezes, and suffers from itchy eyes and a drippy nose every year from mid-August until the first frost, it's a safe bet that allergic rhinitis related to ragweed is the culprit. Testing in this case would be merely confirmatory. However, an unsuspected allergy to dust might coexist and potentiate the ragweed sensitivity. Dust avoidance procedures might reduce ragweed-related symptoms. Testing should be performed to identify all allergens and provide a baseline for therapy if the patient is considering immunotherapy.

The next piece of advice may sound like common sense, but don't make an allergy diagnosis without observing, talking to, and examining the patient. Referred to as the remote practice of allergy, this practice may include making diagnoses, recommending treatment (including immunotherapy), and providing allergenic extracts for immunotherapy based solely on information provided by the referring or personal physician; the results of in vitro assays, total IgE antibody, and allergen-specific IgE antibodies performed on serum that has been mailed in by the personal physician; or the results of skin tests performed by the referring physician, who may be untrained in allergy and whose interpretation of results may not relate appropriately to the patient's history and clinical condition.[2,3] The American Academy of Allergy, Asthma, and Immunology strongly discourages the remote practice of allergy.

Insect Venom Allergies

In the case of suspected insect venom allergy, only test if immunotherapy is being planned. Patients must understand that immunotherapy is unnecessary for purely local reactions to insect bites. It is used only when bites result in systemic reactions, including life-threatening complications such as angioedema, asthma, hypotension, and other symptoms of anaphylaxis. Radioallergosorbent testing (RAST) is not sensitive enough for insect venom allergy; skin testing is required.

Food Allergies

For suspected food allergies, the primary reason for allergy testing is a history of urticaria or anaphylactic reactions. In general, foods are not a cause of respiratory problems—although anecdotal reports of rhinorrhea resolving when certain foods are eliminated are not uncommon. Foods can be a cause, particularly in children, of eczema, which is also a valid reason to test for allergies. But respiratory symptoms in the absence of eczema or other symptoms are not usually due to foods.

For food allergies, elimination diets or double-blind food challenges may be more definitive than skin testing, but challenges are very time-consuming, require special expertise, and should be performed cautiously when a patient has a history of anaphylactic shock to a specific food. With food allergies, both skin testing and RAST sometimes produce false-positive results for a food that can actually be eaten without difficulty. The chance that a positive test represents a true food allergy is only 30-50%. The false-negative rate, however, is very low, with a negative result being correct at least 95% of the time. Some food extracts—especially fruits, berries, and shellfish—are unreliable, so if a patient has a history of anaphylaxis but negative test results using commercial extracts, prick testing with fresh food is indicated before sensitivity is determined to be absent. Intradermal skin tests for food allergy are rarely, if ever, indicated because they only increase the number of false-positive results that occur with puncture skin testing.

Therefore, a negative skin test or RAST can rule out an IgE-mediated food sensitivity, and a positive result can at least warn that a patient may be sensitive to a certain food and that further investigation may be warranted. If a history corroborates the test, trial avoidance of the food is advised to see if symptoms improve. Realize, however, that most cases of milk- or soy-induced enterocolitis are non-IgE-mediated food hypersensitivities. These patients will have negative results on skin tests and RAST. Diagnosis currently relies on a careful history, confirmatory skin testing, and the judicious use of oral challenge tests. Such challenges must be performed with extreme caution because dangerous, even life-threatening, reactions can occur.

Asthma

National Heart, Lung, and Blood Institute guidelines for the diagnosis and management of asthma have been recently revised. The new guidelines recommend that patients with persistent asthma who require daily therapy be evaluated for their sensitivity to perennial indoor allergens. For suspected allergies to inhalants, provocation tests are rarely used except in research protocols. Prick testing is a more effective and time-honored diagnostic test for allergic sensitivity.

The History and Physical Examination

Ask specific questions about symptoms, including congestion, rhinorrhea, the character of nasal discharge, postnasal drip, sneezing, cough, and pruritus of the nose or eyes. Investigate complaints related to the lungs, skin, and GI tract. Explore how long the symptoms last and when they occur. Whenever possible, identify specific triggers. Ask whether the patient has used medications, which ones, and what the response to them was.

The medical history should focus on any suggestion of other atopic conditions. The patient with a history of significant eczema, for example, is at much higher risk of other atopic diseases. Also inquire about any history of drug or food allergy or recurrent infections, especially sinusitis and otitis media.

A negative family history does not rule out allergy but is certainly evidence against it. Conversely, a strongly positive family history increases the odds that your patient's symptoms have an allergic etiology.

Finally, obtain a detailed environmental history, focusing on specific triggers that might be present in the home, work, day-care, or school environments. Exposure to pets or smokers is of particular significance. Inquire about possible cockroach exposure, the age of the home, problems with moisture, the type of heating and cooling systems, the use of humidifiers and dehumidifiers, and the presence of carpets. At least 60% humidity is required year-round to control dust mites. Ask specifically about the patient's bedroom—whether it has carpets and curtains, the type of bed and bedding, and, for children, the number of stuffed animals sharing the bed.

Assess the nose with regard to mucosal edema (boggy in an allergic patient), the color of the mucosa (pale or blue), and the character of the discharge (watery). Check the eyes for conjunctival edema or erythema. The facial exam should focus on the presence of allergic shiners, a transverse nasal crease, or Morgan-Dennie lines (secondary creases in the lower eyelids). Also look for a high, arched palate caused by chronic mouth breathing. Examine the chest for wheezing or other abnormal lung sounds and the skin for evidence of atopic dermatitis or urticaria. Keep in mind that the physical exam can fluctuate greatly in a patient with allergies. A patient who seems completely normal may have had significant symptoms just a day or two earlier.

In many cases, therapy can be started based on the history and physical exam alone. But when the diagnosis is unclear, a trial of therapy has failed, or allergen avoidance techniques are to be provided, some form of allergy testing may need to be initiated.

Types of Allergy Testing

Tests may be classified by name—skin testing, RAST, IgE levels, and so on—or by purpose—either screening or diagnostic. Screening tests help to determine whether a patient has an allergic condition. They assist in identifying a patient as being either atopic or nonatopic, but they do not pinpoint specific allergens. Diagnostic tests identify specific allergic sensitivities.

Table 47.2. Causes of Elevated IgE Levels

- Allergic bronchopulmonary aspergillosis
- Atopic conditions
- Hyper-IgE syndrome
- Malignancy
- Parasitic infections
- Vasculitis (Kawasaki syndrome)
- Wiskott-Aldrich syndrome (and other immunodeficiency syndromes)

Table 47.3. Common Allergens

Age < 3 yr	Age > 3 yr
Cat	Cat
Cockroach	Cockroach
Dog	Dog
Dust mites	Dust mites
Foods	Grasses
Molds	Molds
	Trees
	Weeds (including ragweed)

Screening Tests

IgE levels. The total serum IgE level is neither very sensitive nor very specific, and most allergists prefer to measure specific IgE by skin testing. Serum IgE levels may be similar in atopic and nonatopic persons, making results difficult to interpret. In general, about 20-40% of atopic persons have normal IgE levels, and as many as 20% of nonatopic persons have elevated levels. Although significant elevations-higher than 50 IU/mL in infants or 200 IU/mL in older children and adults—generally correlate with atopy, a variety of nonatopic conditions can be associated with even these levels (see Table 47.2). Nevertheless, elevated IgE levels can be helpful in evaluating suspected immunodeficiency or allergic bronchopulmonary aspergillosis. And as a research tool, the test for IgE levels has some value in predicting future atopy in newborns and infants, though family history is virtually as predictive.

Eosinophil counts. Though patients with atopy tend to have higher eosinophil counts than those without atopy, this test has limited sensitivity and specificity and should not be used as a routine allergy screen. It may be useful to look for eosinophils in nasal secretions, however, particularly when you suspect allergic rhinitis. A smear in which more than 10% of the cells are eosinophils is suggestive of allergy, but eosinophils can also occur in nonallergic rhinitis. The absence of eosinophils in nasal secretions does not rule out allergy but does make it considerably less likely. False-negative results occur most often when infection is present because large numbers of neutrophils may obscure eosinophils.

Multiallergen screening tests. Tests such as the Phadiatop have become widely available in the past few years. They are performed much like RAST, except that multiple allergens, instead of a single allergen, are bound to the disk. Because multiallergen tests are standardized to provide only a positive (atopic) or negative (nonatopic) result, it's not possible to determine which allergens led to a positive reaction. As pure screening tools, the multiallergen tests are probably the most sensitive and specific of all the options currently available. They delay a specific diagnosis, however, and require drawing blood.

RAST. A limited RAST panel including several common allergens can be useful as a screening tool. The advantage of using a RAST panel for screening is that it can also diagnose specific sensitivities—as long as relevant allergens are chosen (see Table 47.3).

Diagnostic Tests

Skin testing. There are two kinds of skin tests: prick or percutaneous testing and intradermal or intracutaneous testing. Scratch tests, where the skin surface beneath the droplet of allergen is scratched by a needle, have been largely replaced by prick tests.

Prick testing involves putting a drop of concentrated antigen on the skin and pricking the most superficial layer with a disposable needle or some kind of lancet device. Testing is performed on the back or the arm. The back is somewhat more reactive and provides a larger area for proper placement of the tests. Use of the arm, however, allows the patient to see the reaction and is the site preferred by many allergists. Prick tests must be placed at least 2 cm apart; 4-5 cm is better to reduce false-positive results.

If prick test results are negative or marginal, selective intradermal tests may be useful. With intradermal testing, a more dilute concentration of allergen is injected into the most superficial layer of the skin. Intradermal tests must be placed 5-6 cm apart.

Both types of skin testing produce wheel and flare reactions. For a prick test to be positive, swelling at the site must be at least 3 mm larger than the negative control (usually saline or another diluent) and accompanied by a red flare. An intradermal skin test positive reaction is 5-10 mm of wheel and a corresponding flare.

Wheal size is often also compared to a positive control (histamine). Control tests are necessary because some patients have false-positive results caused by dermatographism. Others have false-negative results due to prior medication use or skin disease.

Prick testing is preferred initially because it is more rapid, associated with less discomfort, compatible with testing more allergens per session, less expensive per test, and less apt to give rise to systemic reactions. It can be performed with glycerinated, and hence more stable, extracts, and results tend to correlate better with clinical sensitivity than those of intradermal testing.

Intradermal testing, on the other hand, offers somewhat greater reproducibility and much greater sensitivity than prick testing. To produce a wheel equivalent in size to that produced by an intradermal test, the extract used in prick testing must be 1,000-30,000 times more concentrated.

While prick testing results usually correlate very closely with symptoms, intradermal skin tests do not correlate as closely with the results of provocation, with avoidance, or with immunotherapy results. They are of mixed value and are more prone to giving false-positive results, nor do they predict symptoms on natural exposure.[4] Consequently, if a patient has a negative prick test result but a positive intradermal test result, counsel allergy avoidance but hold off on starting immunotherapy.

Generally speaking, skin testing results should correlate with clinical symptoms if you are testing with substances endemic to the area. If you test a patient who lives in New York with European olive, which grows in the Southwest, a positive result will be clinically meaningless.

What Yogi Berra once said about bunting in baseball applies to skin testing in medicine: If you don't do it a lot, don't do it at all. For allergy testing to be worthwhile, the tester must have considerable knowledge about the botany of the surrounding geographic area. The tester must also know quite a bit about the reagents used. Are they potent, too strong, or outdated, for example? Allergenic extracts in aqueous solution progressively lose potency. The loss is accelerated with increasing dilution. Loss of potency can be retarded, but not prevented, by use of preservatives. All extracts must be maintained at refrigerator temperatures when not in use. In addition to extract variables, the site of testing, spacing of tests, and application technique, as well as patient age and medications being taken, can all affect results. Finally, since skin testing carries with it a very small risk of inducing a systemic allergic reaction, it should only be performed with certain equipment readily available.

RAST. The most common kind of serum allergy test, RAST measures allergen-specific IgE. A known quantity of allergen is bound to a paper disk, and the patient's serum is incubated with that disk so that any IgE specific for that allergen will bind to it. The disk is then incubated with radiolabeled anti-IgE antibody, which detects any IgE from the patient that has bound to the allergen on the original disk. Measuring the level of radioactivity on the disk provides a semiquantitative measure of the amount of specific IgE in the patient's serum. These results are then compared to a known standard.

RAST is not as sensitive as skin testing. Even prick testing, which is less sensitive than intradermal testing, is more sensitive than RAST. Therefore, most allergists regard skin testing as the gold standard and use RAST only for patients who have a compelling reason to avoid skin testing—for example, they are morbidly afraid of it, they have diffuse skin disease, or they will not or cannot stop taking a medication with antihistaminic properties. Patients must stop antihistamines and some antidepressants—such as amitriptyline HCl—3-7 days ahead of time for the results of skin testing to be accurate. Astemizole, a very long-acting antihistamine, must be stopped 3-6 weeks before testing.

RAST is simple; the only skill required is blood drawing. Moreover, medications and even severe skin disease do not interfere with results. At $10-$20 per allergen, however, RAST can be expensive—even prohibitive for a patient who needs extensive testing. In addition, RAST results can vary from one lab to another. At least overnight incubation is required with RAST, whereas skin testing results are available in about 15 minutes. And interpretation can be problematic since RAST results are provided in the form of a lab report rather than seeing an actual patient reaction.

Newer variations on the RAST theme include replacing paper disks with plastic beads or cellulose threads, or using a different label for the anti-IgE antibody, as with ELISA (enzyme-linked immunosorbent assay) techniques. These include MAST (multiple-thread allergosorbent test), EAST (enzyme allergosorbent test), and FAST (fluorescent allergosorbent test), among others.

Studies have shown that a significantly positive skin test result and a significantly positive RAST result can occur in the absence of any clinical symptoms. About 40% of people in the general population, if tested, would have positive results, but only about 20% of people in the general population would have clinical symptoms of allergy. This means that if people were treated based on RAST results alone, half of those treated wouldn't need the therapy. Interestingly, however, if those people are followed, one third to one half will eventually show signs of allergies.

Allergen Avoidance and Immunotherapy

If testing confirms sensitivity to allergens, a detailed discussion of allergen avoidance techniques is in order to help the patient reduce exposure to offending agents. Allergen avoidance reduces rhinitis, conjunctivitis, asthma, and other allergic symptoms and reduces airway hypersensitivity as well. Advice should include methods to reduce exposure to pollen, molds, dust, animal dander, cockroaches, and other implicated allergens.

Making a Commitment to Immunotherapy

Patients need to understand that they will be receiving an injection weekly for months, then every other week, then every three weeks, and then every four weeks. The entire course of treatment can last 3-5 years, and patients may not begin to see results until after several months of treatment. Results show, in properly selected patients, somewhere around 86% success. Generally speaking, if improvement isn't significant by two years into treatment, therapy should be stopped.

Once patients have been receiving immunotherapy for 3-6 years, they should be reassessed. About half elect to continue because they are satisfied with the relief provided by immunotherapy and aren't willing to risk having symptoms return without it. The other half decide to stop treatment. At least half of those who stop remain symptom-free, but symptoms recur in the other half within 2-5 years.

Can Patients "Outgrow" Allergies?

True allergies are not outgrown—although about 50% of persons with asthma that started after age 2 years will have a relative remission between age 16 and 25 years. However, asthma tends to recur in the 20s and 30s. There is a tendency for IgE to decline after age 50, so that people older than 50 usually start to notice a lessening of their allergic symptoms and a progressive decline after age 60-70.

Not only do most people not outgrow their allergies, but asthma develops in many people with allergic rhinitis. Some data indicate that allergy exposure in early childhood determines when asthma will manifest itself later in life.

Immunotherapy for Very Young Children

Immunotherapy can be given to properly selected children younger than 5 years, but most allergists would rather avoid it. Pediatric allergists usually say they prefer to treat symptomatically and to wait as long as possible to get a complete picture of all the things the child is allergic to. Also, establishing rapport is difficult with very young children, who end up afraid of medical personnel and needles. Nor can very young children articulate symptoms of reaction to an allergy shot the way older people can. Some experts say too that anaphylactic shock is harder to handle in young children and that this group is at increased risk of systemic reactions.[5]

Working with the Allergist

After you've referred a patient for an allergy workup, you should receive the following in return:

- Clarification of an allergic or other cause for the patient's condition
- A list of specific allergens or other triggers for symptoms

- Assistance in developing an effective treatment plan, including allergy avoidance, pharmacotherapy, and immunotherapy, if this is appropriate

- Provision of immunotherapy extracts, if appropriate

- An understanding of how and at what dosage and dilution to resume interrupted immunotherapy.

Look for an allergist who understands that the patient will reap the greatest benefits if the two of you work as a team.[6]

References

1. Allergen testing in patients with type I hypersensitivity. *DTB* 1995;33:45-46.

2. Position statement: The remote practice of allergy. *J Allergy Clin Immunol* 1986:77:651-652.

3. Nelson HS, Aveson J, Reisman R: A prospective assessment of the remote practice of allergy: Comparison of the diagnosis of allergic disease and the recommendations for allergen immunotherapy by board-certified allergists and a laboratory performing in vitro assays. *J Allergy Clin Immunol* 1993;92: 380-386.

4. Nelson HS, Oppenheimer J, Buchmeier A, et al: An assessment of the rate of intradermal skin testing in the diagnosis of clinically relevant allergy to timothy grass. *J Allergy Clin Immunol* 1998;97:1193-1201.

5. Ownby DR, Adinoff AD: The appropriate use of skin testing and allergen immunotherapy in young children. *J Allergy Clin Immunol* 1994;94:662-665.

6. Kaliner MA: Allergy care in the next millennium: Guidelines for the specialty. *J Allergy Clin Immunol* 1997;99:729-734.

Suggested Reading

Nelson HS: Variables in allergy skin testing. *Allergy Proc* 1994;15:265-268.

Position statement: Allergen skin testing. *J Allergy Clin Immunol* 1993;92:636-637.

Chapter 48

Tests and Treatments to Avoid

You may be tempted to consider alternative remedies for allergies, such as the heavily promoted nutritional therapies. But be aware that no vitamin or mineral supplements or herbal remedies have been proven effective as a treatment for allergies. If you have a pollen allergy, be especially cautious about herbal remedies; some may contain the very allergens that trigger your symptoms.

In fact, unless your have a food allergy, you shouldn't have to change your diet in any way to prevent an allergic reaction. Extra vitamins, minerals, or nutritional supplements are not necessary because an allergy isn't caused by a nutritional deficiency. It's an immune response.

However, if you or your child has food allergies, you'll have to avoid the food that brings on your symptoms. Infants and small children who are allergic to milk will need formula or a milk substitute. Among the available substitutes are soy formula or elemental formulas composed of processed proteins. Both children and adults allergic to milk and milk products such as cheese will need alternative sources of calcium for strong teeth and bones.

A number of controversial food allergy treatments are heavily advertised and promoted, even though scientific studies have found them ineffective. Be wary of the following treatments; none is likely to relieve your allergy symptoms, and each will make a dent in your wallet.

"Tests and Treatments to Avoid," Johns Hopkins Health, October 1, 1998, ©1996-2000 InteliHealth Inc. Reprinted with permission of InteliHealth.

Intradermal Provocation

Food allergens are injected in an attempt to trigger restlessness and fatigue or other symptoms not usually associated with true food allergies. If symptoms develop, treatment consists of weekly (or more frequent) injections of the "allergen" believed responsible. While not dangerous, there's no evidence that this treatment works.

Sublingual Provocation and Neutralization

Provocation and neutralizing tests involve either injecting allergen extracts under the skin or placing them under the tongue. If a low dose doesn't bring on a reaction, higher doses are used. If symptoms of any kind eventually develop anywhere in the body, adherents of these tests diagnose allergy regardless of the nature of the symptoms or whether they are physical or emotional (such as depression or other mood changes). When the "reaction" occurs, additional doses of the allergen are administered to "neutralize" the symptoms. Studies show that this treatment is safe but ineffective.

Anti-Yeast Treatments

Hypersensitivity to *Candida albicans*, a type of yeast normally found in the body, has been blamed for symptoms ranging from headaches to flatulence. Tests for yeast are usually positive because these organisms are almost always present in the body. The treatment is the drug nystatin, used to control vaginal yeast infections, a special diet and avoiding exposure to numerous environmental substances. Although the treatment isn't dangerous, it is worthless and can be expensive.

Cytotoxic Testing

Another widely advertised and heavily promoted test—cytotoxic testing—has never been scientifically proven reliable for allergy diagnosis. Proponents claim that it can identify food or inhalant allergies by combining extracts of suspected allergens with white blood cells taken from a small sample of the patient's blood; the samples are then examined for changes that purportedly demonstrate the presence of allergy.

Studies show that white cell samples from people with known food allergies do not change when submitted for cytotoxic testing, and results of tests of the same blood samples differ from day-to-day and from laboratory to laboratory.

Chapter 49

The Fight against Allergies

Chapter Contents

Section 49.1

Spring into Action against Seasonal Allergies

"Watery Eyes? Runny Nose? Time to Spring into Action Against Seasonal Allergies," by Rebecca D. Williams, in *FDA Consumer*, March-April 1998.

By the time her daughter, Brooke, was 18 months old, Nancy Sander of Fairfax, Va., had discovered the child was allergic to much of the environment around her. Her eyes watered and her nose ran constantly. Worse yet, her allergy symptoms triggered frightening asthma attacks.

Now a 19-year-old college student, Brooke has her dorm room decked out with an air cleaner, dust mite-proof casings on the pillows and mattresses, a stash of prescription eye drops, nose sprays, and antihistamines, and a sympathetic roommate who does the vacuuming (which kicks up the dust that triggers her allergies).

"I realize she's not your typical college student," says Sander, "but she knows her quality of life is better if she does these things. Rather than hide indoors all spring, she increases her medication as needed. She washes her hair every day to keep the allergens out of it, takes her medication before she has symptoms, and she gets out there and enjoys life."

About 26 million Americans endure chronic seasonal allergies, while the number of people with milder symptoms may be as high as 40 million, according to the National Center for Health Statistics. One study puts the annual costs of "hay fever," as it's commonly called, at $2.4 million for medications and another $1.1 billion in doctors' bills.

For most people, allergies to plants that bloom in the spring and fall are merely annoying. For those with asthma or severe allergic reactions, however, these allergies may be life-threatening.

"It's better to get good treatment than to let it go," says William Storms, M.D., an allergist and professor of medicine at the University of Colorado Health Sciences Center in Denver. "We have learned a few things about this disease. First, it does affect a patient's quality of life—productivity, educational performance. Second, it may lead to secondary diseases such as otitis media [ear infections], sinus infections, and asthma."

Spring is traditionally the main season when allergies blossom because of new growth on trees and weeds. But fall, with a whole different set of blooming plants as well as leaf mold, is a close second. In addition, people who are allergic to pollens are also often sensitive to dust mites (microscopic insects that feed on human skin cells), animal dander (tiny skin flakes shed by animals), and molds, which lurk indoors in any season.

The Food and Drug Administration regulates medications and biological products that offer allergy relief. Combined with a number of strategies to minimize a person's contact with allergens, these can make life bearable for even the worst allergy sufferer.

What Is an Allergy?

An allergy is the body's hypersensitivity to substances in the environment. Allergic reactions range from mild itching, sneezing or eczema (inflamed, itchy skin), to severe hives, hay fever, wheezing, and shortness of breath. An extreme allergic reaction can result in anaphylactic shock, a life-threatening situation in which a person's airway swells shut and blood pressure drops.

Scientists believe allergies originated millions of years ago as a way for the human body to rid itself of parasites and invading worms. The body fights these and other invaders by producing an antibody called immunoglobulin E (IgE for short) in the intestines and lungs. Without modern parasites to fight, IgE reacts to other foreign substances in the body. IgE triggers immune cells to release a number of chemicals, one of which is histamine. Histamine produces hives, watery eyes, sneezing, and itching. The more a person is exposed to allergens, the more the body produces IgE; hence, allergies often get worse with age.

The Nose Knows

The most common symptom of seasonal allergies is allergic rhinitis, otherwise known as hay fever. Symptoms of allergic rhinitis closely mimic those of the common cold.

But there are differences. A cold runs its course in 7 to 10 days. Allergic rhinitis can drag on for weeks or months. Despite its nickname, "hay fever" does not cause fever. With a cold, nasal discharge may be thick and yellow. In allergies, it is generally thin and clear. An allergy is often accompanied by eye, skin or mouth itchiness and can often be traced to a specific trigger.

447

The first step in handling chronic allergies is a visit to an allergist. The doctor will begin by taking a detailed medical history. From that, he or she can establish a list of suspected allergens. To confirm the diagnosis or figure out puzzling allergy symptoms, the doctor may order an allergy skin test.

With this test the practitioner makes a series of punctures, each containing a small amount of one suspect allergen in solution, in a grid pattern across the surface of the patient's back. If the patient is allergic to any of the allergens, a raised red spot like a hive, called a "wheal and flare," will appear after about 20 minutes, at that site.

Depending on the patient's history, a person may be tested for as few as six allergens or as many as 80. Beware of physicians who suggest testing for 200 to 300 allergens, says Berrilyn Ferguson, M.D., an associate professor and otolaryngologist (ear, nose and throat doctor) at the University of Pittsburgh School of Medicine. At that quantity, the skin may react to everything and the test will be useless.

A more sensitive test—the intradermal test—works by injecting a drop of extract into the skin. "The intradermal test is advisable if the puncture test is negative, to avoid a serious overdose reaction," says Paul Turkeltaub, M.D., director of the division of allergenic products and parasitology in FDA's Center for Biologics Evaluation and Research.

Extracts for Allergy Serum

FDA has been working to standardize the biological extracts used to test and treat patients with allergies.

"Extracts prepared from natural sources such as pollens, animals, and foods that trigger allergic reactions will vary in potency if they are not standardized," says Paul Turkeltaub, M.D., director of FDA's division of allergenic products and parasitology in the Center for Biologics Evaluation and Research. "Without standardization, each extract is an unknown. One batch could be stronger than the next. It makes it more difficult to treat patients and it also raises safety concerns."

Manufacturers are working to standardize extracts so they are consistent in potency from lot to lot. Currently, FDA has approved standardized allergy extracts for short ragweed, bee and other stinging insect venoms, dust mites, and cats.

Moreover, FDA is requiring that eight grass and pollen extracts be standardized. "The availability of the grass and pollen extracts will enhance their safe and effective use in diagnosis and treatment of grass allergies," says Turkeltaub. Nonstandardized extracts of cockroach (an important cause of inner-city asthma), giant ragweed, mold, peanuts, dog dander, and feathers are proposed for future standardization.

No allergy extracts are approved for sensitivity to foods, latex, or chemicals such as hair sprays, perfumes or cigarette smoke.

Treating the Symptoms

Once the causes and severity of the patient's allergies are determined, the doctor can prescribe a treatment plan. The first, most obvious, step is to avoid the allergen.

The next step in treating allergies is medication. Antihistamines, which interfere with the effect of histamine, are often prescribed. A major side effect of antihistamines is drowsiness, and some types produce more than others. The term "nonsedating" antihistamine is widely used to describe some prescription drugs, but it is not 100 percent accurate and is not a term used by FDA.

"It's really a matter of degrees," says Peter Honig, M.D., a medical officer in FDA's division of pulmonary drug products in the Center for Drug Evaluation and Research. "All the antihistamines produce drowsiness in patients, but some do more so than others." Benadryl (diphenhydramine hydrochloride), for example, is a common brand name oral antihistamine available without a prescription. It is well known to cause drowsiness in about half of people who take it. For those people, it's best taken at night. Two prescription antihistamines that have less sedation are Allegra (fexofenadine) and Claritin (loratidine).

Among nose sprays, there is Astelin (axzelastine hydrochloride), an antihistamine. Other nasal sprays contain steroids to combat congestion. These include Beconase and Vancenase (both contain beclomethasone dipropionate), Flonase (fluticasone propionate), Nasalide (flunisolide), and Nasacort (triamcinolone acetonide). The drawback to these medications is that they may take a week or so to be maximally effective and can sting and even damage the nasal septum (the soft bony division in the middle of the nose) if the spray is directed at it. Tell your doctor if you have any bloody discharge while using these sprays.

Less stinging but still helpful is the nasal spray Nasalcrom (cromolyn sodium). This nasal spray helps turn off the allergic process in the nose before it starts. It must be taken more often than a nasal steroid. Doctors often recommend this for children because it is extremely safe and it is available without a prescription.

Don't be tempted to treat an allergy with an over-the-counter decongestant nasal spray for more than three days. After a few days of use you may get a "rebound" effect, and your nose may become even more congested than before. These drugs are more useful for short-term use to relieve nasal congestion associated with a cold.

Dangerous Side Effects

Two prescription antihistamines, first touted for their effectiveness without causing drowsiness, are now known to have dangerous side effects. Seldane (terfenadine), and Hismanal (astemizole) have been shown to react with a number of other medications to cause life-threatening cardiac arrhythmias.

Seldane's manufacturer, Hoechst Marion Roussel, Kansas City, Missouri, withdrew the medication along with Seldane-D (terfenadine, pseudoephedrine) from the market voluntarily in 1997.

Patients taking antibiotics, antifungal medications, and some medications to treat HIV infection should talk to their doctors about the risks of taking any products containing terfenadine or Hismanal (astemizole).

Allergy Shots

What should you do if you've tried every drug in the pharmacy and still sneeze from January to December? Allergy shots, also known as immunotherapy, can offer long-lasting relief for many people.

Getting allergy shots is a long process. Over the span of three to five years, the allergy patient receives a small injection of the offending allergens usually twice a week at first, then less often with larger doses as time goes by. These small doses desensitize the body's immune system to each allergen. After at least six months to a year, the sneezing, itching, and hives may begin to subside. After about five years, it's possible for many to stop the shots completely.

"I am more productive, less irritable, and less fatigued since taking allergy shots," says Knoxville, Tennessee, resident Beth Crawford, who is allergic to every tree, grass, and pollen outdoors, plus dust mites, mold, and animal dander indoors. Her allergies occur year-round and have plagued her since childhood.

"Now I have more confidence. I don't have to worry about whether I'm going to have a sneezing attack in public," she says. A clinical social worker, Crawford's job requires occasional public speaking; in addition, she sings in her church's choir. "Now I can sing or give a speech without worrying. I know this sounds silly, but I can get ready in the morning much more quickly because I don't have to spend 30 minutes sneezing. And my husband says we have a substantial savings in Kleenex!"

About a third of patients who get allergy shots are cured after treatment, another third have a partial relapse, and the rest will relapse completely. Those not cured may be helped by resuming the shots.

Another approach to allergy shots is called "rush immunotherapy." Patients spend several days receiving repeated shots to desensitize them against allergens. They then go on the maintenance schedule earlier. Studies have suggested rush immunotherapy can be at least somewhat effective under certain circumstances, but more study is needed to show widespread safety and effectiveness. Currently, no allergen extracts are approved by FDA for this approach.

Over-the-Counter and Through the Pharmacy

Hay fever strikes some 10 to 30 percent of Americans, and more than half of them turn to over-the-counter medications instead of a doctor's prescription to control their symptoms. Pharmacy aisles are crowded with dozens of individual allergy drugs featuring various combinations of the half dozen active ingredients approved by FDA for allergy relief. Given the variety, consumers may find themselves posing some common questions:

My hay fever strikes every spring and fall. I sneeze, my eyes water, and my throat itches. How do I choose the best medicine for me?

For typical hay fever symptoms, three over-the-counter options can help: oral antihistamines, decongestants (both oral and nasal sprays), and a nasal spray containing cromolyn sodium.

Brands such as PediaCare, Robitussin, Comtrex, and Benadryl, as well as generic store brands, contain antihistamines, either chlorpheniramine or diphenhydramine. These drugs are effective for runny noses, sneezing, and itching, but can make you drowsy.

"If the OTC antihistamines are effective in relieving symptoms but are too sedating, a newer less sedating antihistamine can be obtained by prescription," says Linda Hu, M.D., a medical reviewer in FDA's division of OTC drugs. Antihistamines work on a runny nose, but not as well on a stuffy one, so many brands combine an antihistamine with a decongestant (for example, pseudoephedrine). Decongestants can also be found in fast-acting nasal sprays, but these may have a rebound effect and after about three days they'll make your nose even more congested. They are better used for a short-lived cold than an ongoing allergy. One nasal spray that doesn't cause a rebound effect is Nasalcrom (cromolyn sodium). This drug is helpful to prevent your symptoms if started a few days before the allergy season begins and taken continuously. It causes few side effects and will not make you drowsy.

Remember that it's the active ingredient that is important, and many products contain more than one. Read the labels to make sure you're not combining drugs with the same ingredients. Look at the ingredients in the drug product and choose the type of ingredient that will best treat the symptoms you have.

My job requires a lot of driving. Is it safe to take an antihistamine in the morning before I go to work?

Probably not. Antihistamines may affect your ability to drive or use machinery even if you don't feel sleepy.

"Drowsiness is the most common side effect of antihistamines and may be a problem for users who need to remain alert," says Hu. "Also, alcohol should be avoided because it may increase the drowsiness caused by antihistamines. If you need to be alert, some prescription antihistamines are less sedating."

I have emphysema and high blood pressure. Can I take an over-the-counter allergy medicine?

Antihistamines should not be used by anyone with breathing problems such as emphysema or bronchitis, anyone with glaucoma, by those taking sedatives or tranquilizers, or anyone with difficulty in urination unless directed by their doctors. These drugs dry up secretions and may cause urinary retention and drowsiness, according to Hu.

Antihistamines may also cause dryness of the mouth and eyes and blurred vision.

Decongestants, which are in many OTC allergy medicines, can raise blood pressure. Ask your doctor what, if anything, you can take. Decongestants should not be used by people with heart disease, thyroid disease, or diabetes unless a doctor says it's OK. If you're taking a drug containing an MAO inhibitor (sometimes used to treat depression), never use a decongestant.

I've tried every medicine on the shelves, and I'm still miserable each spring. What else can I do?

See your doctor. There may be prescription drugs that are more helpful to you, you may need allergy testing or shots, or your symptoms may be caused by something else entirely.

Keep It Clean

You can reduce your allergic misery if you take steps to keep the culprits out of your house.

For seasonal allergies caused by plants and trees, keep windows shut and the air conditioner on. Purchase an air filter to clean out pollens, molds, and dust. Use a dehumidifier in damp areas like the basement. Install wood, tile, or vinyl floors rather than carpet because they can be mopped regularly. If you do have carpets, have someone else do the vacuuming or buy a machine designed to reduce dust emissions.

Minimize clutter, book collections, and bric-a-brac, which collect dust and pollens. Keep pets outside or bathe them regularly if they're indoors, and don't let them sleep in your bed. Wash your hair every day to rinse off dust and pollen, and if you've been in the yard, leave shoes at the door and wash your clothes in hot water as soon as possible.

Since many hay fever sufferers are also allergic to dust mites, "The most cost effective thing is to buy a mattress cover," advises Berrilyn Ferguson, M.D. Mattress and pillow covers can provide a barrier between you and the dust mites in your bed, where they live and breed. In addition, treat carpets with an anti-allergen spray that kills dust mites.

You won't be able to eliminate every allergen from your home, but with these steps you can make it a comfortable place even during the peak of allergy season.

In the Nose, Not the Head

Allergies can certainly be life-threatening, but for most people they are merely annoying. For many, occasional sneezing, itching and watery eyes is no big deal. Others grow accustomed to the inconvenience and accept it as part of spring or fall, even if their symptoms are more severe.

"It's a quality of life issue," says Ferguson. "It's interesting how impaired people with allergies are. Some are just a little bit, but others have serious effects. I think if you are a productive person, you would want to treat your allergies and be as productive as possible."

"I didn't seek treatment earlier because my allergies had just become a way of life," remembers Crawford. "You just get used to it—I had severe allergies and I didn't even know it. Now I realize how much treatment has improved my quality of life. I should have done it years earlier—it was definitely worth it."

—section by Rebecca D. Williams,
writer in Oak Ridge, Tennessee

Section 49.2

Take Care with Over-the-Counter Allergy Medicine

© National Consumers League, 815 15th Street, NW, Washington, DC 20005; 202-639-8140; reprinted with permission.

Your nose is running, you are sneezing, and your head feels stuffy. It may be allergy time.

Some people have an allergy to grass, cats, dogs, flowers, and other things. If you have an allergy to something, over-the-counter allergy medicine can help you feel better. You can buy over-the-counter allergy medicine without a doctor's prescription at a drug store, food store, or other store.

Be Careful

1. Some over-the-counter allergy medicines should not be taken with other medicines. If you have questions about this, ask your doctor or pharmacist before you take allergy medicine.

2. When you take over-the-counter allergy medicine, read the label and follow directions. Do not take more than the label tells you.

3. Be careful if you drive or use machines. Some over-the-counter allergy medicines may make you sleepy.

4. Do not drink alcohol (beer, wine, liquor) when you take over-the-counter allergy medicine.

5. Do not take over-the-counter allergy medicine for more than seven days. If you do not get better, call your doctor.

6. If you have a fever, call your doctor.

Always Remember

1. If you have questions about over-the-counter allergy medicine, ask your doctor or pharmacist before you take the medicine.

2. If you are pregnant or nursing a baby, talk to your doctor before you take any medicine.

3. Keep all medicines away from children. Always keep the bottle cap locked.

Chapter 50

Common Allergy Medications

Dozens of drugs—both over-the-counter and prescription—are available to treat allergy symptoms. These include antihistamines, which combat symptoms by blocking the action of histamine, the chemical released by the body in response to an allergen; decongestants to control nasal symptoms; steroids and leukotriene inhibitors to control inflammation; and topical (skin) ointments to treat eczema.

Many antihistamines and decongestants used to treat allergy symptoms are available without a prescription; prescriptions are required for other drugs, such as steroid medications. Some antihistamines (both over-the-counter and by prescription) can slow reaction times, impair judgment and make you sleepy. So don't drive (or operate machinery) while taking drugs with these side effects. Here's a list of common allergy medications.

Drugs to Prevent Allergy Symptoms

Antihistamines

These drugs combat allergy symptoms including sneezing, runny or itchy nose, watery or itchy eyes, and hives. They work by blocking the action of histamine, the chemical released by the body in response to an allergen producing the reaction.

Johns Hopkins Health Information, InteliHealth, online at http://www.intelihealth.com, ©2000 InteliHealth Inc. Reprinted with permission of InteliHealth.

Histamine has many actions within the body—including stimulating salivation and dilating blood vessels and making them leaky (which helps explain why a rash is often part of an allergic reaction). Antihistamines work to counter these reactions.

Most antihistamines are available over-the-counter. Some, but not all, newer prescription products don't cause one of the best-known side effects—drowsiness—that occurs with over-the-counter antihistamines in about 15% of patients, but they are more expensive.

Common Drugs—Nonprescription: [tablets/capsules] Benadryl Allergy Antihistamine; Chlor-Trimetron Allergy Antihistamine; Comtrex; Contac 12-hour Allergy; Eficac 24 Antihistamine; Tavist-1 Antihistamine; Tylenol Allergy/Sinus.

Common Drugs—Prescription: Loratadine (Claritin tablets and syrup), cetirizine (Zyrtec tablets and syrup), fexofenadine (Allegra).

Common Side Effects: Both prescription and nonprescription drugs can cause drowsiness; impaired coordination; and dry nose, mouth, and throat. Make certain that you read the information provided with either over-the-counter antihistamines or those available only by prescription.

Precautions: All antihistamines, including those touted as being "non-sedating" have the potential to cause drowsiness. Sedation and drowsiness are more common with over-the-counter antihistamines. Don't drive or operate heavy machinery when taking these drugs; tell your doctor about any drugs you are taking and about any other physical disorder you may have, especially urinary or prostate problems and glaucoma. Drinking alcohol can magnify the sedating effects of antihistamines.

For Prescription Antihistamines: Some drugs can interact with prescription (non-sedating) antihistamines and lead to a risk of irregular heart beats.

What You Need To Know: Whether by prescription or purchased over-the-counter at any drugstore or supermarket, antihistamine medications are an effective way to keep hay fever reactions at bay and make allergy season a little more tolerable. As the name implies, antihistamines work by blocking the action of histamine, the chemical released by the body in response to an allergen that produces the sneezing, runny nose or other reactions. Here's what you need to know about taking these popular pills:

- *Make it a routine:* Too often, a hay fever sufferer takes one anti-histamine pill, feels better, and then waits until the symptoms get bad again before taking another. This can make you feel worse in days to come. So if your doctor advises that you go the antihistamine route, take your medicine regularly during an allergy season to prevent hay fever problems. If you know the season when your allergies occur, start to take your medication at least two weeks before symptoms start.

Anti-Allergy Nasal Sprays

If simple antihistamines don't adequately relieve nasal symptoms, corticosteroids represent the next treatment option. Nasal corticosteroids are anti-inflammatory drugs that inhibit allergic reactions and reduce nasal swelling and mucous secretions. These sprays work to relieve congestion caused by allergic and nonallergic rhinitis and nasal polyps. In clinical trials they are consistently better than antihistamines at relieving the nasal symptoms of runny, stuffy and itchy nose. Instead of waiting until allergic symptoms develop, these medications must be used daily.

Cromolyn (Nasalcrom, Opticrom) is a non-steroid agent used in spray form that interferes with the release of histamine and other chemicals from mast cells, and thereby prevents sneezing and itchy, runny nose.

Common Drugs: Corticosteroid: beclomethasone (Beconase, Vancenase), budesonide (Rhinocort), flunisolide (Nasalide), fluticasone (Flonase) and triamcinolone. Cromolyn (Nasacort, Opticrom).

Common Side Effects: Sneezing, an itchy, mild dryness or burning in the nose, and unpleasant taste, thrush infection in the mouth; nosebleeds; headaches.

Precautions: Tell your doctor if you have glaucoma, liver disease, or tuberculosis.

Drugs Used to Treat Allergy Symptoms

Decongestants

These drugs relieve nasal congestion by shrinking swollen nasal tissues. Most are available without a prescription, as tablets, syrups, and nasal sprays. Some of these drugs are combined with an antihistamine.

Common Drugs—Nonprescription [Tablets and Syrups]:
Phenyleprine (Dimetapp, Sinex); Phenylpropanolamine[1] (Alka-Seltzer Plus, Allerest, Sine-Aid, Triaminix); Pseudoephedrine (Actifed, CoTylenol Tablets, Drixoral, Sudafed).

Common Drugs—Prescription [Tablets and Syrups]: Entex.

Common Drugs—Nonprescription [Nasal Sprays]: Oxymetazoline (Afrin; Dristan Long Lasting), NeoSynephrine (Sinex)

Common Side Effects: Nervousness, restlessness, insomnia. Nasal sprays may dry or irritate the nose.

Precautions: Consult your doctor before using oral decongestants if you are taking antidepressants or have high blood pressure, diabetes, or heart disease. Long term use of nonprescription decongestant nasal sprays can lead to a "rebound" effect in which the drug stops working and symptoms return, worse than before. For this reason, decongestant sprays should not be used for longer than three days.

Antihistamine/Decongestants

These combination drugs work on two fronts: They block the action of histamine and relieve nasal congestion, sneezing, and other allergy symptoms. Many are available over the counter.

Common Drugs—Nonprescription: Actifed Cold & Allergy; Allerest; Benadryl Allergy/Sinus; Contac Day & Night Allergy/Sinus; Dimetapp Allergy/Sinus; Drixoral Allergy/Sinus; Sudafed Plus; Tavist D; Tylenol Allergy/Sinus.

Common Drugs—Prescription: Claritin-D; Allegra D; Trinalin; Entex LA.

Common Side Effects: Drowsiness, nervousness.

Precautions: Ask the pharmacist about interactions with any other drugs you are taking.

Medications for Asthma

Treatment for asthma typically involves a "step" approach in which asthma is treated by stepping up the number of medications and the number of times the medications is taken as a person's asthma gets worse. During times that the asthma is well controlled, medications are stepped down.

There are a range of asthma medications. Some work to relieve symptoms, typically during an acute episode, and others work to keep asthma in check. Medications that are used to relieve acute symptoms are called inhaled short-acting beta-agonists. Those that are prescribed to control the asthma include inhaled anti-inflammatory agents, oral corticosteroids, long-acting bronchodilators, and oral anti-leukotrienes.

Drugs Used to Treat Asthma Symptoms

Inhaled Short-Acting Beta Agonists

These medications relax the muscles around the airways, and therefore prevent or reverse them from narrowing. Administered by metered-dose inhaler or, for some patients, by nebulizer, they typically make breathing easier within 5 minutes. Usually the effect lasts for 4 to 6 hours. Short-acting beta agonists act as reliever medicines to reverse symptoms that have already started or, when used just before exercise, to prevent exercise-induced asthma.

Common Drugs: albuterol (Proventil, Ventolin), bitolterol (Tornalate), pirbuterol (Maxair), terbutaline (Breathaire).

Common Side Effects: Nervousness or restlessness, trembling, dry mouth, or rapid or irregular heart beat; tend to become less frequent or severe as the body adapts to the medicine.

Drugs Used to Prevent Asthma Symptoms

Inhaled Anti-Inflammatory Agents

These medications act to avert or reduce airway inflammation and to diminish airway sensitivity to irritants. Inhaled anti-inflammatory agents work only when they are taken regularly—it usually takes between 4 and 6 weeks before the effect can be felt. Strictly controller medications, these cannot stop an asthma attack once it has started.

Common Drugs: Cromolyn sodium (Intal), Nedocromil sodium (Tilade) [Metered-dose or nebulizer inhalation]. [Metered-dose inhaled corticosteroids] Beclomethasone (Beclovent, Vanceril), Flunisolide (AeroBid), Fluticasone (Flovent) Triamcinolone (Azmacort).

461

Common Side Effects: Cough, headache, unpleasant taste; Corticosteroids can cause thrust (yeast infection) in the throat and headache. A spacer attachment on the inhaler and rinsing with the mouth out with water after using the medication can reduce some of the side effects. When used according to directions, inhaled corticosteroids do not cause serious side effects associated with regular use of oral steroids.

Oral Corticosteroids

These drugs work to reverse and inhibit airway inflammation. Administered orally in tablet or liquid form, they begin to work in about three hours; the peak effectiveness is between 6 to 12 hours. They are used for short-term relief from severe asthma episodes, and to control some forms of severe, persistent asthma.

Common Drugs: Prednisone (Cortan, Deltasone, Orasone Prednicen-M, Sterapred), Prednisolone (Delta-Cortef, Pediapred, Prelone), Methylprednisolone (Medrol).

Common Side Effects: [short-term use] increased appetite, fluid retention, weight gain, rounding of the face, mood changes, increased blood pressure; [long-term use] loss of bone density, cataracts, and high blood pressure; [long-term use in children] growth retardation.

Precautions: Start and stop an oral corticosteroid as instructed by your physician. This is true for any medication, but proper use of corticosteroids in asthma is especially important. If, while taking oral corticosteroids, an asthma attack does not clear up with the use of a bronchodilator, contact your doctor. Also contact your doctor if you have a serious case of the flu or other illness, or if you are considering surgery. Corticosteroid dosages may need to be adjusted.

Note: Although corticosteroids are sometimes called steroids, they are not the same as anabolic steroids.

Long-Acting Bronchodilators

These medications relax the muscles around the airways for about 10 to 12 hours. They work only if taken consistently. They are often given for long-term management of asthma symptoms or to control symptoms at night. They may also be useful in preventing exercise-induced asthma. Salmeterol is often coupled with an inhaled corticosteroid.

Common Drugs: [Beta agonists—metered-dosage inhaler or prolonged release tablets] Salmeterol (Serevent), Albuterol (Volmax, Proventil Repetabs), [Methylxanthines—tablets and syrups], Theophylline (Theo-Dur, Slo-Phyllin; Uniphyl; Slo-Bid).

Common Side Effects: Nervousness, restlessness, trembling, dry mouth, rapid or irregular heart beat, insomnia, nausea, heartburn. Salmeterol, which is longer acting, may also cause fewer side effects than oral prolonged release albuterol.

Precautions: Theophylline may cause diarrhea or bloody or black stools, rapid breathing, vomiting, confusion, increased urination or difficulty urinating, convulsions or seizures, muscle twitching. Should you experience any of these, contact your doctor at once. If you are taking theophylline and develop a high fever or symptoms of the flu, serious side effects may also develop. Finally, you should contact your physician before getting a flu shot.

In addition, directions for salmeterol (Serevent) should be followed closely and should not be used to relieve acute attacks.

Oral Anti-Leukotrienes

These medications are the latest in asthma control. They belong to a new class of oral anti-inflammatory agents known as antileukotrienes and appear to produce fewer long-term side effects than oral corticosteroids. They prevent and reduce airway inflammation. Administered on a regular basis—even when no symptoms are present—in tablet form, they prevent constriction of airway muscles and reduce sensitivity to triggers. In addition, they seem to reduce a person's need for short-acting bronchodilators. However, these medications work strictly to control asthma symptoms and can not stop an asthma attack that has already begun.

Common Drugs: Zafirlukast(Accolate); Zileuton (Zyflo) Montelukast (Singulair).

Common Side Effects: Dyspepsia (upset stomach), increased infections, nausea, and diarrhea.

Precaution: Because some people who take zileuton and monteukast may show elevated liver function, they should have their liver function tested prior to taking this medication, and periodically while on this medication.

Medications to Treat Anaphylaxis

If you are allergic to insect venom or have a food allergy and have had an anaphylactic reaction in the past, you may have another. For this reason, you should carry an emergency kit with a syringe containing the drug epinephrine (adrenaline) to use if you are stung or inadvertently eat the food to which you are allergic. Two emergency kits are on the market: Epi Pen and AnaKit:

- EpiPen is an automatic injector. You merely pull off the safety cap, place the tip against your outer thigh and push against the skin. The pen will automatically inject a pre-measured dose of epinephrine. EpiPen Jr. is available for children. However, discuss the use of epinephrine with your child's pediatrician, because infants and children may be especially sensitive to the effects of epinephrine.

- Ana-Kit contains a syringe with a preloaded, measured dose of epinephrine. To use it, you remove the protective sheath surrounding the syringe and inject the epinephrine into your outer thigh or upper arm.

These emergency measures may head off your reaction, but the kits are not designed to replace medical treatment. Instead, they should be used as a holding action until you can get to a hospital emergency room. There is a danger of a recurrence later in the day, and you may need oxygen or medications to improve your breathing, as well as intravenous fluids to restore your blood pressure to normal. Remember to replace your emergency epinephrine kit after using it. And be sure to check the expiration dates on the kits; after expiration, the medication may not be effective.

Note

1. Phenylpropanolamine (PPA) was withdrawn from the U.S. market by the Food and Drug Administration in the fall of 2000. Brand name products still offered for sale have been reformulated using alternate ingredients.

Chapter 51

Medication Updates

Zyrtec® Approved for Allergic Rhinitis in Children Two to Five Years Old

The U.S. Food and Drug Administration (FDA) has approved Pfizer Inc. and UCB Pharma's antihistamine Zyrtec® (cetirizine HCl) for the treatment of seasonal allergic rhinitis, perennial allergic rhinitis, and chronic idiopathic urticaria in children down to the age of two years old.

Zyrtec was initially approved for patients 12 years and older in January 1996 and was subsequently approved down to the age of six years in September 1996. Zyrtec is the first and only once-daily prescription antihistamine indicated for use in pediatric patients under the age of six years.

Zyrtec is available in a 1 mg per 1 ml alcohol-free and dye-free fruity banana-grape flavor syrup. The recommended initial dose of Zyrtec Syrup in children aged two to five years is 2.5 mg (1/2 teaspoon) once daily. The dosage in this age group can be increased to a maxi-

Excerpted from "Zyrtec Approved for Allergic Rhinitis in Children Two to Five Years Old," "FDA Grants Atrovent Nasal Spray Pediatric Indication for Rhinorrhea," "FDA Approves Rhinocort for Once-A-Day Relief of Allergy Symptoms," "FDA Approves Nasonex for Use in Children as Young as Three," and "Loteprednol Offers Relief of Ocular Allergy Symptoms with Fewer Side Effects," in *Doctor's Guide to the Internet*, 1998, 1999. ©1998, 1999 by P\S\L Consulting Group Inc. Reprinted by permission. *Doctor's Guide to the Internet* is at http://www.docguide.com.

mum dose of 5 mg per day given as 1 teaspoon (5 mg) once daily, or as 1/2 teaspoon (2.5 mg) given every 12 hours, depending on symptom severity and patient response. Zyrtec is also available as 5 mg and 10 mg tablets.

The effectiveness of Zyrtec for the treatment of seasonal and perennial allergic rhinitis and chronic idiopathic urticaria in this pediatric age group of two to 11 years is based on an extrapolation of the demonstrated efficacy of Zyrtec in adults in these conditions and the likelihood that the disease course, pathophysiology, and the drug's effect are substantially similar between these two populations.

Clinical studies support the safety of Zyrtec in children in this age group. In studies, side effects were mild or moderate including drowsiness, fatigue, and dry mouth in adults and drowsiness, headache, sore throat, and stomach pain in children. Drowsiness occurred in between 11 percent and 14 percent in adults, depending on dose, compared to six percent taking placebo. In children, drowsiness occurred in between two percent and four percent, depending on dose, compared to one percent taking placebo.

Approximately six million children suffer from seasonal allergies. If one parent has allergies, chances are one in three that each child will have an allergy. If both parents have allergies, it is much more likely (seven in 10) that their children will have allergies.

"Because it may be difficult to discern the difference between cold and allergy symptoms, many parents frequently mistake allergy symptoms for those associated with a cold and do not seek appropriate medical attention," said James Kemp, M.D., clinical professor, department of pediatrics, University of California, San Diego. "Once a diagnosis is made, avoidance of allergy triggers, such as pollen and animal dander, along with treatment, can play a key role in controlling nagging symptoms."

FDA Grants Atrovent® Nasal Spray Pediatric Indication for Rhinorrhea

Boehringer Ingelheim Pharmaceuticals, Inc.' s Atrovent® (ipratropium bromide) Nasal Spray .03% for the treatment of rhinorrhea (runny nose) associated with allergic and nonallergic perennial rhinitis has now been granted an indication for use in children six years and up by the [U.S. FDA].

It is not indicated for the relief of nasal congestion, sneezing, or postnasal drip.

Atrovent Nasal Spray .03% is an anticholinergic agent that blocks the action of acetylcholine, which causes a runny nose. It provides significant relief from the first day of therapy, with no nasal rebound.

In clinical trials, the most frequently reported nasal adverse events were transient episodes of epistaxis [(nosebleed)] (9.0 percent vs. 4.6 percent with vehicle) or nasal dryness (5.1 percent vs. 0.9 percent with vehicle). The most frequently reported non-nasal adverse events were transient episodes of headache (9.8 percent vs. 9.2 percent with vehicle) or upper respiratory tract infections (9.8 percent vs. 7.2 percent with vehicle).

FDA Approves Rhinocort for Once-A-Day Relief of Allergy Symptoms

The U.S. FDA has approved its water-based, corticosteroid medication, Rhinocort Aqua™ (budesonide) Nasal Spray, for the treatment of seasonal and perennial allergic rhinitis in adults and children six years of age and older. Rhinocort Aqua provides for once-a-day dosing with a recommended starting dose regimen requiring only one spray per nostril for children and adults.

The active medication is budesonide, a corticosteroid, in a fragrance-free aqueous formula that contains no alcohol and no benzalkonium chloride preservative. Rhinocort Aqua uses potassium sorbate as a preservative.

In some clinical trials, Rhinocort Aqua provided a significant reduction in the severity of nasal allergy symptoms—congestion, runny nose, and sneezing—in as few as 24 hours after initial therapy. Maximum benefit generally takes two weeks to achieve. Product effectiveness depends on use at regular intervals. The recommended once-daily starting dose regimen is one spray per nostril for both adults and children. The maximum recommended dose regimen is two sprays per nostril (children) or four sprays per nostril (adults) administered once-daily.

"We are pleased that Rhinocort Aqua will offer allergy sufferers and physicians a new aqueous once-daily, nasal spray that provides a patient-friendly therapeutic option for allergy relief," said Frank Casty, M.D., Global Medical Director for Respiratory and Inflammation at AstraZeneca.

Safety and Efficacy of Rhinocort Aqua

The safety and efficacy of Rhinocort Aqua was evaluated in seven placebo-controlled clinical trials, which included over 1500 patients aged six years and older with seasonal allergic or perennial allergic rhinitis. The key findings of these trials were that, overall, Rhinocort Aqua significantly reduced the severity of the nasal symptoms—runny nose, sneezing, and congestion. The studies demonstrated that Rhinocort Aqua is effective and well-tolerated in both adults and children suffering from seasonal allergic and perennial allergic rhinitis.

Rhinocort Aqua showed a low incidence of side effects in clinical trials

The most commonly reported adverse events for Rhinocort Aqua and vehicle placebo (a formulation with no active drug) respectively were: epistaxis (nosebleed)—8 percent vs. 5 percent; pharyngitis (sore throat)—4 percent vs. 3 percent; bronchospasm—2 percent vs. 1 percent; nasal irritation—2 percent vs. <1 percent; and coughing—2 percent vs. <1 percent.

Patients previously treated with oral corticosteroids (e.g., pills) and transferred to nasal corticosteroids should be carefully monitored for adrenal insufficiency. As with other nasal corticosteroids, after symptomatic relief is achieved, the dose should be reduced to the least amount necessary to control symptoms. Physicians should routinely monitor the growth of children taking intranasal corticosteroids to detect possible growth effects.

Combining Convenience and Efficacy

"Convenient dosing is critical with allergy treatments because effective symptom relief is dependent on consistent use of the medication," said Robert Overholt, M.D., president of The Allergy, Asthma & Sinus Center in Knoxville, Tennessee. "Given this, patients and physicians should find Rhinocort Aqua to be a useful treatment option combining convenience and efficacy."

Rhinocort Aqua is contained in a pocket-sized bottle with each metered dose delivered through a hand-held, wing-tipped applicator. The bottle contains 60 metered sprays. Each spray provides 32 mcg of budesonide mixed in water.

Since its introduction in 1986, the intranasal, aqueous formulation of budesonide has been approved for allergic rhinitis relief in over sixty countries, including the United Kingdom and Canada. Budesonide belongs to a class of anti-inflammatory medications known as corticosteroids. Leading U.S. allergy specialists' organizations—the American Academy of Allergy, Asthma and Immunology, the American College of Allergy, Asthma and Immunology and the Joint Council on Allergy, Asthma and Immunology—consider nasally inhaled corticosteroids to be the most effective medication class for controlling the nasal congestion associated with allergic rhinitis.

Seasonal and Perennial Allergic Rhinitis Takes Its Toll

Approximately 20 to 40 million Americans suffer from seasonal and perennial allergic rhinitis. Allergic rhinitis, sometimes known as hay fever, is believed to be the most common chronic allergic disease in the U.S. Although not life-threatening, allergic rhinitis can be serious enough to interfere with daily life—resulting in school absences, lost work days, loss of sleep, and a decreased ability to perform everyday activities.

Symptoms, such as congestion, sneezing, and runny nose, can often be mistaken for the common cold, but unlike a cold can last anywhere from a few weeks to all year. The cost of treating this medical condition and the indirect costs related to lost workplace productivity are significant. In 1995 alone, the estimated costs of allergic rhinitis based on direct and indirect costs were 2.7 billion dollars.

Rhinocort Aqua represents a new formulation of the active ingredient, budesonide, which was first launched in the U.S. in 1994 as an aerosolized metered dose inhaler for rhinitis patients six years of age and older. Known as Rhinocort® (budesonide) Nasal Inhaler, it is today the number one prescribed, nasally-inhaled, aerosol-based corticosteroid in the U.S. (based on IMS Health National Prescription Audit Data, from September 1996 to June 1999). AstraZeneca will continue to market its aerosolized nasal spray—giving patients and physicians a choice of budesonide therapies.

Both aerosolized and aqueous formulations provide budesonide in a fragrance-free mixture with a once-a-day dosing schedule.

FDA Approves Nasonex for Use in Children as Young as Three

Schering-Plough Corporation announced that Nasonex® (mometasone furoate monohydrate) Nasal Spray 50 mcg has received marketing approval from the U.S. FDA for the treatment of the nasal symptoms of seasonal and perennial allergic rhinitis in children as young as 3 years of age. Nasonex is the only drug in its class to be indicated for children as young as age three.

Nasonex is currently marketed for the treatment of nasal symptoms of seasonal and perennial allergic rhinitis in adult and adolescent patients 12 years and older. It is also approved for the prevention of nasal symptoms of seasonal rhinitis in adult and adolescent patients 12 years and older, and is the only nasal inhaled steroid approved in the United States for this indication.

The new approval follows the FDA's review of clinical trials specifically designed to evaluate the safety and efficacy of Nasonex Nasal Spray in pediatric populations and represents the youngest indication for any prescription nasal inhaled corticosteroid.

"A growing child has medical considerations quite different from those of a mature adult," said Dr. Eric J. Schenkel, director, Valley Clinical Research Center, Easton, Pa. "Assumptions about pediatric pharmacology should be validated in clinical studies that account for the developmental stages of a child. This approval demonstrates that Nasonex is a safe and effective medicine for treating allergies even in children as young as age three," he said.

Allergic rhinitis affects more than six million children each year and accounts for two million missed school days, with indirect costs reaching $4 billion. Day care centers and schools are environments where exposure to allergens such as dust mites, mold, and pet dander carried from home on children's clothing can be particularly high.

The FDA in 1998 reviewed data that some nasal corticosteroids may have an adverse effect on growth in children, but it is uncertain whether there is a long-term effect on ultimate height or whether all nasal steroids have such an effect. In support of this newest indication for Nasonex for young children, long-term clinical studies were conducted that showed no statistically significant effect on growth velocity in children ages three to nine compared to placebo. Controlled clinical studies have shown intranasal corticosteroids may cause a reduction in growth velocity in pediatric patients. The growth of pediatric patients receiving intranasal corticosteroids, including Nasonex, should be monitored routinely (e.g., by stadiometry).

Nasonex has a virtually undetectable level of absorption into the bloodstream. The overall incidence of adverse events was comparable to placebo and did not differ significantly based on age or sex. The most commonly reported adverse events, not necessarily drug-related were, for Nasonex and vehicle placebo, respectively: headache (17 percent vs. 18 percent), viral infection (8 percent vs. 9 percent), pharyngitis (10 percent vs. 10 percent), epistaxis/blood-tinged mucus (8 percent vs. 9 percent) and coughing (13 percent vs. 15 percent).

The usual recommended dose of Nasonex Nasal Spray for children three to 11 years of age is one spray (50 mcg per spray) in each nostril once daily. For adults and children 12 years of age and older, the usual recommended dose is two sprays (50 mcg per spray) in each nostril once daily. Nasonex is available nationwide by prescription only.

Loteprednol Offers Relief of Ocular Allergy Symptoms with Fewer Side Effects

Results of a recently published study show seasonal allergy sufferers may have another option to taking traditional corticosteroid drugs used to relieve the redness, itching, and swelling of the eyes.

Corticosteroids such as fluorometholone or prednisolone are effective in treating eye problems experienced by seasonal allergy sufferers. However, drugs derived from the steroid, cortisone, can increase pressure inside the eye, possibly leading to optic nerve damage.

A study published in the American Academy of Ophthalmology's Journal, *Ophthalmology,* showed loteprednol etabonate, the first site-active corticosteroid, to be safe and effective in treating ocular allergy symptoms.

"The advantage of loteprednol etabonate is that it is site-active," said one of the study's investigators, David G. Shulman, M.D., of San Antonio, Texas. "This means it is not absorbed into the body and, as a result, does not cause side effects associated with steroids such as increased intraocular pressure. This is particularly good news for people concerned about taking steroid medications, including those suffering from glaucoma."

Of the 135 patients participating in the six-week study, 67 were given eye drops containing loteprednol etabonate 0.2 percent ophthalmic suspension and 68 received the placebo. The loteprednol etabonate-treated patients experienced significant improvement in their symptoms over the placebo group.

Only one patient each from each group experienced elevated intraocular pressure, far below the 33 to 44 percent of patients taking other corticosteroid drugs.

Chapter 52

Immunotherapy (Allergy Shots)

Immunotherapy was first used successfully in 1911 by Leonard Noon, who noticed that in many people the onset of allergic symptoms coincided with the pollination of grass in England. He found that intradermal injections of an extract of grass pollen relieved the signs and symptoms that patients experienced during the grass pollen season.

Since that time, the use of immunotherapy has greatly increased. According to the American Academy of Allergy and Immunology, approximately 33 million injections are given per year in the United States. Immunotherapy appears to be effective for the treatment of allergic rhinoconjunctivitis and for insect sting allergies. (The use of immunotherapy for insect sting allergies is not discussed in this chapter.) There is healthy debate on the effectiveness of immunotherapy in the treatment of asthma, with opinions varying from "effective" to "completely ineffective." However, some authorities argue that the risks of immunotherapy exceed the benefits in patients with unstable asthma.

At present, no evidence points to the effectiveness of immunotherapy for urticaria, atopic dermatitis, and food allergy. Although preliminary data suggest that immunotherapy may be effective for the treatment of food allergy, use of immunotherapy for this purpose is fraught with danger. Until further data are available, immunotherapy for food allergy should probably not be undertaken outside of research settings.

Indications

Table 52.1. summarizes the indications for immunotherapy. Immunotherapy has traditionally been attempted in patients with a history of IgE-mediated disease that correlates with positive results on skin testing or radioallergosorbent testing (RAST). Before the decision is made to administer immunotherapy, environmental control measures, including avoidance of the offending agents, should have been tried and should have been shown not to result in improvement of symptoms. In addition, either an incomplete response to medications has been observed or the patient has made the decision not to take medications. A trial of immunotherapy is warranted if these criteria are met and contraindications do not exist.

The cost of the buildup phase during the first year of immunotherapy varies, depending on the number of injections required and the extracts used. Maintenance therapy may range from $200 to $1,000 per year, depending on the number of injections given and physician fees.

Table 52.1. Indications for Immunotherapy for Allergic Rhinitis and Conjunctivitis

- IgE-mediated disease
- Skin test or RAST (radioallergosorbent) test positive for IgE to a specific antigen
- Correlation between allergic symptoms and test results
- No relief of symptoms with environmental changes or avoidance of exposure to precipitators
- Failure to obtain relief with medications, failure to tolerate medications, or unwillingness to take medications

Immunotherapy in Allergic Rhinitis

Biochemical changes in the mucosa and the nasal secretions occur following immunotherapy for allergic rhinitis.[1] When compared with placebo, immunotherapy has been shown to be associated with decreased concentrations of histamine, tosyl-L-arginine methyl esterase (or TAME, the esterase that can activate the bradykinin system) and prostaglandin G_2. This effect suggests that, as a result of immunotherapy, there is a reduction in the release of mediators by mast cells, an important component during the early phases of the immune reaction in allergic rhinitis.[1]

Immunotherapy can also inhibit the influx of inflammatory cells, such as eosinophils. Eosinophils are thought to be a key component in the late phase of allergic rhinitis. The late phase seems to be responsible for the priming effect, which causes worsening of symptoms from day to day in the face of similar antigen exposure. Thus, immunotherapy not only decreases mast cell mediator release but also the inflammatory response associated with allergic rhinitis.[2]

Changes in the immune system also occur with immunotherapy. Early in therapy, the IgE level increases, prior to the increase of the IgG level. It is at this time that patients may be at the greatest risk of anaphylaxis and other adverse effects of immunotherapy.[3] Later, IgG levels specific to the allergen used for treatment increase as total IgE and specific IgE levels decrease.

Studies of immunotherapy for allergy to ragweed in the eastern part of the United States and to grasses in the western United States have demonstrated a reduction in symptoms and medication use when patients receive immunotherapy as compared with placebo injections.[4,5] Improvement in symptoms is limited only to the pollen season for the particular extract that is being administered—thus, the reaction is specific. This effect persists during the course of immunotherapy and, probably, for years after completion of a full course of immunotherapy.[6]

Immunotherapy in Asthma

Asthma is a multifactorial disease. Exercise, industrial and occupational agents, weather changes, viral infections, medications (for example, aspirin), emotions, tobacco smoke, and particulate matter may all trigger symptoms of asthma. Allergens are an important aspect to consider in the management of asthma, but allergens are not the only triggers that need to be controlled.

In patients with asthma, there is a trend toward a lower correlation between asthma symptoms and allergy with increasing age. It is estimated that 90 percent of children with asthma have allergic disease; sensitivities include house-dust mites (52 percent of patients), animal dander (29 percent), pollens (20 percent), molds (14 percent), and cockroaches.[7] Therefore, when possible, skin testing or RAST testing is essential to define the allergic component of asthma, and these data should be used to direct appropriate environmental changes. Multiple studies have been performed stressing the importance of avoidance measures and techniques to accomplish avoidance in persons with asthma.[1-9] However, data to support the use of immunotherapy in asthma are less concrete.

A recent study investigated the effectiveness of immunotherapy in patients with asthma.[10] Screening for ragweed allergy was conducted in 1,000 patients with asthma, and 77 patients (7.7 percent) were found to have ragweed sensitivities that met criteria for inclusion in the study. Overall symptom improvement and decreased use of medications were noted in the group receiving immunotherapy, but only in the first year of therapy. Peak flow values improved, as did the response to an inhalation challenge with ragweed. As would be expected, IgE levels decreased and an increase was noted in the IgG level that is specific for ragweed. This finding suggests that there is benefit from immunotherapy in patients with asthma. However, the study revealed no cost savings with the use of immunotherapy compared with drug therapy.

There have been two recent attempts to perform a meta-analysis on immunotherapy studies.[11,12] Abramson and colleagues[11] conducted a meta-analysis on studies that were randomized and properly controlled. The studies were performed between 1966 and 1990. Some of them were done without high-dose therapy (antigen levels that have been demonstrated in the literature to be effective in inducing desensitization) or standardized extracts (extracts with a defined level of a specific antigen that can be reproduced from lot to lot). Of the studies reviewed, nine focused on house-dust mites, five on pollens, five on animal dander and one on mold allergy. The meta-analysis demonstrated that immunotherapy is associated with a reduction in symptoms, a decreased need for asthma medications, and a reduction in bronchial hyperreactivity. The authors concluded from this meta-analysis that immunotherapy is effective for the treatment of asthma, but it should be used with caution because it may also exacerbate asthma symptoms in some patients.

The second meta-analysis, performed by Sigman and Mazer,[12] focused on the use of immunotherapy in children with asthma. Twelve studies were reviewed. The authors found a lack of uniformity across the studies, which limited the ability to do a true meta-analysis. The analysis indicated that four of five studies showed some effectiveness of immunotherapy in mite-allergic persons. The data available for animal dander and fungi were limited, and no conclusion could be drawn. The benefit of pollen immunotherapy was also questionable.

Because of the safety factors associated with the use of immunotherapy, Sigman and Mazer were unable to conclude that immunotherapy should be used in asthma. They stated that well-performed, well-controlled clinical studies are needed to define whether immunotherapy is an effective treatment in children with asthma.

Adverse Effects

Adverse effects from immunotherapy are common. Fortunately, the vast majority of these effects are minor and mainly consist of local swelling at the site of injection. One study[13] revealed that 1 to 50 percent of patients receiving immunotherapy injections experience some type of adverse effect. The incidence of adverse effects per 1,000 injections is between one and 17. Our experience suggests that approximately 15 percent of patients experience adverse effects. The risk increases under each of the following circumstances: "rush" therapy (desensitization accomplished over one day to a few days), the use of high doses, and immunotherapy introduced without premedication.

Patients at risk of adverse effects include those with a history of frequently large local reactions, asthma, a recent use of steroids, and a recent hospitalization or emergency department visit for asthma therapy. The risk is also increased in patients with signs or symptoms of asthma before their injection[13] (Table 52.2).

Table 52.2. Indicators of Increased Risk of Adverse Effects from Immunotherapy

- Large local reactions to injections
- High-dose therapy
- Use of standardized extracts
- Signs or symptoms of asthma before injection
- Recent hospitalization for asthma
- Administration of injections in the allergen season
- Strongly positive skin tests
- Buildup phase of treatment
- Vial changes
- Prior anaphylaxis to immunotherapy
- Peak flow or FEV_1, below 70% of predicted value in patients with asthma

FEV_1 = forced expiratory volume in one second.

A review[14] of data on immunotherapy related fatalities in the United States shows that there were 24 deaths from 1959 to 1984 and 17 deaths from 1985 to 1989. Asthma had been diagnosed in 13 of the cases, and most of these patients had unstable asthma during the time they were receiving immunotherapy.

A more recent review 15 of adverse effects of immunotherapy revealed that patients at highest risk of adverse effects were those with strongly positive skin tests, those receiving immunotherapy during the season in which they were allergic, those with a history of prior anaphylaxis, and those with a diagnosis of asthma. Adverse effects were also increased when vials were changed, independent of whether the change in vials occurred during the buildup or the maintenance phase of the program. A risk-benefit analysis should be done in such patients to determine whether immunotherapy should be started or continued.

To decrease the risks associated with immunotherapy, it should be administered cautiously in all patients with asthma. A peak flow test should be done prior to injection and should be above 70 percent of the predicted value (or above 70 percent of the patient's personal best) before an injection is administered. For patients who are at high risk of adverse effects, a peak flow value should be determined before the patient leaves the office to ensure that there is no decrement after the injection. Some authors have suggested that children under the age of five should not receive immunotherapy because of the increased risk associated with bronchospasm in this age group.[16]

Guidelines for the Use of Immunotherapy

Because of the risk of anaphylaxis, recent guidelines have been published to properly identify patients who should (or should not) receive immunotherapy.[17,18] The Canadian Society of Allergy and Clinical Immunology published guidelines in 1995.[17] The consensus is that immunotherapy should be administered only with a specific allergen when patients have documented IgE disease and have not improved following avoidance techniques. Before immunotherapy is initiated, a failure of control of symptoms with medications should be documented. Patients who have autoimmune disease or uncontrolled asthma or who are under the age of five should not receive immunotherapy because the risks of such therapy exceed the benefits. If immunotherapy failed to alleviate the symptoms in the past, a second trial should not be attempted. If the patient's symptoms do not respond within the first two years of immunotherapy, the attempt should be discontinued. Lastly, the guidelines suggest that high-dose therapy should only be used for a maximum of five years.

The American Academy of Allergy and Immunology published immunotherapy guidelines in 1994.[18] This consensus suggests that immunotherapy should not be self-administered by the patient. Rather, it should be administered in a physician's office, with a physician in the immediate vicinity. The physician should be knowledgeable in both the treatment of anaphylaxis and the administration of immunotherapy. Patients with asthma should be observed for 30 minutes after an immunotherapy injection. The suggested emergency equipment that should be available in the office is listed in Table 52.3. Of note, defibrillation equipment is not considered essential.

Even though alternate routes of administration are being investigated, the standard of care is still the use of subcutaneous immunotherapy. High-potency and, in most cases, standardized extract should be used. Appropriate dose reductions should be made if local reactions are large, systemic adverse effects are noted, delays in therapy occur, or the vials are changed. One or two nurses who are knowledgeable in immunotherapy administration should be responsible for the program, and informed consent should be obtained before starting immunotherapy. As with any other injection, universal precautions should be maintained.

Table 53.3. Equipment Needed to Avert Immunotherapy Complications

- Intravenous equipment and needles
- Equipment to establish an oral airway
- Epinephrine
- Tourniquet
- Injectable antihistamine
- Injectable steroids
- Aminophylline
- Oxygen
- Vasopressors

Contraindications

Relative and absolute contraindications to immunotherapy are listed in Table 52.4. Pregnancy is not an absolute contraindication. Once a patient is receiving maintenance therapy, the risk of anaphylaxis is minimal and, thus, immunotherapy can be continued during pregnancy as long as there is no prior history of adverse effects.

Initiation of immunotherapy during pregnancy is too risky, however, and should not be done.[17]

Although no evidence suggests an increased incidence of autoimmune diseases in patients who are receiving immunotherapy, the concern is that an increased production of IgG stimulated by immunotherapy may be a risk factor for the development of immune complex-mediated disease. Thus, most authorities recommend not administering immunotherapy in patients with a history of autoimmune disease.[17]

Patients who have unstable coronary artery disease or who are receiving beta-adrenergic blockers are at increased risk of death from anaphylaxis and are also at risk from the intervention (epinephrine) needed to treat anaphylaxis. Such patients should not receive immunotherapy.[14]

Children under the age of five also should not receive immunotherapy. Small-caliber airways result in a smaller respiratory reserve; therefore, children younger than age five are at increased risk of respiratory problems associated with immunotherapy. Similarly, patients with unstable asthma who have a forced expiratory volume in one second (FEV_1) or a peak flow value below 70 percent of predicted value should not receive immunotherapy because of their decreased respiratory reserve secondary to the underlying disease.[16]

Patients who repeatedly exhibit large local reactions should be given a reduced dose to decrease the risk of systemic reactions. If a patient has had systemic reactions in the past, immunotherapy is potentially dangerous and should be avoided.

Table 52.4. Relative and Absolute Contraindications to Immunotherapy

- Pregnancy*
- Autoimmune disease
- Unstable coronary artery disease
- Use of beta-adrenergic blocking agents
- Unstable asthma
- FEV_1 or peak flow below 70% of predicted value
- Age under 5 years

FEV_1 = forced expiratory volume in one second.

*Immunotherapy can be continued during pregnancy if the patient is receiving maintenance therapy and there are no adverse effects.

Preparation of Extracts

Immunotherapy doses should be mixed only by those well trained and experienced in the preparation and dilution of immunotherapy. Extracts that are used to formulate immunotherapy can be obtained from multiple pharmaceutical companies. In most cases, patients present to the office with the dilutions already prepared. The physician prescribing the immunotherapy should instruct the physician who is administering immunotherapy on the storage of the preparation, precautions, dose adjustments and emergency procedures to follow if adverse effects occur. An alternative to mixing the extract is to directly order pre-diluted extract from a pharmaceutical company. In this case, the physician should prescribe the dosing schedule, dilutions, and concentrations of the extract. Pharmaceutical companies should not prepare extract from RAST data, because clinical correlation is necessary to determine if a positive test is of significance. For example, a patient who has a positive test to ragweed but has never had symptoms during the ragweed season should not be desensitized to ragweed.

To decrease liability, deviation from the dosing schedule is not recommended. If the immunotherapy schedule needs to be adjusted or temporarily changed, an allergist or other physician who prepared the extract should be consulted. Immunotherapy schedules vary significantly, from very aggressive desensitization protocols, referred to as "rush protocols," which can achieve maintenance levels in days, to conservative protocols in which maintenance may take months to achieve. The dosing schedule varies, depending on the extract concentration, the number of serial dilutions prepared, the expected risk for adverse effects, and the patient's health.

To decrease the risks associated with immunotherapy, a quality assurance program should be in place. All vials should be appropriately labeled, and instructions should be easy to follow and read. Patients who have asthma should bring a peak flow meter with them to each appointment. As mentioned previously, their peak flow value should be above 70 percent of their expected value. Because of the small risk of a delayed reaction, patients may want to have self-injectable epinephrine, such as an EpiPen, available at home. This is especially true for people who are at high risk of adverse reactions. Extending the waiting period from the usual 20 minutes to 30 minutes for patients most likely to experience adverse events may also decrease the risk of complications from a delayed reaction at home. Patients who are symptomatic, especially with signs and symptoms of asthma, should not receive their allergy injection that day.

A dose of subcutaneous epinephrine should be readily available in each room where immunotherapy is given so that the response to anaphylaxis can be rapid, to avert the progression of side effects associated with the use of immunotherapy.

Duration of Immunotherapy

Studies have demonstrated both short- and long-term benefits of immunotherapy. These benefits persist even after discontinuation of the immunotherapy. One study demonstrated that the IgE level, the signs and symptoms and the response to a histamine challenge showed continued improvement three to five years after discontinuation of immunotherapy.[6] In general, immunotherapy is administered for three to five years. A trial of discontinuing immunotherapy should be attempted after three to five years of therapy.[17]

Alternative Forms of Immunotherapy

Recently, three alternative routes of immunotherapy have been attempted. These include sublingual, oral, and intranasal immunotherapy.[19-21] In the United States, all three alternate routes of immunotherapy are considered experimental and are limited to use in research projects.

References

1. Creticos PS. Immunotherapy in asthma. *J Allergy Clin Immunol* 1989;83(2 Pt 2):554-62.

2. Van Bever HP, Stevens WJ. Evolution of the late asthmatic reaction during immunotherapy and after stopping immunotherapy. *J Allergy Clin Immunol* 1990;86:141-6.

3. Creticos PS, Van Metre TE, Mardiney MR, Rosenberg GL, Norman PS, Adkinson NF Jr. Dose response of IgE and IgG antibodies during ragweed immunotherapy. *J Allergy Clin Immunol* 1984;73(1 Pt 1):94-104.

4. Reid MJ, Moss RB, Hsu YP, Kwasnicki JM, Commerford TM, Nelson BL. Seasonal asthma in northern California: allergic causes and efficacy of immunotherapy. *J Allergy Clin Immunol* 1986;78(4 Pt 1):590-600.

5. Van Metre TE, Adkinson NF Jr, Amodio FJ, Lichtenstein LM, Mardiney MR, Norman PS, et al. A comparative study of the effectiveness of the Rinkel method and the current standard method of immunotherapy for ragweed pollen hay fever. *J Allergy Clin Immunol* 1980;66:500-13.

6. Hedlin G, Heilborn H, Lilja G, Norrlind K, Pegelow KO, Schou C, et al. Long-term follow-up of patients treated with a three-year course of cat or dog immunotherapy. *J Allergy Clin Immunol* 1995;96(6 Pt 1):879-85.

7. Ostergaard PA, Kaad PH, Kristensen T. A prospective study on the safety of immunotherapy in children with severe asthma. *Allergy* 1986;41:588-93.

8. Peat JK, Tovey E, Toelle BG, Haby MM, Gray EJ, Mahmic A, et al. House dust mite allergens. A major risk factor for childhood asthma in Australia. *Am J Respir Crit Care Med* 1996; 153:141-6.

9. Adinoff AD. Environmental controls and immunotherapy in the treatment of chronic asthma, *J Asthma* 1990-27:277-89.

10. Creticos PS, Reed CE, Norman PS, Khoury J, Adkinson NF Jr, Buncher CR, et al. Ragweed immunotherapy in adult asthma. *N Engl J Med* 1996;334: 501-6.

11. Abramson MJ, Puy RM, Weiner JM. Is allergen immunotherapy effective in asthma? A meta-analysis of randomized controlled trials. *Am J Respir Crit Care Med* 1995; 151:969-74.

12. Sigman K, Mazer B. Immunotherapy for childhood asthma: is there a rationale for its use? *Ann Allergy Asthma Immunol* 1996;76;299-305.

13. Hejjaoui A. Ferrando R, Dhivert H, Michel FB, Bousquet J. Systemic reactions occurring during immunotherapy with standardized pollen extracts. *J Allergy Clin Immunol* 1992;89:925-33.

14. Reid MJ, Lockey RF, Turkeltaub PC, Platts-Mills TA. Survey of fatalities from skin testing and immunotherapy 1985-1989. *J Allergy Clin Immunol* 1993; 92(1 Pt 1): 6-15.

15. Wells JH. Systemic reactions to immunotherapy: comparisons between two large allergy practices. *J Allergy Clin Immunol* 1996;97:1030-2.

16. Bousquet J, Michel FB. Specific immunotherapy in asthma. *Allergy Proc* 1994; 15:329-33.

17. Canadian Society of Allergy and Clinical Immunology. Guidelines for the use of allergen immunotherapy. *Can Med Assoc J* 1995; 152:1413-9.

18. American Academy of Allergy and Immunology. Guidelines to minimize the risk from systemic reactions caused by immunotherapy with allergenic extracts. *J Allergy Clin Immunol* 1994;93-811-2.

19. Nelson HS, Oppenheimer J, Vatsia GA, Buchmeier A. A double-blind, placebo-controlled evaluation of sublingual immunotherapy with standardized cat extract. *J Allergy Clin Immunol* 1993;92:229-36.

20. Bordignon G, DiBerardino L. Efficacia di una nuova immunoteropia per graminacee ad assorbimento orale. Studio parallelo esequito pertre anni. *Giornace It Allergol Immunol Clin* 1994;4:153-9.

21. Andri L, Senna G, Andri G, Dama A, Givanni S, Betteli C, et al. Local nasal immunotherapy for birch allergic rhinitis with extract in powder form. *Clin Exp Aller* 1995;25:1092-9.

— by Timothy Craig,
Amy M. Sawyer, and
John A. Fornadley

Timothy Craig, D.O., is presently an associate professor and chief of the allergy service in the Department of Medicine at Milton S. Hershey Medical Center, Hershey, Pennsylvania. He graduated from the New York College of Osteopathic Medicine, New York City, and received training in allergy and immunology at Walter Reed Medical Center, Washington, DC, and in internal medicine at San Diego Naval Hospital. His research interests are asthma, rhinitis, and hypersensitivity pneumonitis.

Amy M. Sawyer, R.N., M.SC.N., is a pulmonary clinical nurse specialist at Milton S. Hershey Medical Center. She is a graduate of Johns Hopkins University School of Nursing, Baltimore. Her clinical background includes medical and surgical critical care nursing and management of special care areas, including the emergency department, critical care, and prehospital systems.

John A. Fornadley, M.D., is an otolaryngologist at Milton S. Hershey Medical Center. He is a graduate of Pennsylvania State University College of Medicine, Harrisburg. Following an internship at Bethesda (Maryland) Naval Hospital, he served as a medical officer with Submarine Squadron Six in Norfolk, Virginia, before entering an otolaryngology residency at Portsmouth Naval Hospital. He has a particular interest in sinonasal disease, allergy, and Eustachian tube function.

Chapter 53

Anti-Immunoglobulin E (IgE) Therapy for Asthma

Some people with allergic asthma can experience improvement in their symptoms even as they reduce or completely eliminate the need for oral or inhaled corticosteroids by using anti-IgE, according to the latest issue of the *New England Journal of Medicine*.

"This is a completely new approach to therapy, one that may greatly improve the treatment outlook for people with allergic asthma. It's unlike anything that's been used before," said Henry Milgrom, M.D., lead author of the article and a pediatric asthma specialist at National Jewish Medical and Research Center. The study information published in the *New England Journal of Medicine* is the result of Phase II clinical trials.

Thirty-three percent of patients in the high dose anti-IgE group and 43 percent in the low dose group completely eliminated the use of oral corticosteroids, which come in syrup and pill form. Seventeen percent taking the placebo stopped using oral corticosteroids, as well. (Researchers believe that patient education throughout the study encouraged better self-management of asthma, leading to the drop in medication use in the placebo groups.)

"Oral corticosteroids suppress the swelling and inflammation of the airways that are responsible for asthma symptoms. These drugs have serious long-term side-effects, such as osteoporosis, high blood pressure, cataracts, and, in children, slowed growth. The ability to eliminate or reduce the need for this medicine would be a very favorable development in the treatment of allergic asthma," Dr. Milgrom said.

Anti-IgE medication has minimal side effects. "Anti-IgE therapy may reduce steroid use in some patients and eliminate it in others," he added.

Dr. Milgrom and other researchers around the United States were involved in a multi-center study of more than 300 adolescents and adults with moderate to severe allergic asthma. All patients used inhaled and/or oral corticosteroids to control the disease, which can be triggered by allergies to pollen, animal dander, mold, or dust mites.

Patients received a high or low dose of anti-IgE or placebo throughout the study. During the first 12 weeks, patients took anti-IgE or a placebo as well as their inhaled and/or oral corticosteroids. For the next eight weeks patients continued to take anti-IgE or placebo while they were weaned from corticosteroids.

IgE, an antibody in the immune system, causes allergic symptoms by attaching to certain cells in the body. When these cells come in contact with an allergen, a substance to which an allergy sufferer is sensitive, allergic symptoms such as coughing, wheezing, nasal congestion, hives, and swelling begin. Anti-IgE binds IgE and removes it from circulation. In the study, IgE in patients' blood was reduced by more than 95 percent. IgE was discovered by National Jewish researchers in 1966.

Symptoms, such as chest tightness, wheezing, or excessive coughing, improved by 42 percent in people receiving high [doses] and 40 percent in those on low doses of anti-IgE. In people receiving the placebo, asthma symptoms improved by 30 percent.

For those using oral corticosteroids, 78 percent on high dose anti-IgE and 57 percent on low dose were able to reduce corticosteroid use by more than 50 percent. Thirty-three percent on placebo had a 50 percent reduction in oral corticosteroid use.

In addition to a reduced requirement for corticosteroids, patients had markedly improved scores on quality-of-life questionnaires that assessed their activities, asthma symptoms, emotional functioning, and symptoms induced by environmental exposures.

Anti-IgE is being developed jointly by Genentech, Inc., Novartis Pharma AG, and Tanox, Inc. The companies are collaborating in the evaluation of the safety and efficacy of this drug in the therapy of asthma and seasonal allergic rhinitis.

Chapter 54

How to Use Your Inhaler Effectively

Using an inhaler seems simple, but most patients do not use it the right way. When you use your inhaler the wrong way, less medicine gets to your lungs. (Your doctor may give you other types of inhalers.)

For the next 2 weeks, read these steps aloud as you do them or ask someone to read them to you. Ask your doctor or nurse to check how well you are using your inhaler.

Use your inhaler in one of the three ways pictured (Figures 54.1 or 54.2 are best, but Figure 54.3 can be used if you have trouble with Figures 54.1 and 54.2).

Steps for Using Your Inhaler

Getting ready:

1. Take off the cap and shake the inhaler.

2. Breathe out all the way.

3. Hold your inhaler the way your doctor said (Figure 54.1, 54.2, or 54.3 on pages 430–431).

Excerpted from "How to Use Your Metered-Dose Inhaler the Right Way," in *Practical Guide for the Diagnosis and Management of Asthma,* based on the *Expert Panel Report 2: Guidelines for the Diagnosis and Management of Asthma.* Produced by U.S. Department of Health and Human Services, National Heart, Lung, and Blood Institute (NHLBI), NIH Publication No. 97-4053, October 1997.

Breathe in slowly:

4.   As you start breathing in slowly through your mouth, press down on the inhaler one time. (If you use a holding chamber, first press down on the inhaler. Within 5 seconds, begin to breathe in slowly.)

5.   Keep breathing in slowly, as deeply as you can.

Hold your breath:

6.   Hold your breath as you count to 10 slowly, if you can.

7.   For inhaled quick-relief medicine (beta$_2$-agonists), wait about 1 minute between puffs. There is no need to wait between puffs for other medicines.

Figure 54.1. Hold inhaler 1 to 2 inches in front of your mouth (about the width of two fingers).

Figure 54.2. Use a spacer/ holding chamber. These come in many shapes and can be useful to any patient.

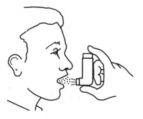

Figure 54.3. Put the inhaler in your mouth. Do not use for steroids.

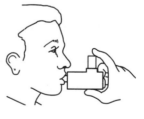

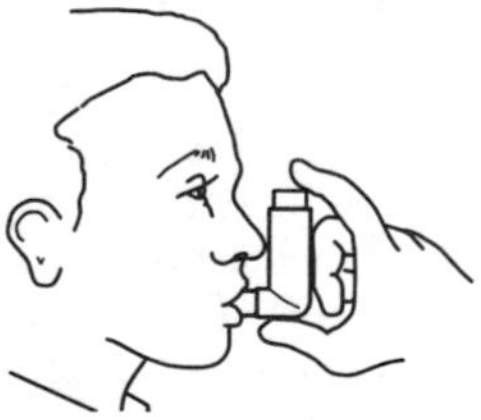

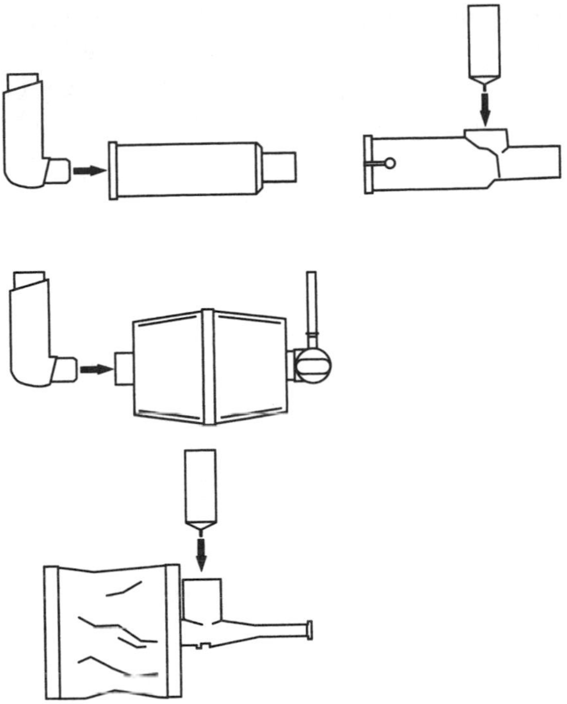

Figure 54.4. Examples of spacer/holding chamber devices.

Clean Your Inhaler as Needed

Look at the hole where the medicine sprays out from your inhaler. If you see "powder" in or around the hole, clean the inhaler. Remove the metal canister from the L-shaped plastic mouthpiece. Rinse only the mouthpiece and cap in warm water. Let them dry overnight. In the morning, put the canister back inside. Put the cap on.

Know When to Replace Your Inhaler

For medicines you take each day, [follow this example]. Say your new canister has 200 puffs (number of puffs is listed on canister) and you are told to take 8 puffs per day. [Divide 200 puffs by 8 puffs to find the number of days this canister will last. The answer is 25.] So this canister will last 25 days.

If you started using this inhaler on May 1, replace it on or before May 25. You can write the date on your canister.

For quick-relief medicine take as needed and count each puff.

Do not put your canister in water to see if it is empty. This does not work.

Chapter 55

Preservatives in Certain Asthma Medications May Be Harmful

Preservatives used in certain asthma medications may be doing more harm than good in some patients. Researchers say that the stabilizer edetate disodium (EDTA) and the preservative benzalkonium chloride (BAC), which are commonly used in nebulizer solutions for the treatment of asthma and chronic pulmonary disease, actually counteract the effects of the medications in many patients.

Approximately 15 million people in the United States are affected by asthma, 5 million of whom are children, according to the Department of Health and Human Services. There was an overall increase of 75% in the number of cases of asthma between 1980 and 1994, with an increase of 160% among preschool children for the same period. Many researchers feel there is a strong link between environmental conditions and the development of asthma.

The treatment of asthma usually involves two medication options, according to Phillip Korenblat, a professor of clinical medicine at Washington University in St. Louis, Missouri, and a spokesman for the American College of Allergy, Asthma, and Immunology—rapid relievers, or bronchodilators, and long-term controllers. Korenblat says that asthma patients should keep a rapid reliever available at all times in the case of an asthma attack, but they should not rely on such a medication for long-term treatment. There are two types of bronchodilators—multidose inhalers, which administer medicine by means of a propellant or dry powder, and nebulizer solutions, which

"Not Breathing Easier," *Environmental Health Perspectives*, Volume 106, Number 8, August 1998.

are delivered by an air compressor in the form of a spray designed to be inhaled. Korenblat says a very small minority of asthma patients use the nebulizer solutions. However, they are often administered to patients in hospitals and in emergency situations.

An article by asthma researchers at the Wellington College of Medicine in New Zealand and the University of Florida in Gainesville, published in the January-February 1998 issue of *Pharmacotherapy*, offers a review of studies conducted on nebulizer solutions both with and without the preservatives. The preservatives BAC and EDTA are added to nebulizer solutions that are dispensed in multidose dropper bottles and unit-dose screw-cap products in order to keep them sterile. The medications contained in nebulizer solutions are designed to open the bronchial tubes leading to the lungs, but the authors contend that at standard doses BAC constricts these airways, working against the medications and sometimes worsening the lung function in patients. They say EDTA causes the same effects in higher doses.

The authors also state that the addition of the preservatives was not preceded by safety studies, and they cite evidence that, indeed, the preservatives do not prevent bacterial contamination. Leslie Hendeles, a professor of pharmacy and pediatrics at the University of Florida who coauthored the study, says, "The preservatives don't prevent bacterial contamination, so they don't appear to have any benefits, and can actually cause harm."

The authors recommend that patients avoid the preservatives by using nebulizer solutions that are dispensed in preservative-free, sterile, single-dose vials, which have been shown to remain free of significant bacterial contamination. They point out that these single-dose vials are either the preferred product or the only nebulizer solutions available in most Western countries.

Current U.S. regulations do not require manufacturers to list on the label the concentration of preservatives contained in a product, and the amount of preservatives varies greatly between products. Also, it is legal for pharmacists to substitute these medications for one another so that even when a doctor has prescribed a preservative-free product, one containing high concentrations of BAC may be dispensed. The authors of the *Pharmacotherapy* study recommend that U.S. regulatory agencies ban the use of preservatives. In the meantime, Hendeles says he hopes the risks associated with the preservatives are communicated to pharmacists. He has worked with the Florida State Board of Pharmacy to issue a warning about the preservatives in its newsletter.

Even though a small number of patients use nebulizer solutions, Korenblat says the new information is cause for concern, and the medications should be studied further. He also says that patients should be aware of this information. "This should not raise alarm for people who have been doing well," Korenblat says, "but it is significant enough that asthma patients should know about it."

At this time, the FDA is not planning to take action on the issue, according to Robert Meyer, a medical team leader in the Division of Pulmonary Drug Products at the FDA. He says, "This is an issue that we had already been familiar with for quite a while." Because there is concern, he says the FDA recommends that the use of preservatives be avoided wherever possible, and if preservatives are necessary, they should be used in the lowest amounts possible. "We don't feel like this is a major public health problem," Meyer says. "The bottom line is that an individual who has been known to have adverse reactions should be careful to avoid the preservatives."

Chapter 56

Alternate Therapies for Allergies: Insufficient Data

Chapter Contents

Section 56.1

Researching Unusual Remedies for Asthma, Allergies, and Immunology

"OAM-Supported CAM Clinical Research Center Studies Unusual Remedies for Asthma, Allergies, and Immunology," *CAM Newsletter*, National Center for Complementary and Alternative Medicine, (NCCAM), Fall 1998.

Each year, increasing numbers of Americans seek relief in doctor's offices and pharmacies across the country for their wheezing, itching, sneezing, and difficulty breathing—symptoms caused by allergies and asthma.

According to the National Institute of Allergy and Infectious Diseases (NIAID), as many as 50 million Americans have allergies and more than 14.6 million battle asthma. Among inner city populations, asthma has been called epidemic: the death rate among African American children and teenagers resulting from asthma nearly doubled between 1980 and 1993, according to the NIAID. The Institute is a component of the National Institutes of Health (NIH) that conducts and supports research to prevent, diagnose, and treat illnesses such as sexually transmitted diseases, asthma, and allergies.

Over-the-counter and prescription drugs are the treatments used most commonly to alleviate symptoms. Now, with help from a clinical research center funded by the OAM, [Office of Alternative Medicine] additional relief could be on the way. Researchers at the Center for Complementary and Alternative Medicine Research in Asthma, Allergy, and Immunology at the University of California at Davis are studying a range of unlikely sources, from ancient Chinese health practices to grass juice.

One current study is examining whether people with hay fever will improve after taking the very thing that ails them: a juice made from wheat and rich in pollen, the substance that actually causes hay fever. According to Merrill Eric Gershwin, M.D., the principal investigator at the Center, recent pilot research suggests that oral immunotherapy, the ingestion of pollen allergens and particularly the main IgE-binding protein found in grasses, may be a promising complementary therapy

498

for people with seasonal allergic rhinitis or hay fever. The protein is also present in the blood of many people with hay fever.

"It's a 'like cures like' theory that the immune system can build a resistance to these allergens," says Dr. Gershwin. "Oral immunotherapy may be a very promising, safe, and low-cost option for managing seasonal hay fever and asthma."

To test this theory, Dr. Gershwin and Judith S. Stern, Sc.D., R.D., the Center's co-principal investigator, designed a randomized, double-blind, placebo-controlled trial in which researchers are determining whether people with hay fever who drink the juice every day for a year will "desensitize" their immune systems to the allergen.

The grass juice trial is just one of several small-scale but scientifically rigorous studies the Center is conducting on complementary and alternative medicine (CAM) therapies. With a nearly $1 million grant from the OAM, the Center began 3 years ago as one of the 13 OAM-funded research centers that investigate CAM.

Review of Scientific Literature

Researchers began by reviewing thousands of research papers on asthma and allergies; they found few solid scientific trials about complementary and alternative medicine treatments published in reputable, peer-reviewed publications, according to Dr. Gershwin. Next, the Center conducted a national survey of physicians, CAM practitioners, and their asthma and allergy patients to determine which CAM therapies were used most and the therapies about which patients most frequently asked their doctors.

Dietary changes and nutritional and botanical supplements were the therapies most frequently asked about, the survey found. Dr. Gershwin says that many of the alternative treatments people in the survey reported using have not been tested and probably don't work.

"We are hoping that we've identified the most promising therapies to scientifically evaluate," he adds. "We want to one day tell consumers what works and what doesn't, but it will not be overnight. These conditions are complex."

After the findings from the literature search and survey were evaluated, the Center called for proposals from scientists to conduct research. More than 50 applications underwent extramural executive committee reviews at the University of California at Davis Medical School. Five projects on promising therapies for treating asthma and allergies were selected: acupressure, biofeedback, botanical and glandular extracts, grass juice, and vitamin C.

"There is a tremendous interest in all of these studies," Dr. Gershwin says. "We get inquiries from patients and physicians alike. We have to tell them to wait until we thoroughly test these therapies."

Section 56.2

Questioning the Efficacy of Homeopathic Allergy Remedies

From "What's the Alternative?" by Fred Gebhart, in *Drug Topics,* Vol. 141, No. 7, April 7, 1997, p. 72. Copyright © 1997 Medical Economics Publishing Co. Reprinted with permission.

Patients who use homeopathic or other alternative remedies may not be harming themselves, but they probably aren't doing themselves much good either. That's the conclusion of a small pilot study conducted by James DeMasi, associate professor of pediatrics at Albany Medical College in Albany, N.Y.

"I wouldn't try to push these results very far at all," DeMasi told an audience at the American Academy of Allergy, Asthma, and Immunology's annual meeting in San Francisco last month. "This at least indicates that alternative medicines are safe, if not very effective."

DeMasi tested the antihistamine effect of an over-the-counter homeopathic remedy in seven patients suffering from seasonal allergic rhinitis. The four-week trial included a one-week baseline followed by random double blinded crossover treatment with an active and a placebo homeopathic product. Histamine prick skin tests were performed before treatment as well as one day into treatment and one week after treatment.

Homeopathy is based on the premise that "like cures like," DeMasi explained. A major difference between homeopathy and more traditional immunotherapy, he noted, is the level of allergen present to challenge the immune system. Injections designed to desensitize patients to specific allergens contain a measurable quantity of the target substance. Homeopathic products, by contrast, are diluted to the point that they contain no measurable allergen.

DeMasi said he chose his test product, Doliosos Energy, on the recommendation of a homeopathic pharmacist for the treatment of seasonal allergic rhinitis. The label listed *Allium cepa* (red onion), *Apis mellifica* (honey bee), *Arsenicum album* (arsenic), *Euphrasia officinalis* (eyebright), and *Nux vomica* (poison nut) as active ingredients.

There was no change in skin test reactivity in any of the patients, indicating that neither the active product nor the placebo had any effect on histamine levels, DeMasi reported.

"It's not even a valid scientific method," charged Bill Nicholetti, a pharmacist and president of Doliosos USA. "Using histamine levels to determine the efficacy of a homeopathic product makes as much sense as using orange juice to test for the presence of apples. Too many allopathic practitioners don't want to accept that alternative medicines can work."

DeMasi said he began looking at the safety and efficacy of alternative remedies because Americans spend as much on alternative medicine as they do on traditional allopathic treatments. Many herbal, homeopathic, and other alternative medicines are accepted by medical communities, insurers, and government-sponsored health plans in Europe and elsewhere.

Lack of proven efficacy doesn't mean that homeopathic products will fail in all patients, DeMasi emphasized. One patient dropped out of the study because all of his rhinitis symptoms disappeared soon after taking the initial dose. "This patient was absolutely convinced that one dose of the homeopathic product had cured him of rhinitis," said DeMasi. "He couldn't see any reason to continue in the study when it was obvious that homeopathy worked. When we broke the code, it turned out that he had received the placebo."

Section 56.3

If You Are Considering Complementary and Alternative Therapies for Allergies

"Considering CAM?" an undated fact sheet produced by the National Center for Complementary and Alternative Medicine, (NCCAM). Available at http://www.nccam.nih.gov.

The decision to use complementary and alternative treatments is an important one. The following are topics to consider before selecting an alternative therapy: the safety and effectiveness of the therapy or treatment; the expertise and qualifications of the healthcare practitioner; and the quality of the service delivery. These topics should be considered when selecting any practitioner or therapy.

Assess the Safety and Effectiveness of the Therapy

Generally, safety means that the benefits outweigh the risks of a treatment or therapy. A safe product or practice is one that does no harm when used under defined conditions and as intended. Effectiveness is the likelihood of benefit from a practice, treatment, or technology applied under typical conditions by the average practitioner for the typical patient. Many people find that specific information about an alternative and complementary therapy's safety and effectiveness may be less readily available than information about conventional medical treatments. Research on these therapies is ongoing, and continues to grow.

You may want to ask a healthcare practitioner, whether a physician or a practitioner of complementary and alternative healthcare, about the safety and effectiveness of the therapy or treatment he or she uses. Tell the practitioner about any alternative or conventional treatments or therapies you may already be receiving, as this information may be used to consider the safety and effectiveness of the entire treatment plan.

The practitioner may have literature with information about the safety and effectiveness of the therapy. Credible information may be found in scientific research literature obtained through public libraries, university libraries, medical libraries, and online computer services, such as "CAM on PubMed" and the U.S. National Library of Medicine at the National Institutes of Health (http://www.nlm.nih.gov).

CAM on PubMed

CAM on PubMed (http://www.nlm.nih.gov/nccam/camonpubmed.html), developed jointly by the National Library of Medicine and the National Center for Complementary and Alternative Medicine, contains bibliographic citations (1966-present) related to complementary and alternative medicine. These citations are a subset of the National Library of Medicine's PubMed system that contains over 11 million journal citations from the MEDLINE database and additional life science journals important to health researchers, practitioners and consumers. CAM on PubMed also displays links to publisher web sites offering full text of articles.

For information about researching alternative medical therapies using the NLM, please contact the National Center for Complementary and Alternative Medicine (NCCAM) Clearinghouse (http://nccam.nih.gov/fcp/clearinghouse/index.html) and request the fact sheet, "Alternative Medicine Research Using MEDLINE."

Additional Sources of Information

For general, nonscientific information, thousands of articles on health issues and complementary and alternative medicine are published in books, journals, and magazines every year. Articles that appear in popular magazines and journals may be located by using the *Reader's Guide to Periodical Literature* available in most libraries. For articles published in more than 3,000 health science journals, consult the *Index Medicus*, found in medical and university libraries and some public libraries.

Be an informed health consumer and continue gathering information even after a practitioner has been selected. Ask the practitioner about specific new research that may support or not support the safety and effectiveness of the treatment or therapy. Ask about the advantages and disadvantages, risks, side effects, expected results, and length of treatment that you can expect.

Speak with people who have undergone the treatment, preferably both those who were treated recently and those treated in the past.

Optimally, find people with the same health condition that you have and who have received the treatment.

Remember that patient testimonials used alone do not adequately assess the safety and effectiveness of an alternative therapy, and should not be the exclusive criterion for selecting a therapy. Controlled scientific trials usually provide the best information about a therapy's effectiveness and should be sought whenever possible.

Examine the Practitioner's Expertise

Health consumers may want to take a close look into the background, qualifications, and competence of any potential healthcare practitioner, whether a physician or a practitioner of alternative and complementary healthcare.

First, contact a state or local regulatory agency with authority over practitioners who practice the therapy or treatment you seek. The practice of complementary and alternative medicine usually is not as regulated as the practice of conventional medicine. Licensing, accreditation, and regulatory laws, however, are increasingly being implemented.

Local and state medical boards, other health regulatory boards or agencies, and consumer affairs departments provide information about a specific practitioner's license, education, and accreditation, and whether there are any complaints lodged against the practitioner. Check to see if the practitioner is licensed to deliver the services the practitioner says he or she delivers.

Appropriate state licensing of education and practice is the only way to ensure that the practitioner is competent and provides quality services. Most types of complementary and alternative practices have national organizations of practitioners that are familiar with legislation, state licensing, certification, or registration laws.

Some organizations will direct medical consumers to the appropriate regulatory agencies in their state. These organizations also may provide referrals and information about specific practitioners. The organizations usually do not function as regulatory authorities, but promote the services of their members.

Second, talk with those who have had experience with this practitioner, both health practitioners and other patients. Find out about the confidence and competence of the practitioner in question, and whether there have ever been any complaints from patients.

Third, talk with the practitioner in person. Ask about the practitioner's education, additional training, licenses, and certifications, both unconventional and conventional. Ask about the practitioner's approach to treatment and patients. Find out how open the practitioner is to communicating with patients about technical aspects of methods, possible side effects, and potential problems.

When selecting a healthcare practitioner, many medical consumers seek someone knowledgeable in a wide variety of disciplines. Look for a practitioner who is easy to talk to. You should feel comfortable asking questions. After you select a practitioner, the education process and dialogue between you and your practitioner should become an ongoing aspect of complementary healthcare.

Consider the Service Delivery

The quality of the service delivery, or how the treatment or therapy is given and under what conditions, is an important issue. However, quality of service is not necessarily related to the effectiveness or safety of a treatment or practice.

Visit the practitioner's office, clinic, or hospital. Ask the practitioner how many patients he or she typically sees in a day or week, and how much time the practitioner spends with the patient. Look at the conditions of the office or clinic.

Many issues surround quality of service delivery, and each one individually does not provide conclusive and complete information. For example, are the costs of the service excessive for what is delivered? Can the service be obtained only in one place, requiring travel to that place? These issues may serve as warning signs of poor service.

The primary issue to consider is whether the service delivery adheres to regulated standards for medical safety and care.

Contact regulatory boards or agencies described in the previous section to obtain objective information. You also may gather information by talking with people who have used the service, and through healthcare consumer organizations.

Consider the Costs

Costs are an important factor to consider as many complementary and alternative treatments are not currently reimbursed by health insurance. Many patients pay directly for these services. Ask your practitioner and your health insurer which treatments or therapies are reimbursable.

Find out what several practitioners charge for the same treatment to better assess the appropriateness of costs. Regulatory agencies and professional associations also may provide cost information.

Consult Your Healthcare Provider

Most importantly, discuss all issues concerning treatments and therapies with your healthcare provider whether a physician or practitioner of complementary and alternative medicine.

Competent healthcare management requires knowledge of both conventional and alternative therapies for the practitioner to have a complete picture of your treatment plan.

Chapter 57

Home Control of Allergies

Air Particles We Breathe

Many particles of different types and sizes are carried in the air we breathe. Some large particles may settle on the walls and furniture in your home. Other large particles are removed by your nose and mouth when you inhale. Smaller particles are breathed deep into the lungs.

Asthma may be triggered by both the large and small particles. Some air particles come from the indoors. Others are carried in the outdoor air. Outdoor particles come into your home through windows, doors, and heating systems.

For most people, the indoor air particles cause no problems. But people with allergic symptoms including asthma can have problems, right in their own home.

Asthma and Allergy "Triggers"

If you or someone you know have allergic symptoms or asthma, you are sensitive to "triggers," including particles carried in the air. These "triggers" can set off a reaction in your lungs and other parts of your body. Triggers can be found indoors or outdoors. They can be simple things like:

- Cold air.

- Tobacco smoke and wood smoke.

- Perfume, paint, hair spray, or any strong odors or fumes.

- Allergens (particles that cause allergies) such as dust mites, pollen, molds, pollution, and animal dander (which are tiny scales or particles that fall off hair, feathers or skin) from any pets.

- Common cold, influenza, and other respiratory illnesses.

You may be able to add more triggers to this list. Other things may also trigger your asthma or allergies. It's important to learn which triggers are a problem for you. Ask your doctor to help. Your doctor may suggest:

- Keeping an asthma diary.

- Skin testing to test for allergies.

- A special diet to look for food allergies.

- Cold air.

Finding triggers isn't always easy. If you do know your triggers, cutting down exposure to them may help avoid asthma and allergy attacks.

If you don't know your triggers, try to limit your exposure to one suspected trigger at a time. Watch to see if you get better. This may show you if the trigger was a problem for you.

Outdoor Air, Indoor Air, and Air-Conditioning

Controlling your exposure to triggers outdoors is hard. You may have to avoid outdoor air pollution, pollen, and mold spores. Any time air pollution and pollen levels are high, it's a good idea to stay indoors.

The air at home is easier to control. Some people with asthma and allergies notice that their symptoms get worse at night. Trigger controls in the bedroom or wherever you sleep need the most care.

Air-conditioning can help. It allows windows and doors to stay closed. This keeps some pollen and mold spores outside. It also lowers indoor humidity. Low humidity helps to control mold and dust mites.

Avoid too much air-conditioning or too much heat. Room air temperature should be comfortable for someone with allergies or asthma. Some people can't tolerate a big change in temperature, particularly from warm to cold air.

There are some devices that effectively remove particles from air. Their usefulness in reducing allergy symptoms is under study.

Trigger Controls

Here are some common triggers and some ways to help control them at home:

Tobacco Smoke

Smoke should not be allowed in the home of someone with asthma or allergies. Ask family members and friends to smoke outdoors. Suggest that they quit smoking. Your local American Lung Association can help. Ask your Lung Association how you can help a family member or friend quit smoking.

Wood Smoke

Wood smoke is a problem for children and adults with asthma and allergies. Avoid wood stoves and fireplaces.

Pets

Almost all pets can cause allergies, including dogs and especially cats. Small animals like birds, hamsters and guinea pigs can cause problems, so all pets should be removed from the home if pets trigger asthma and allergy symptoms.

Pet allergen may stay in the home for months after the pet is gone because it remains in house dust. Allergy and asthma symptoms may take some time to get better.

If the pet stays in the home, keep it out of the bedroom of anyone with asthma or allergies. Weekly pet baths may help cut down the amount of pet saliva and dander in the home.

Sometimes you hear that certain cats or dogs are "non-allergenic." There really is no such thing as a "non-allergenic" cat or dog, especially if the pet leaves dander and saliva in the home. Goldfish and other tropical fish may be a good substitute.

Cockroaches

Even cockroaches can cause problems, so it's important to get rid of roaches in your home. The cockroach allergen comes from dead roaches and roach droppings. It collects in house dust and is hard to remove. Careful cleaning (see tips under "Dust Mites") of your home will help.

Indoor Mold

When humidity is high, molds can be a problem in bathrooms, kitchens, and basements. Make sure these areas have good air circulation and are cleaned often. The basement in particular may need a dehumidifier. And remember, the water in the dehumidifier must be emptied and the container cleaned often to prevent forming mildew.

Molds may form on foam pillows when you perspire. To prevent mold, put the pillow in an airtight cover and tape the cover shut. Wash the pillow every week, and make sure to change it every year.

Molds also form in house plants, so check them often. You may have to keep all plants outdoors.

Strong Odors or Fumes

Perfume, room deodorizers, cleaning chemicals, paint, and talcum powder are examples of triggers that must be avoided or kept to very low levels.

Dust Mites

Dust mites are tiny, microscopic spiders usually found in house dust. Several thousand mites can be found in a pinch of dust. Mites are one of the major triggers for people with allergies and asthma. They need the most work to remove.

Use an allergy control solution, a cleaner that can kill the mite allergen. Check with your doctor or pharmacist about what cleaner to buy.

Following these rules can also help get rid of dust mites:

- Put mattresses in airtight covers. Tape over the length of the zipper.

- Put pillows in airtight covers. Tape over the length of the zipper. Or wash the pillow every week.

- Wash all bedding every week in water that is at least 130 degrees F. Removing the bedspread at night may help.

- Don't sleep or lie down on upholstered (stuffed) furniture.

- Remove carpeting in the bedroom.

- Clean up surface dust as often as possible. Use a damp mop or damp cloth when you clean. Don't use aerosols or spray cleaners in the bedroom. And don't clean or vacuum the room when someone with asthma or allergies is present.

- Window coverings attract dust. Use window shades or curtains made of plastic or other washable material for easy cleaning.

- Remove stuffed furniture and stuffed animals (unless the animals can be washed), and anything under the bed.

- Closets need extra care. They should hold only needed clothing. Putting clothes in a plastic garment bag may help. (Do not use the plastic bag that covers dry cleaning).

- Dust mites like moisture and high humidity. Cutting down the humidity in your home can cut down the number of mites. A dehumidifier may help.

- Air filters may be of limited help by keeping your home cleaner and more comfortable. Ask your doctor for advice about air filters.

- Cover bedroom air vents with several layers of cheesecloth to lower the number of large-size allergen particles coming into the bedroom.

General Rules to Help Control the Home Environment

Controlling the home environment is a very important part of asthma and allergy care. Some general rules for home control for all members of the family are:

- Reduce or remove as many asthma and allergy triggers from your home as possible.

- If possible, use air filters and air conditioners to make your home cleaner and more comfortable.

- Pay attention to the problem of dust mites. Work hard to control this problem in the bedroom.

- Vacuum cleaners stir up dust and allergens in the air. A vacuum cleaner with an air filter or a central vacuum cleaner with a collection bag outside the home may be of limited value. Anyone with asthma or allergies should avoid vacuuming. If vacuuming must be done, a dust mask may help.

Chapter 58

Photocatalytic Air Cleaning System

Allergy and asthma sufferers soon may have a new weapon in their fight against airborne enemies: an indoor-air cleaning system that uses light and simple chemicals to destroy the dust mites and mold spores that cause many allergies.

Developed at the University of Florida's Solar Energy and Energy Conversion Laboratory, the photocatalytic air filtration system has been tested in medical and industrial settings and already has proven successful at zapping odors and impurities caused by chemicals, viruses, and bacteria. It soon will be available for home use, said Yogi Goswami, professor and director of the laboratory.

"This technology will revolutionize our notions about the quality of indoor air," Goswami said. "With people spending more and more time indoors, it becomes increasingly important to provide clean air."

The system uses light, which reacts with a titanium dioxide-based chemical catalyst as air passes through. The result is oxidation, which attacks and destroys microbes by disintegrating their DNA. The reaction also kills dust mites and mold.

Goswami said the photocatalytic process is superior to conventional techniques using filters, which must be changed and disposed of.

"With this system, contaminants are destroyed rather than transferred. No toxic chemicals are employed," Goswami explained. Allergy

From "Photocatalytic Air Cleaning System Promises to Help Allergy Sufferers," in *Doctor's Guide to the Internet*, October 14, 1997. © 1999 by P\S\L Consulting Group Inc. Reprinted by permission. *Doctor's Guide to the Internet* is at http://www.docguide.com.

and asthma suffers may find great relief once dust mites and mold spores are eliminated from the air they breathe.

"Dust mites in the air cause allergic reactions in an estimated 15 to 20 percent of the population and have been linked to the development of childhood asthma. The droppings of dust mites live in bedding and carpeting, but they also circulate in the air," Goswami said. "Inhaled mold spores are also responsible for many allergy symptoms and aggravate asthma. Mold seeds are microscopic and need to be 100 percent destroyed. Otherwise they lie dormant and grow back."

"Because mold spores also circulate in the air, cleaning an environmental surface is not an efficient way of eliminating molds. This system eliminates molds altogether."

Goswami said the system has been tested successfully in medical research settings where the air in laboratories must be microbe-free.

"We've tested the photocatalytic air cleaning system on a variety of indoor air problems, including toxic bacteria, such as those found to cause Legionnaire's disease," Goswami explained. "Surgical suites and hospital nurseries are just two obvious places for this system. Sick building syndrome will be a thing of the past where this system is used. The photocatalytic system can quickly kill off 100 percent of bacteria in indoor air."

The technology is being readied for the market by Universal Air Technology at the Sid Martin Phototechnology Development Institute, a biotechnical business incubator of the University of Florida.

Chapter 59

Ventilation/Cleaning System for Dust Mites

An aggressive effort to reduce levels of house dust mites and house dust allergens can have the same effect as a 400 microgram dose of inhaled steroids in improving asthma symptoms over a year, according to a new study.

The study, presented at the British Thoracic Society [BTS] winter meeting in London found that a new eradication technique combining dry and moist heat with a special ventilation system, can eradicate virtually all house dust mites (and mite allergens). Mites and mite allergens have long been identified as a key trigger to asthma attacks but long-term eradication has proved to be difficult to achieve.

The new home system described in the trial could provide an alternative to medication for some allergy sufferers, including those with asthma, rhinitis, and eczema, according to researchers from the University of Sheffield, England.

The researchers carried out a one-year, double-blind controlled trial of 30 adult asthmatics' homes in Sheffield where all soft furnishings, including mattresses, were treated with moistened air. Levels of house dust mites were measured four times within four months and showed a significant reduction at the end of the trial.

The researchers also looked at peak flow measurements and tests for bronchial hyper-responsiveness at five intervals over the same period. They found corresponding improvements equivalent to that of a patient taking a 400 microgram dose of inhaled corticosteroids.

Professor Tim Higenbottam, lead researcher on the Sheffield study said: "The technique combines two types of treatment so you knock out the mites and the vast majority of the allergens caused by the mites. The study shows that it is possible to convert a mite ridden home in a city suburb to conditions more readily found in homes in the Swiss Alps."

"This one off treatment is relatively inexpensive at around UK pounds 400 (about U.S. dollars 650) per year. That is the equivalent to the supply of a patient's inhalers for a year."

—by Mark Pownall

Chapter 60

Synthetic Pillows and Allergy

Doctors may have to proffer new advice to patients with allergies, including asthmatics, in the wake of a new study which has found more allergens on synthetic pillows than on feather ones. It seems that it is not so much what is inside the pillow that matters, than it is the fabric that covers the pillow.

Traditionally, physicians have advised asthma sufferers and others with atopic disease to avoid feather pillows because of possible sensitization from feather particles. The research, from the North West Lung Centre in Manchester, England, presented to the winter meeting of the British Thoracic Society [BTS] in London, found much higher levels of pet allergens on synthetic pillows than feather pillows which had been on the same bed for more than two years.

Patients in the study were not pet owners. The allergens are easily brought into the home on clothing and can be picked up when patients come into contact with animals in other homes. For the cat allergen, Fel d 1, there was seven times more allergen on synthetic as on feather pillows—9.14 nanograms compared to 1.37 nanograms. For the dog allergen, Can f 1, the difference was eight-fold: 18.48 nanograms compared to 2.31 nanograms. In a previous study, the same researchers found that synthetic pillows contained much higher levels of dust mite allergens (another major trigger for asthma) than feather pillows.

From "BTS: Synthetic Pillows May Not Be Best for Allergies," in *Doctor's Guide to the Internet*, December 13, 1999. © 1999 by P\S\L Consulting Group Inc. Reprinted by permission. *Doctor's Guide to the Internet* is at http://www.docguide.com.

Researchers say the difference between the two types of pillow could be explained by the material cover. Feather pillows are encased in a densely woven fabric meant to stop feathers pushing through. More research is needed to identify the best pillows for asthmatics.

One of the researchers, Dr. Adrian Custovic, said: "Tightly woven or allergen proof materials should be used to encase both synthetic and feather filling in pillows to provide an effective barrier against allergens. It is possible this could be of real benefit to asthma sufferers."

—by Mark Pownall

Part Six

Additional Help and Information

Chapter 61

Glossary of Allergy Terms

Airway: The part of the respiratory system between the mouth and lungs.

Allergen: Allergy-provoking substance. Common allergens include:

* Foods, the most common are milk, fruit, fish, eggs and nuts.
* Pollen, especially ragweed, which causes hay fever.
* Mold from plants and food, which are most likely to cause asthma.
* House dust, which contains mites as well as dander from house pets.
* Venom from insects (such as bees, wasps and mosquitoes) or scorpions.
* Plant oils, especially poison ivy, oak, or sumac.
* Additionally, feathers, wool, dyes, cosmetics, and perfumes may also act as allergens.

Allergic Cascade: The allergic cascade is like a domino reaction — once the first domino falls, or an IgE/allergen bond is made, a chain of chemical reactions takes place which eventually results in the release of histamines and other toxic chemicals from the mast cell.

Excerpted from "Allergy Glossary," produced by Health on the Net Foundation (HON); © 2000 HON, reprinted with permission. The full document is available on the internet at http://hon.ch/Library/Theme/Allergy/Glossary.

Allergic Responses: Allergic responses consist of:

1. *Primary Responses:* The immune response (cellular or humoral) to a first encounter with antigen. The primary response is generally small, has a long induction phase or lag period, consists primarily of IgM antibodies, and generates immunologic memory.

2. *Secondary Responses:* The immune response which follows a second or subsequent encounter with a particular antigen. Can be severe in certain cases (for example, anaphylactic shock).

Allergic Rhinitis: Characterized by an inflammation of the nasal mucous membranes due to an allergic response. The most common of all atopic diseases in the United States, affecting up to 10% of the adult population. Clinically, information is gained from a nasal examination which may reveal pale, boggy turbinate as well as clear to greenish rhinorrhea. When colored nasal secretions are stained and examined, they typically reveal large numbers of eosinophils as the main inflammatory cell. In many instances (particularly in children) complications such as chronic otitis media, rhinosinusitis, and conjunctivitis can be traced to chronic obstruction from allergic rhinitis. Concerning the treatment of allergic rhinitis, corticosteroid nasal sprays are very effective agents, especially for symptoms of congestion, sneezing, and runny nose. The main causes of seasonal allergic rhinitis are tree, grass, or weed pollens.

Allergy: Allergies are hypersensitivity reactions of the immune system to specific substances called allergens (such as pollen, stings, drugs, or food) that, in most people, result in no symptoms. The most severe form of allergy is anaphylactic shock, which is a medical emergency. Common allergies include: asthma, house dust mite allergy, food allergy, pet allergy, pollen allergies, and insect sting allergy.

Amino Acid: Small organic molecule containing both a carboxyl group and an amino group bonded to the same carbon atom. For example: histamine; serotonin; epinephrine; norepinephrine.

Analgesic: A drug that reduces pain without reducing consciousness. There are three main categories of analgesic:

1. *Opioid Analgesics:* Chemically related to morphine, a substance extracted from poppies. Very effective in relieving pain

but have many side effects. These include: tolerance; risk of withdrawal symptoms; constipation; sleepiness; and nausea. Overdose results in coma and eventually death.

2. *Nonopioid Analgesics:* All of this class of analgesics, except acetaminophen, are nonsteroidal anti-inflammatory drugs (NSAIDs). These drugs work by interfering with the system responsible for pain—the prostaglandin system—as well as reducing inflammation and irritation around a wound. Aspirin is the classic example of this class of drugs. NSAIDs have the side effects of causing peptic ulcers and stomach irritation.

3. *Adjuvant Analgesics:* Usually given for reasons other than pain relief, but may relieve pain in certain circumstances. For example, some antidepressants are also nonspecific pain relievers and are used to treat chronic pain such as lower back pain and headaches.

Anaphylactic Shock: The severest form of allergy which is a medical emergency. An often severe and sometimes fatal systemic reaction in a susceptible individual upon exposure to a specific antigen (such as wasp venom or penicillin) following previous sensitization. Characterized especially by respiratory symptoms, fainting, itching, urticaria, swelling of the throat or other mucous membranes and a sudden decline in blood pressure.

Anaphylactoid Reactions: Anaphylactoid reactions have symptoms similar to those of anaphylaxis, but are triggered instead by non-IgE mechanisms which directly cause the release of these mediators. These include reactions to nonsteroidal anti-inflammatory drugs (for example, aspirin, ibuprofen), radiocontrast dye (used for x-ray studies) and exercise.

Anaphylatoxin: Substance capable of releasing histamine and other mediators from mast cells or eosinophils.

Anaphylaxis: Anaphylaxis is a medical emergency which involves an acute systemic (affecting the entire body) allergic reaction. It occurs following exposure to an antigen (allergen), to which a person was previously sensitized. Anaphylaxis can be caused by any allergen. However, the most common antigens to cause such a reaction are drugs, insect stings, certain foods, and allergen immunotherapy injections.

An anaphylactic reaction starts when the allergen enters the bloodstream and reacts with an IgE class antibody. This causes cells to release histamine, which in turn causes the airways to constrict (causing difficulty in breathing), blood vessels to constrict (lowering blood pressure) and the walls of the blood vessels to leak fluid (resulting in hives and swelling). The person may also go into shock.

Anaphylaxis occurs immediately or at most within 2 hours of exposure to the allergen. Treatment is an epinephrine injection, which usually stops the reaction. Those who are allergic to bee stings or certain foods should carry a dose of epinephrine with them at all times.

Animal Allergy: Many people are allergic to animals. Most people are not allergic to the animal's fur or feathers. The allergy is more usually an immune reaction to a protein (an allergen) found in the saliva, dander (dead skin flakes), or the urine of an animal. The allergen gets carried in the air or in dust on very small, invisible particles. It then lands on the lining of the eyes (conjunctiva) and nose. It may also be inhaled directly into the lungs, causing allergic symptoms. Allergen contact with an allergic person's skin may also cause itching and hives.

Antigen: A substance that elicits an antibody response.

Antigen-Processing Cell (APC): T lymphocytes are part of the immune system involved in identifying antigens. However, for an antigen to be recognized by a T-lymphocyte, it must be first processed and "presented" in a form the antigen can recognize. This is the function of an APC; also referred to as accessory cells.

Antihistamine: Drugs which block the action of histamine, thus preventing or alleviating the major symptoms of an allergic response. Antihistamines are typically combined with a decongestant to help relieve nasal congestion. Examples include: Alkylamines (Chlorpheniramine, Brompheniramine); Ethanolamines (Diphenhydramine, Dimenhydranate, Clemastine); Piperazines (Hydroxyzine, Meclozine, Compazine); Piperadines (Azatadine, Triprolidine); Ethylenediamines (PBZ); Phenothiazines (Thorazine, Temaril); Tricyclic antidepressants (Imipramine, Doxopin, Amitryptoline); and others (Terfenadine, Astemizole, Loratadine, Acrivastine).

Asthma: Asthma can be defined clinically as a condition of intermittent, reversible airway constriction, due to a hyperreactivity to certain substances producing inflammation. In an asthma attack the smooth muscles of the lungs go into spasm with the surrounding tissue inflamed and secreting mucus into the airways. Thus, the diameter of the airways is reduced causing the characteristic wheezing as the person affected breathes harder to get air into the lungs. Attacks can vary in intensity and frequency. Asthma can be divided into two principal types:

- *Extrinsic Asthma:* Asthma triggered by external agents such as pollen or chemicals. Most cases of extrinsic asthma have an allergic origin and are caused by an IgE mediated response to an inhaled allergen. This is the type of asthma commonly diagnosed in early life. Many patients with extrinsic asthma may respond to immunotherapy.

- *Intrinsic Asthma (Bronchial Asthma, Exercise-Induced Asthma):* Asthma triggered by boggy membranes, congested tissues, and other native causes such as adrenaline stress or exertion. Intrinsic asthma generally develops later in life and virtually nothing is known of its causes. It carries a worse prognosis than extrinsic asthma and tends to be less responsive to treatment. Intrinsic bronchial hyperactivity can be triggered by infection, exercise, or drugs such as aspirin.

Atopic Dermatitis: Atopic dermatitis is a chronic, itchy inflammation of the upper layers of the skin. Often develops in people who have hay fever or asthma or who have family members with these conditions. Most commonly displayed during infanthood, usually disappearing by the age of 3 or 4.

Atopy: A type of inherited allergic response involving elevated immunoglobulin E (IgE). Sometimes called a reagin response, it means that you have hay fever, bronchial asthma, or skin problems like urticaria or eczema. It can also be acquired, sometimes following hepatitis or extended contact with solvents or alcohol.

Basophil: A type of leukocyte (white blood cell), also called a granular leukocyte, filled with granules of toxic chemicals, that can digest micro-organisms. Basophils are responsible for the symptoms of allergy. Despite similarities, basophils appear to be a distinct cell type from mast cells. When basophils are triggered, they release two kinds of mediators:

1. Preformed granule-associated mediators such as histamine, serotonin, bradykinin, heparin, cytokines.

2. Newly-generated mediators, prostaglandins and leukotrienes, made from arachidonic acid in surrounding tissues.

B-Cell (B Lymphocyte): White blood cells which develop from B stem cells into plasma cells which produce immunoglobulins (antibodies).

Bronchiole: The branching airways connecting the bronchi with the alveolar ducts. Bronchiolitis is an inflammation of the bronchioles.

Bronchitis: Bronchitis is an inflammation of the bronchus usually caused by an infection. This often includes the trachea and the bronchioles. Generally a mild condition that eventually heals totally, however, bronchitis can also be chronic. In this condition there is diffused inflammation of the air passages in the lungs, leading to decreased uptake of oxygen by the lungs and increased mucus production. Two main types of bronchitis exist:

- *Infectious Bronchitis:* Caused by viruses and bacteria (for example, *Mycoplasma pneumoniae* and *Chlamydia*). Most frequent in winter. Smokers and those with chronic sinusitis, bronchochietasis, allergies and children with enlarged tonsils and adenoids may experience recurrent infections.

- *Irritative Bronchitis:* Caused by dust, pollen, strong acid fumes, ammonia, chlorine, hydrogen sulfide, sulfur dioxide, ozone, tobacco smoke.

Bronchoconstriction: An airflow limitation due to contraction of smooth airway muscle.

Bronchodilator: Anything that opens or expands the bronchi (that part of the body that conveys air to and from the lungs). Bronchodilating drugs are usually prescribed if a cough occurs with airway narrowing, and they can reduce coughing, wheezing, and shortness of breath. Bronchodilators can be taken orally, injected or inhaled and begin to act almost immediately but with the effect only lasting 4-6 hours. The most common bronchodilators are:

- *Beta-adrenergic receptor agonists:* These are the drugs used most commonly to relieve a sudden asthma attack or to prevent an attack during exercise. This type of bronchodilator stimulates beta-adrenergic receptors to widen the airways. Beta-adrenergic receptor agonists act either on all beta-adrenergic receptors (for example, adrenaline) which can cause side effects such as headache, muscle tremors and restlessness. However, there also exist drugs of this class that act only on beta2-adrenergic receptors in the lungs, thus causing less side effects.

- *Anticholinergic drugs:* Drugs of this class, such as ipratropium bromide and atropine, block acetlycholine from causing smooth muscle contractions and from producing excess mucus in the bronchi. These drugs further widen the airways of people who are already taking beta2-adrenergic receptor agonists.

- *Theophylline:* Drug used in asthma treatment and prevention.

Bronchospasm: A bronchospasm is an acute bronchoconstriction.

Bronchus: The air passage between the trachea and the bronchioles (air passages between the throat and the lungs). The inflammation of the bronchus is called bronchitis.

Casein Intolerance: An intolerance to casein, a milk protein, where the immune system of the body produces immunoglobulin A (IgA) and Immunoglobulin G (IgG) against casein. Casein peptides are absorbed through the intestine and collect in the kidneys. These antibodies can be detected with a relatively simple, highly accurate blood serum test called ELISA.

Catecholamine: A class of hormones, two of which are known to be important in a medical emergency. These are epinephrine and norepinephrine. All the catecholamines stimulate high blood pressure and can trigger symptoms usually associated with threatening situations leading to a panic attack.

Celiac Disease: Celiac disease, or celiac sprue, is a malabsorption disorder characterized by a permanent gluten-sensitive enteropathy resulting in malabsorption, failure to thrive, and other gastrointestinal manifestations. However, it should not be confused with a food allergy or hypersensitivity to food products.

Celiac disease is an inherited cell-mediated hypersensitivity involving a tissue-bound immune cell, often delayed, reaction to a food allergen such as wheat, rye, oats, or barley. Gluten, a protein in these grains, is thought to be the offending agent. The onset of the disease has no age restriction but there are many hypotheses related to possible causative factors. In some adults, symptoms leading to a diagnosis of celiac disease have been observed to appear following severe emotional stress, pregnancy, an operation, or a viral infection.

Clusters of Differentiation (CD): Cluster of antigens, with which antibodies react, that characterize a cell surface marker. Lymphocytes can be divided into subsets either by their functions or by surface markers.

Conjunctivitis (Pink Eye): Conjunctivitis is an inflammation of the conjunctiva, a membrane that lines the inside of the eyelid and touches the white part of the eye, secreting a mucous that lubricates the eyeballs. There are many different causes of conjunctivitis. The main causes are the following:

- *Infectious:* resulting from bacterial or viral infections.

- *Noninfectious:* due to certain allergies (such as pollen or animal dander) and chemical irritants (such as smoke, preservatives in contact lens solutions and some eye drops, or the chlorine in swimming pools).

Allergic conjunctivitis is usually accompanied by intense symptoms (itching, redness, tearing, and swelling of the eye membranes). It is frequently seasonal, and is accompanied by other typical allergic symptoms such as sneezing, itchy nose, or scratchy throat.

Contact Dermatitis: Contact dermatitis is a reaction which occurs when skin comes in contact with certain substances. Two mechanisms exist by which substances can cause skin inflammation: irritation (irritant contact dermatitis) or allergic reaction (allergic contact dermatitis). Common irritants include soap, detergents, acids, alkalis and organic solvents (as are present in nail varnish remover). Contact dermatitis is most often seen around the hands or areas that touched or were exposed to the irritant/allergen. Contact dermatitis of the feet also exists but differs in that it is due to the warm, moist conditions in the shoes and socks. An allergic reaction does not generally occur the first time one is exposed to a particular substance but on subsequent exposures, which can cause dermatitis in 4 to 24 hours.

Corticosteroid: Corticosteroids are a group of anti-inflammatory drugs similar to the natural corticosteroid hormones produced by the cortex of the adrenal glands. Among the disorders that often improve with corticosteroid treatment are asthma, allergic rhinitis, eczema, and rheumatoid arthritis. How these anti-inflammatory agents inhibit late phase allergic reactions occurs via a variety of mechanisms, including decreasing the density of mast cells along mucosal surfaces, decreasing chemotaxis and activation of eosinophils, decreasing cytokine production by lymphocytes, monocytes, mast cells and eosinophils, inhibiting the metabolism of arachidonic acid and other mechanisms. But for the side effects, corticosteroids would be the only drug needed for treating most allergic reactions. Much effort is underway to develop safer corticosteroids including topical application and modifying the molecules to preserve the anti-inflammatory properties while minimizing the undesirable side effects.

Cross-Reactivity: The ability of an immunoglobulin, specific for one antigen, to react with a second antigen. A measure of relatedness between two different antigenic substances.

Cytokine: Cytokines are soluble glycoproteins released by cells of the immune system, which act nonenzymatically through specific receptors to regulate immune responses. Cytokines resemble hormones in that they act at low concentrations bound with high affinity to a specific receptor. Common cytokines in allergology include: interleukins, lymphokine, interferon, colony stimulating factor, platelet-activating factor, and tumor necrosis factor.

Decongestant: The three most common oral decongestants are pseudoephedrine, phenylpropanolamine and phenylephrine. [Note: Phenylpropanolamine was withdrawn from the U.S. market by the Food and Drug Administration in 2000.] These work by shrinking blood vessels in the nose, thus reducing congestion. Unfortunately, their effect is not confined to the nose as decongestants can worsen hypertension (high blood pressure), Raynaud's phenomenon, and can act as a stimulant. Due to this last side effect, decongestants are frequently combined with sedating antihistamines. However, the stimulant and sedative effects do not always cancel each other out, resulting in an upset in one's daily cycle.

Dermatitis: Dermatitis is an inflammation of the upper layers of the skin causing rash, blisters, scabbing, redness and swelling. There are many different types of dermatitis, these include: acrodermatitis, allergic contact dermatitis, atopic dermatitis, contact dermatitis, diaper rash (diaper dermatitis), exfoliative dermatitis, herpetiformis dermatitis, irritant dermatitis, occupational dermatitis, perioral dermatitis, photoallergic dermatitis, phototoxic dermatitis, seborrheic dermatitis, and toxicodendron dermatitis.

Desensitization Therapy: A method where the body is repeatedly exposed to small amounts of an allergy causing substance, an allergen, in order to reduce the allergic reaction. For instance, if a person with diabetes has a bad reaction to taking a full dose of beef insulin, the doctor gives the person a very small amount of the insulin at first. Over a period of time, larger doses are given until the person is taking the full dose. This is one way to help the body get used to the full dose and to avoid an allergic reaction.

Drug Allergy: Certain drugs can cause a severe allergic reaction, known as an anaphylactic reaction. First exposure to a drug does not cause this reaction but subsequent exposure may. However an anaphylactoid reaction can occur following the first injection of certain drugs (for example, polymyxin, Pentamidine, opioids, and contrast media used for x-rays). Although many organ systems can be involved in an allergic drug reaction, the skin is most commonly affected. Dermatologic reactions include urticaria, angioedema, dermatitis (allergic contact dermatitis, photodermatitis, exfoliative dermatitis), fixed drug eruption, and erythema multiforme (characterized by a rash and patches of red skin all over the body).

Common antibiotics that can cause allergic reactions include: penicillins, cephalosporins, sulfonamides, and miscellaneous others, including Aztreonam, Isoniazid, and Nitrofurantoin.

Dust: Dust is a common allergen. House dust contains mites (which are the primary cause of dust-related allergies), microscopic particles of animal dander, pollen, mold, fibers from clothing and other fabrics, and detergents. Dust mites, the primary cause of dust allergy, are microscopic organisms found in homes. It is actually the excrement of these mites to which people are allergic, thus dust mites can cause allergic reactions even when dead.

Eczema: A skin hypersensitivity due to hereditary influences. The term eczema comprises a number of pathogenetically different conditions, all with the histologic hallmark of intercellular edema of the epidermis (spongiosis). Examples include: atopic eczema (atopic dermatitis), adult seborrheic eczema, infantile seborrheic eczema, allergic contact dermatitis, and irritant contact dermatitis.

Edema: An accumulation of fluid between cells, causing swelling of the involved area. Edema is most often seen in the lower legs, the feet, and around the eyes.

Eosinophil: One of the five different types of white blood cell (WBC) belonging to the subgroup of WBCs called polymorphonuclear leukocytes. Characterized by large red (that is "eosinophilic") cytoplasmic granules.

Eosinophil function is incompletely understood. They are prominent at sites of allergic reactions and with parasitic larvae infections (helminths). Eosinophil secretory products inactivate many of the chemical mediators of inflammation and destroy cancer cells. This phenomenon is most obvious with mast cell-derived mediators. Mast cells produce a chemotactic factor for eosinophils.

Produced in the bone marrow, eosinophils then migrate to tissues throughout the body. When a foreign substance enters the body, lymphocytes and neutrophils release certain substances to attract eosinophils which release toxic substances to kill the invader.

Epinephrine (Adrenaline): An hormone released by the adrenal gland, which is the drug of choice for the treatment of anaphylaxis. Indeed, those who are allergic to insect stings and certain foods should always carry a self-injecting syringe of epinephrine. Epinephrine increases the speed and force of heart beats and, therefore the work that can be done by the heart. It dilates the airways to improve breathing and narrows blood vessels in the skin and intestine so that an increased flow of blood reaches the muscles and allows them to cope with the demands of exercise. Usually treatment with this hormone stops an anaphylactic reaction. Epinephrine has been produced synthetically as a drug since 1900.

Food Allergy: A food allergy is any adverse reaction to a food or food component involving the body's immune system. Some adverse reactions to foods do not involve the immune system and are known as food intolerance (for example, food poisoning or the inability to properly digest certain food components such as lactose or gliadin). A true allergic reaction to a food involves two primary components:

1. Contact with food allergens (part of the food that stimulates the immune system)

2. Immunoglobulin E (IgE: an antibody in the immune system that reacts with allergens) and mast cells (tissue cells) as well as basophils (blood cells), which release histamine or other substances causing allergic symptoms when IgE antibodies attach onto these cells.

Although most Americans consume a wide variety of food additives daily, only a small number have been associated with reactions. These reactions do not involve the immune system and therefore are examples of food intolerance rather than food allergy. While most allergic reactions to food are relatively mild, a small percentage of food-allergic individuals have severe reactions that can be life-threatening.

Anaphylaxis is a rare but potentially fatal condition in which several different parts of the body experience food-allergic reactions simultaneously, causing hives, swelling of the throat, and difficulty in breathing. Food allergies can cause a host of symptoms, including: swelling of the lips, tongue, or throat; hoarseness; cough; hives; skin rashes; a runny nose and watering eyes; and asthma. Sometimes symptoms are limited to nausea, vomiting, or cramping diarrhea. Symptoms of a food allergy are highly individualistic and usually begin within minutes to a few hours after having eaten the offending food.

The most common food allergens involved in food allergy are shellfish, milk, fish, soy, wheat, peanuts, egg, and tree nuts such as walnuts. Pharmacologically active substances found in food include histamine, tyramine, tryptamine, and serotonin, which may be consumed in foods such as red wine, cheese, yeast extract, avocados and bananas. In susceptible people, these foods can trigger urticaria, facial flushing, and headaches. Patients with hypersensitivity to avocados, bananas, kiwis or chestnuts sometimes exhibit clinical reactions to latex. This is termed cross-reactivity.

Food Intolerance: Food intolerance is an adverse reaction to food which does not involve the body's immune system. It can be caused by a metabolic reaction to an enzyme deficiency such as the inability to digest milk properly (lactose intolerance), by food poisoning such as ingesting contaminated or spoiled fish, or a food idiosyncrasy such as sulfite-induced asthma.

Fungus: A general term used to describe a group of eukaryotic protists, which include mushrooms, yeasts, rusts, molds, and smuts. All are characterized by the absence of chlorophyll and by the presence of a rigid cell wall, composed of chitin, mannans, and sometimes cellulose. They are usually of simple morphological form or show some reversible cellular specialization, such as the formation of pseudo-parenchymatous tissue in the fruiting body of a mushroom. The dimorphic fungi grow, according to environmental conditions, as molds or yeasts.

Gell and Coombs Classification of Hypersensitive Reactions: Allergic reactions are classified depending on the type of tissue damage that develops.

- *Type I (atopic or anaphylactic) Hypersensitivity (Immediate Hypersensitivity):* A Type I reaction occurs when an antigen entering the body encounters mast cells or basophils. These types of immune defense cells have antibodies attached to their surfaces and the antigen binds to this. The result is the release of histamine, causing blood vessel dilation and a narrowing of the airways. Examples include: allergic rhinitis, intrinsic asthma, and anaphylactic shock.

- *Type II Hypersensitivity (Cytotoxic Hypersensitivity):* Type II hypersensitivity reactions destroy cells because the antibody-antigen combination activates toxic substances. An example is Goodpasture's syndrome.

- *Type III Hypersensitivity (Immune Complex Initiated Hypersensitivity, Immune Complex Hypersensitivity, Immune Complex Reaction):* This type of reaction occurs when large numbers of antibody-antigen complexes accumulate. This may cause widespread inflammation that damages tissue. Systemic lupus erythematosus is an example of a Type III reaction.

- *Type IV (delayed or cell-mediated) Hypersensitivity (Delayed Type Hypersensitivity):* This type of hypersensitive (allergic) reaction occurs when an antigen interacts with antigen-specific lymphocytes that release inflammatory and toxic substances, which attract other white blood cells and results in tissue injury. Three examples of Type IV reaction are:

  - *Contact Hypersensitivity.* This is characterized by a reaction at the site of contact with the allergen. It is an epidermal response most often elicited by small molecules called haptens. The cell involved in antigen presentation at this site is the Langerhans cell. The pathway from initial exposure involves sensitization and exposure, followed by aggregation of mononuclear cells around blood vessels and glands in the epidermis and edema. The reaction decreases 48-72 hours following exposure.

  - *Tuberculin Hypersensitivity.* This response was first observed when soluble antigens from organisms such as mycobacteria were administered subcutaneously. In these individuals, fever, general unwellness, plus an area of red, hard swelling was observed. The skin test for Tuberculosis is of this nature.

- *Granulomatous Hypersensitivity.* This type of reaction is characterized by persistence of the antigen within macrophages as well as of the lesion. Such antigens are particulate matter such as talc and silica but also mycobacteria. The characteristic cells found in the lesion are epitheloid cells (probably macrophages) and giant-cells (multi-nucleated macrophages). The granuloma consists of a hard core of cells sometimes with a necrotic core. This is surrounded by lymphocytes with a deposition of collagen fibers.

- *Type V Hypersensitivity (Stimulating Antibody):* IgG antibodies reacting with tissue receptors like, for example, in Graves disease.

- *Type VI Hypersensitivity (Antibody Dependant Cell Mediated Cytotoxicity):* A phenomenon in which target cells, coated with antibody, are destroyed by specialized killer cells (NK cells, Killer T-cells and macrophages). These receptors allow the killer cells to bind to the antibody-coated target. Eosinophils kill helminths (parasitic larvae infections) by antibody dependant cell mediated cytotoxicity (ADCC).

Gliadin: A glycoprotein fraction of gluten. Gliadin is present in wheat, oats, rye, and barley and, it seems, millet.

Gluten: A protein in cereal grains. Wheat, rye, barley, and oats contain the gliadin subfraction of gluten that is toxic to persons with celiac disease.

Glycoprotein: A protein coated with sugars. For example, cytokines.

Histamine: A hormone/chemical transmitter (biogenic monoamine, similar to serotonin, epinephrine, norepinephrine) involved in local immune responses, regulating stomach acid production, and in allergic reactions as a mediator of immediate (Type I) hypersensitivity. When released from mast cells, histamine causes vasodilation and an increase in permeability of blood vessel walls. These effects, in turn cause the familiar symptoms of allergy including a runny nose and watering eyes. When released in the lungs, histamine causes the airways to swell shut in an attempt to close the door on offending allergens and keep them out. Unfortunately, the ultimate result of this response is the wheezing and difficulty in breathing seen in people with asthma.

Hormone: Hormones are substances released into the bloodstream by glands or organs, which affect activity in cells at another site. Most are proteins composed of amino-acid chains of various lengths. Others are steroids. Hormones (similar to the cytokines and other mediators) act at low concentrations with very large responses in the body and bind with high affinity to specific receptors. These receptors are on the surface or inside the cell and the result of such binding causes an alteration in the cell's functioning.

Hormones control growth and development, reproduction, and sexual characteristics as well as exercising a large influence over the body's use of energy. Examples include the catecholamines (such as epinephrine and norepinephrine) and the corticosteroids released by the adrenal glands.

Humoral Immunity: Any immune reaction that can be transferred with immune serum is termed humoral immunity (as opposed to cell-mediated immunity). In general, this term refers to resistance that results from the presence of specific antibodies (immunoglobulins). These antibodies circulate through the blood and lymph system. When blood is spun in centrifuge, the red blood cells fall to the bottom of the tube, leaving behind a straw-colored liquid called the serum. Antibodies are located in the blood serum and thus can be transferred with an immune serum.

Hymenoptera: Hymenoptera are the most common insects which cause allergy. Scientists estimate that there are more than 300,000 species of Hymenoptera in the world, though only 120,000 have been identified and named so far. Examples include: Bees; Honey-bees; Yellow jackets; Yellow hornets; Wasps and White-faced hornets.

Immunoglobulin (Ig): Immunoglobulins (antibodies) are proteins produced by plasma cells (or B-cells, a type of lymphocyte), which are designed to control the immune response in extracellular fluids by binding to substances in the body that are recognized as foreign antigens (often proteins on the surface of bacteria and viruses). Each Ig unit is made up of two heavy chains and two light chains and has two antigen-binding sites. Antibodies are diverse, with more than 1010 possible variations, yet each antibody is designed to recognize only a specific antigen.

Initially bound to B-cells, upon encountering its specific antigen, an antibody/antigen complex stimulates the B-cell to produce copies of the antibody with the aid of helper T-cells. The new antibodies, which are all designed to recognize the infecting antigen, are released into the intercellular fluid where they bind to the infecting antigen, identifying it for destruction by phagocytes and the complement system.

Immunoglobulins also play a central role in allergies when they bind to antigens that are not necessarily a threat to health and provoke an inflammatory reaction. There are five main types of antibody: IgA; IgD; IgE; IgG and IgM, of which IgA, IgG, and IgM are the most common.

Immunoglobulin A (IgA): One of the five classes of immunoglobulins produced by humans (the others being IgE, IgD, IgG and IgM). IgA is found circulating and secreted on all defended body surfaces, as the primary defense against invaders. Secretory (sIgA) is found in large amounts in breast milk, saliva, and gastrointestinal secretions. IgA may also be an important and effective antibody in sites other than mucosal tissues, such as the central nervous system. IgA inhibits the binding of micro-organisms to mucosal surfaces, thus preventing entry. sIgA deficiency is associated with increased gastrointestinal tract permeability and increased manifestations of delayed patterns of food allergy.

Immunoglobulin E (IgE): One of five classes of immunoglobulins made by humans (the others being IgA, IgD, IgG and IgM). Main function seems to be to protect the host against invading parasites. While parasitic disease may not be a major clinical issue in most industrialized nations, it is a major public health problem in developing nations. The antigen-specific IgE interacts with mast cells and eosinophils to protect the host against the invading parasite. However, the same antibody-cell combination is also responsible for typical allergy or immediate hypersensitivity reactions such as hay fever, asthma, hives, and anaphylaxis. Reagin is the allergist's term for IgE antibodies.

Immunoglobulin M (IgM): The "big" multivalent antibody, capable of capturing and binding antigens to form large insoluble complexes which are then readily cleared from the blood. Usually the first antibody to appear after initial exposure to an antigen. IgM levels may be elevated in patients with delayed patterns of food allergy and probably manifest a protective defense response.

Immunotherapy (Allergy Shots): When an allergen can not be avoided, allergen immunotherapy is often the only viable solution. Here, tiny amounts of the allergen are injected under the skin in gradually increased doses until a maintenance level is reached. This stimulates the body to block or neutralize certain antibodies that are produced in response to the allergen and are thus responsible for the allergic symptoms experienced.

Multiple theories have been advanced to explain the mechanism of how allergen immunotherapy works. Most researchers agree that three major events commonly occur in patients who receive a course of allergen immunotherapy:

1. The production and release of many of the proinflammatory mediators (particularly cytokines) are diminished. This may be via a direct effect on mast cells and eosinophils or an immunoregulatory effect mediated by specific populations of lymphocytes.

2. It is common to find increasing amounts of allergen-specific IgG circulating in the plasma of patients receiving allergen immunotherapy. Such IgG could also bind to the specific allergen and prevent its interaction with mast cell-bound IgE.

3. Finally, it can be demonstrated that, after an initial rise, allergen-specific IgE levels in the plasma fall with allergen immunotherapy. This is thought to be due to active immunoregulatory mechanisms that alter how a specific individual responds to a particular allergen.

Not all mechanisms are likely to be active in every treated patient. Also, this form of treatment varies in efficacy among different types of allergy and between individuals. Dust, pollen, mite, dander, and insect venom allergic reactions usually respond best. Researchers are trying to determine exactly which mechanisms are active in a specific patient so allergen immunotherapy can be better tailored to the individual. Also, work is ongoing to better chemically define the treating allergens, make allergen immunotherapy safer, and safely increase the interval between injections.

Insect Sting Allergy: Allergic reactions to insect stings can be so severe that death may occur within the few minutes following a sting. Even if not fatal, sting allergy symptoms can be frightening, including dizziness, itchy welts or massive swelling of the body, inability to breathe, swallow or speak, fainting from low blood pressure, and shock.

Insulin Allergy: An allergic reaction can result from insulin made from pork or beef due to the fact that this insulin is not exactly the same as human insulin or because it contains impurities. The allergy can be of two forms. Sometimes an area of skin becomes red and itchy around the place where the insulin is injected. This is called a local allergy. In another form, the whole body can have a bad reaction. This is called a systemic allergy. Hives or red patches all over the body or changes in heart and breathing rate may result. A doctor can treat this allergy by either prescribing purified insulin or through desensitization therapy.

Lactase: An intestinal enzyme that is needed to digest lactose. The lack of lactase results in what is called lactose intolerance.

Lactose: A complex sugar found in milk and milk products (also the principal sugar found in these products). Lactose must be broken down by lactase into the simple sugars galactose and glucose in order to be absorbed.

Lactose Intolerance: Intolerance to milk and milk products due to a lactase deficiency. The digestive system does not produce enough of this enzyme to break down the lactose into simpler sugars (glucose and galactose). Thus, the lactose sugar ferments in the small intestine producing gas, bloating, cramps, abdominal cramping, and diarrhea after drinking milk or eating dairy products. This problem is present in over 80 percent of nonwhite adults. Lactose intolerance can be diagnosed by certain tests such as a Lactose Intolerance Test, Breath Hydrogen Level test, and Stool Acidity Test. Lactose intolerance is not the same as a milk allergy.

Leukocyte (White Blood Cell): Leukocytes or white blood cells (WBC) are cells in the blood that are involved in defending the body against infective organisms and foreign substances. Like all blood cells, they are produced in the bone marrow. There are 5 main types of white blood cell, subdivided between two main groups:

1. *Polymorphonuclear leukocytes (granulocytes):* neutrophils, eosinophils, and basophils

2. *Mononuclear leukocytes:* monocytes and lymphocytes

White blood cells are the principal components of the immune system and function by destroying "foreign" substances such as bacteria and viruses. When an infection is present, the production of WBCs increases. If the number of leukocytes is abnormally low (a condition known as leukopenia), infection is more likely to occur, and it is more difficult for the body to get rid of the infection.

Lymphocyte: A white blood cell of the mononuclear leukocyte sub-group (like macrophage/monocytes). Lymphocytes identify foreign substances and germs (bacteria or viruses) in the body and produce antibodies and cells that specifically target them. It takes from several days to weeks for lymphocytes to recognize and attack a new foreign substance. The main lymphocyte sub-types are:

- *B-Cells:* Special B cells produce specific antibodies, proteins that help destroy foreign substances.

- *T-Cells:* T-cells attack virus-infected cells, foreign tissue, and cancer cells. They also produce a number of substances that regulate the immune response.

- *NK Cells:* Among other functions, natural killer cells destroy cancer cells and virus-infected cells through phagocytosis and by producing substances that can kill such cells.

- *Null cells:* An early population of lymphocytes bearing neither T-cell nor B-cell differentiation antigens.

Mast Cell Stabilizers (Cromolyn Salts, Cromolyn Sodium, Nedocromil Sodium): One way to stop histamine from being released would be to stop mast cells from degranulating—even if IgE was crosslinked. Several drugs have this property. Cromolyn was the first drug licensed as a mast cell stabilizer, that is, inhibit degranulation and activation. It is available for use in the nose, lungs, and gastrointestinal (GI) tract. Its major limitation is a short duration of action (approximately 6 hours) and lack of available systemic preparation. Recently, a related compound called nedocromil has been released in the U.S for use in asthmatics. It appears to have a longer action duration and may have more anti-inflammatory properties than cromolyn.

Since the process of mast cell activation, mediator production and chemotaxis takes longer than mast cell degranulation, allergic reactions often have two distinct phases—the first or early phase occurs in minutes. The second or late phase occurs some 3-12 hours later and is an inflammatory reaction due to mast cell and eosinophil products. Antihistamines have no effect on late phase reactions while corticosteroids have little direct effect on early phase reactions. Cromolyn and nedocromil appear to be effective against both reaction phases.

Mast Cells: Large tissue cells that resemble basophils (which are blood cells) but lack some of the chemical components of basophils.

They are important in producing the symptoms of an immediate hypersensitivity reaction.

Milk Allergy: This is an allergic reaction by the body's immune system to one or more of milk's proteins, such as casein or lactoglobulin. The resulting symptoms typically include swelling, itching, bronchospasm, hives, hypotension or shock, abdominal cramps, and diarrhea. One of the more common food allergies.

Mold: Molds are naturally occurring clusters of microscopic fungi which reproduce by releasing airborne spores. Certain individuals will develop asthma and nasal symptoms if they breathe in these spores and thus have a mold allergy.

Mold Allergy: Many people are allergic to mold. Mold spores are carried in the air and may be present all year long. Mold is most prevalent indoors in damp locations (in bathrooms, washrooms, fabrics, rugs, stuffed animals, books, wallpaper, and other "organic" materials). Outdoors, mold lives in the soil, on compost, and on damp vegetation.

Nonsteroidal Anti-Inflammatory Drugs (NSAID): NSAIDs are of the class of analgesics known as nonopioid or non-narcotic. Anti-inflammatory medications reduce the symptoms and signs of inflammation, however, anaphylactoid reactions can be provoked by nonsteroidal anti-inflammatory drugs.

Norepinephrine (Noradrenaline): A hormone released by the adrenal gland. Norepinephrine is released, along with epinephrine, from the adrenals and from nerves when heart failure takes place. These hormones are the first line of defense during any sudden stress. The release of these hormones cause the heart to pump faster, making up for the pumping problem caused by heart failure.

Oral Allergy Syndrome: In some children, food allergies often produce flares of atopic dermatitis. Another common manifestation of food allergy is the "oral allergy syndrome," in which certain foods cause itching or hives where they touch the lips and mouth. Fresh fruits and vegetables are often associated with this kind of reaction. These reactions are believed to be due to pollen protein cross-reactions (responses to fruits and vegetables frequently occurring as clusters of hypersensitivity to members of the same botanical family, for which the immunologic basis lies in a number of common allergens) in the fruits, which are inactivated by cooking. For example, persons sensitive to ragweed pollen may develop hives on the lips while eating melon. Similarly, people sensitive to birch tree pollen may react to fresh apples. The same people, however, might tolerate cooked apples, as in apple pie.

Peptide: A molecule formed by joining two or more amino acids.

Placebo: An inactive compound having no physiological effect; an inert substance identical in appearance to the treatment drug used in clinical studies. A form of safe but non-active treatment frequently used as a basis for comparison with pharmaceuticals in research studies.

Placebo Effect: An apparently beneficial result of therapy that occurs because of the patient's expectation that the therapy will help.

Pollen: Microscopic grains produced by plants in order to reproduce. Each plant has a pollinating period. These can vary depending on the plant, climate, and region.

Pollen Allergy: A hypersensitive reaction to pollen. While grass pollens are generally the most common cause of hay fever (seasonal allergic rhinitis), other pollen types are also important. These include tree pollens such as alder, hazel, birch, beech, cypress, pine, chestnut, and poplar, and weed pollens such as plantain, mugwort, and ragweed. The relative importance of the kinds of pollen that can cause hay fever varies between different climatic and vegetation zones. For example, ragweed pollen, although very common in North America, is present in Europe only in the French Rhône valley and some areas of Eastern Europe, while the pollen most associated with seasonal allergy in Mediterranean regions is the olive tree. A person allergic to one pollen is generally also allergic to members of the same group or family. Pollen induced reactions include extrinsic asthma, rhinitis, and bronchitis.

Polypeptide: Many peptides joined together. For example, insulin.

Protein: A molecule composed of many amino acids and with a complex structure. For example, immunoglobulin, casein.

Respiratory System: The respiratory system is the system by which oxygen, essential for life, is taken into the body and the waste product, carbon dioxide, is expelled from the body. The respiratory system consists of the mouth and nose, airways, and lungs.

Rhinitis: Rhinitis is an inflammation of the nasal mucosa (the mucous membrane that lines the nose and the sinus), often due to an allergic reaction to pollen, dust, or other airborne substances (allergens). Although the pathophysiology of many types of rhinitis is unknown, an accurate diagnosis is necessary, since not all types of rhinitis will respond to the same treatment measures. Types of chronic rhinitis include: atopic rhinitis, seasonal allergic rhinitis (also known as hay fever), perennial rhinitis (year-round) with allergic triggers, perennial rhinitis with non-allergic triggers, idiopathic non-allergic rhinitis, infectious rhinitis, rhinitis medicamentosa, mechanical obstruction, and hormonal.

Seborrheic Dermatitis: An inflammation of the upper layers of the skin where scales appear on the scalp, face and sometimes in other areas. Usually more common in cold weather and often runs in families.

Serum Sickness: A hypersensitivity reaction consisting of fever, rashes, joint pain and glomerulonephritis, resulting from localization of circulating, soluble, antigen-antibody complexes, which induce inflammatory reactions. Serum sickness was originally induced following therapy with large doses of antibody from a foreign source (for example, horse serum).

Shock: A life-threatening condition where blood pressure is too low to sustain life. Occurs when a low blood volume (due to severe bleeding, excessive fluid loss, or inadequate fluid uptake), inadequate pumping action of the heart, or excessive dilation of the blood vessel walls (vasodilation) causes low blood pressure. This in turn results in inadequate blood supply to body cells, which can quickly die or be irreversibly damaged.

Sinusitis: Inflammation of the sinuses, with causes ranging from dust to hay fever. Obstinate cases can be caused by chronic sinus infections or the continued exposure to allergens from food, pets or environmental irritants. The most commonly affected sinus is the maxillary sinus.

Specificity: The property of antibodies which enables them to react with some antigenic determinants and not with others. Specificity is dependent on chemical composition, physical forces, and molecular structure at the binding site.

Stasis Dermatitis: A chronic redness, scaling, warmth, and swelling on the lower legs. Often results in dark brown skin due to a pooling of blood and fluid under the skin, thus usually displayed by those with varicose veins and edema.

Stevens-Johnson Syndrome: A severe allergic drug reaction characterized by blisters breaking out on the lining of the mouth, throat, anus, genital area, and eyes. A severe form of erythema multiforme. Drugs that can cause this reaction include the penicillins, antibiotics containing sulfa, barbiturates, and some drugs used to treat high blood pressure and diabetes.

T-Cell (T-Lymphocyte): A lymphocyte (white blood cell) that develops in the bone marrow, matures in the thymus, and expresses what appear to be antibody molecules on their surfaces but, unlike B-cells, these molecules cannot be secreted. Works as part of the immune system in the body. Produces cytokine to help B-Lymphocytes produce immunoglobulin.

Theophylline: A drug used in asthma treatment and prevention. Theophylline is a bronchodilatory drug and comes in various forms such as short-acting tablets and syrups, as well as longer-acting sustained release capsules and tablets. It can also be given intravenously if a serious asthma attack is taking place. The dose of Theophylline must be closely monitored as too little has little effect, while too much can cause side effects such as abnormal heart rhythms, nausea, insomnia, and seizures.

Toxicodendron Dermatitis: When people get urushiol, the oil present in poison ivy, poison oak and poison sumac on their skin, it causes a form of allergic contact dermatitis. This is a T-cell-mediated immune response, also called delayed hypersensitivity, in which the body's immune system recognizes as foreign, and attacks, the complex of urushiol-derivatives with skin proteins. The irony is that urushiol, in the absence of the immune attack, would be harmless.

Urticaria (Hives): Urticaria is a skin symptom that accompanies many allergic disorders. It is a relatively common disorder caused by localized mast-cell degranulation, with resultant dermal venular hyperpermeability culminating in pruritic wheals. Mostly results from an antigen-induced (pollens, foods, drugs, insect venom) release of histamine and other vasoactive amines via sensitization with specific IgE antibodies. Most individual lesions develop and fade within 24 hours.

Allergic skin diseases such as urticaria and angioedema as well as atopic dermatitis are not clearly defined as true allergic diseases. Urticaria and angioedema are both due to excessive mast cell activity in the skin. Chronic urticaria and angioedema are seldom due to a definable IgE mechanism (as is the case with all allergies) but, when determined, is generally due to a drug, food or food additive.

White Blood Cell (WBC) Count: Measures the number of white blood cells in a microliter of blood. Normal values range from 4100/ml to 10900/ml but can be altered greatly by factors such as exercise, stress and disease. A low WBC may indicate viral infection or toxic reactions. A high WBC count may indicate infection, leukemia, or tissue damage. An increased risk of infection occurs once the WBC drops below 100/ml.

Chapter 62

Allergy Information Resources

Allergy and Asthma Network/Mothers of Asthmatics
2751 Prosperity Avenue
Suite 150
Fairfax, VA 22031
Toll Free: 800-878-4403
Phone: 703-641-9595
Fax: 703-573-7784
Internet: http://www.aanma.org
E-Mail: aanma@aol.com

Allergy Society of South Africa
P.O. Box 88
Observatory, 7935
Cape Town, RSA
Phone: +27 (0) 21-4479019
Fax: +27 (0) 21-4480847
Internet: http://allergysa.org

American Academy of Allergy, Asthma, and Immunology
611 East Wells Street
Milwaukee, WI 53202
Toll Free: 800-822-ASMA
Phone: 414-272-6071
Internet: http://www.aaaai.org
E-Mail: info@aaaai.org

American Academy of Dermatology
930 N. Meacham Rd.
Schaumburg, IL 60168-4014
Toll Free: 888-462-DERM
Phone: 847-330-0230
Fax: 847-330-0050
Internet: http://www.aad.org

Information in this chapter was compiled from several sources deemed accurate; contact information was updated and verified in June 2001.

**American Academy of
Family Physicians**
11400 Tomahawk Creek
Parkway
Leawood, KS 66211
Phone: 913-906-6000
Fax: 913-906-6090
Internet: http://
www.familydoctor.org
E-Mail: fp@aafp.org

**American Academy of
Otolaryngic Allergy**
1990 M Street, N.W., Suite 680
Washington, DC 20036
Phone: 202-955-5010
Fax: 202-955-5016
Internet: http://www.allergy-
ent.com
E-Mail: info@aaoaf.org

**American Academy of
Otolaryngology-Head and
Neck Surgery, Inc.**
One Prince Street
Alexandria, VA 22314-3357
Phone: 703-836-4444
Internet: http://www.entnet.org

**American Allergy
Association**
1259 El Camino, No. 254
Menlo Park, CA 94025
Phone: 650-855-8036
E-Mail: allergyaid@aol.com

**American Association of
Certified Allergists**
85 W. Algonquin Rd., Suite 550
Arlington Heights, IL 60005
Phone: 847-427-8111
Fax: 847-427-1294
Internet: http://www.acaai.org
E Mail. mail@acaai.org

**American Board of Allergy
and Immunology**
510 Walnut, Suite 1701
Philadelphia, PA 19106
Phone: 215-592-9466
Fax: 215-592-9411
Internet: http://www.abai.org
E-Mail: abai@abai.org

**American College of
Asthma, Allergy, and
Immunology**
85 W. Algonquin Road, Suite 550
Arlington Heights, IL 60005
Toll Free: 800-842-7777
Phone: 847-427-1200
Fax: 847-427-1294
Internet: http://allergy.mcg.edu
E-Mail: mail@acaai.org

**American College of Chest
Physicians**
3300 Dundee Road
Northbrook, IL 60062
Toll Free: 800-343-2227
Phone: 847-498-1400
Fax: 847-498-5460
Internet: http://
www.chestnet.org
E-Mail: accp@chestnet.org

The American Dietetic Association
216 W. Jackson Blvd.
Chicago, IL 60606-6995
Toll Free: 800-877-1600
Phone: 312-899-0040
Internet: http://www.eatright.org

American Lung Association
1740 Broadway
New York, NY 10019-4374
Toll Free: 800-586-4872
Phone: 212-315-8700
Internet: http://www.lungusa.org
E-Mail: info@lungusa.org

American Osteopathic College of Allergy and Immunology
7025 E. McDowell Road
Suite 1B
Scottsdale, AZ 85257
Phone: 480-585-1580
Fax: 480-585-1581

Asthma All-Stars™
Toll Free: 888-825-5249
Internet: http://www.asthmaallstars.org

Asthma and Allergy Foundation of America
1233 20th Street, N.W., Suite 402
Washington, DC 20036
Toll Free: 800-727-8462
Phone: 202-466-7643
Fax: 202-466-8940
Internet: http://www.aafa.org
E-Mail: info@aafa.org

Environmental Protection Agency
Indoor Air Quality Information
P.O. Box 37133
Washington, DC 20013-7133
Toll Free: 800-438-4318
Internet: http://www.epa.gov/iaq

Food Allergy and Anaphylaxis Network
10400 Eaton Place, Suite 107
Fairfax, VA 22030-2208
Toll Free: 800-929-4040
Phone: 703-691-3179
Fax: 703-691-2713
Internet: http://www.foodallergy.org
E-Mail: faan@foodallergy.org

Food and Drug Administration
For information about extracts used in allergy testing:

Center for Biologics Evaluation and Research
1401 Rockville Pike, Suite 200N
Rockville, MD 20852-1448
Toll Free: 800-835-4709
Phone: 301-827-1800
Fax: 888-CBER-FAX (Within the U.S.) or 301-827-3844 (Outside the U.S. and local to Rockville, MD)
Internet: http://www.fda.gov/cber

Healthy Environment Information and Referral Service
P.O. Box 580
Chimayo NM 87522
Phone: 505-351-2968

Indoor Air Quality Information Clearinghouse
Environmental Protection Agency
P.O. Box 37133
Washington, DC 20013-7133
Toll Free: 800-438-4318
Phone: 703 356 4020
Internet: http://www.epa.gov/iaq/iaqinfo.html

International Food Information Council Foundation
1100 Connecticut Avenue NW, Suite 430
Washington, DC 20036
Phone: 202-296-6540
Fax: 202-296-6547
Internet: http://ificinfo.health.org
E-Mail: foodinfo@ific.org

National Arthritis, Musculoskeletal and Skin Diseases Information Clearinghouse
One AMS Circle
Bethesda, MD 20892-3675
Toll Free: 877-22-NIAMS
Phone: 301-495-4484
Fax: 301-718-6366
TTY: 301-565-466-2966
Internet: http://www.nih.gov/niams

National Asthma Education and Prevention Program
NHLBI Health Information Network
P.O. Box 30105
Bethesda, MD 20824-0105
Phone: (301) 251-8573
Fax: 301 503 8567
Internet: http://www.nhlbi.nih.gov/about/naepp/index.htm

National Digestive Diseases Information Clearinghouse
2 Information Way
Bethesda, MD 20892-3570
Toll Free: 800-891-5389
Phone: 301-654-3810
Fax: 301-907-8906
Internet: http://www.niddk.nih.gov/health/digest/nddic.htm
E-Mail: nddic@info.niddk.nih.gov

National Eczema Association for Science and Education
1220 S.W. Morrison, Suite 433
Portland, OR 97205
Toll Free: 800-818-7546
Phone: 503-228-4430
Fax: 503-244-3363
Internet: http://www.eczema-assn.org
E-Mail: nease@teleport.com

National Heart, Lung, and Blood Institute
P.O. Box 30105
Bethesda, MD 20824-0105
Phone: (301) 496-4236
Internet: http://www.nhlbi.nih.gov
E-Mail: nhlbiinfo@rover.nhlbi.nih.gov

National Institute of Allergy and Infectious Diseases
Office of Communications
Building 31, Room 7A-50
31 Center Drive MSC 2520
Bethesda, MD 20895
Phone: 301-496-5717
Internet: http://www.niaid.nih.gov
E-Mail: 1f7j@nih.gov

National Institute of Environmental Health Sciences
Office of Communications
P.O. Box 12233
Research Triangle Park, NC 27709
Phone: 919-541-3345
Internet: http://www.nichs.nih.gov/airborne/home.htm

National Jewish Medical and Research Center
1400 Jackson Street
Denver, CO 80206
Toll Free: 800-222-LUNG (5864)
Phone: 303-388-4461
Internet: http://www.njc.org
E-Mail: lungline@njc.org

Pan-American Allergy Society
P.O. Box 947
Fredericksburt, TX 78624
Phone: 830-977-9853
Fax: 830-977-8625
Internet: http://www.paas.org
E-Mail: info@paas.org

Parents of Asthmatic/Allergic Children
1412 Marathon Drive
Ft. Collins, CO 80524
Phone: 970-842-7395

Practical Allergy Research Foundation
P.O. Box 60
Buffalo, NY 14226
Toll-Free: 800-787-8780
Phone: 716-875-5578
Fax: 716-875-5399

U.S. Department of Agriculture
For information about food contents:

Food and Nutrition Information Center
10301 Baltimore Avenue
Beltsville, MD 20705-231
Phone: 301-504-5719
Fax: 301-504-6409
TTY: 301-504-6856
Internet: http://www.nalusda.gov/fnic
E-Mail: fnic@nal.usda.gov

World Allergy Organization
International Association of
Allergology and Clinical
Immunology
611 E. Wells Street
Milwaukee, WI 53202
Phone: 414-276-1791
Fax. 414-272-0049
Internet: http://
www.worldallergy.org
E-Mail: info@worldallergy.org

Chapter 63

Resources for Patients Living with Allergies

Specialized Information Resources

For Information about Air Filtering Devices

Environmental Protection Agency
1200 Pennsylvania Avenue, N.W.
Washington, DC 20460
Toll Free: 800-438-4318
Phone: 202-260-2090
Internet: http://www.epa.gov

For Information about Cosmetics

FDA Office of Cosmetics and
Colors
HFS-100
200 C St., S.W.
Washington, DC 20204
Phone: 202-401-9725
Internet: http://
www.cfsan.fda.gov/~dms/cos-
pol.html

Food and Drug Administration
5600 Fishers Lane
Rockville, MD 20857-0001
Toll Free: 800-463-6332
Internet: http://www.fda.gov

Adapted from "Living with Allergies: Resources for Patients," National Institute of Allergy and Infectious Diseases, May 2001. All contact information verified and updated in July 2001.

For Information about Extracts for Allergy Testing Regulated by the Food and Drug Administration

Center for Drug Evaluation and Research
5600 Fishers Lane
Rockville, MD 20857
Phone: (301) 827-4573
Internet: http://www.fda.gov/cder

For Online Information about Allergic Diseases and Clinical Research Studies

MEDLINEplus
U.S. National Library of Medicine
8600 Rockville Pike
Bethesda, MD 20894
Internet: http://www.nlm.nih.gov/medlineplus

Products, Services, and Publications

For Pollen Maps

National Allergy Bureau
American Academy of Allergy, Asthma and Immunology
611 East Wells Street
Milwaukee, WI 53202
Toll-Free: 800-9-POLLEN (pollen information)
Phone: 414-272-6071
Internet: http://www.aaaai.org
E-Mail: nab@aaaai.org

For Doctor Referrals

American Academy of Allergy, Asthma and Immunology
611 East Wells Street
Milwaukee, WI 53202
Toll-Free: 800-822-ASMA (doctor referrals)
Phone: 414-272-6071
Internet: http://www.aaaai.org
E-Mail: info@aaaai.org

For a Listing of Products, Services, and Publications

Products Directory
The American Allergy Association
1259 El Camino #254
Menlo Park, CA 94025
Phone: 650-855-8036
E-Mail: allergyaid@aol.com

Allergy and Asthma Research Centers Supported by the National Institute ofAllergy and Infectious Diseases (NIAID)

NIAID is a component of the National Institutes of Health (NIH). NIAID supports basic and applied research to prevent, diagnose, and treat infectious and immune-mediated illnesses, including HIV/AIDS and other sexually transmitted diseases, tuberculosis, malaria, autoimmune disorders, asthma and allergies.

California

La Jolla Institute for Allergy and Immunology
10355 Science Center Drive
San Diego, CA 92121
Phone: 858-558-3500
Fax: 858-558-3526
Internet: http://www.liai.org

University of California School of Medicine
405 Hilgard Avenue
Box 951361
Los Angeles, CA 90095-1361
Toll Free: 800-825-2888
Phone: 310-825-4321
TDD: 310-825-2833
Internet: http://
www.medsch.ucla.edu
E-Mail: access@mednet.ucla.edu

Maryland

National Institute of Allergy and Infectious Diseases
National Institutes of Health
31 Center Drive
Bethesda, MD 20892
Phone: 301-496-8973
Internet: http://
www.niaid.nih.gov

Massachusetts

Beth Israel Deaconess Medical Center
330 Brookline Avenue
Boston, MA 02215
Phone: 617-667-7000
Internet: http://
www.bidmc.harvard.edu

Massachusetts, continued

Boston University
121 Bay State Road
Boston, MA 02215
Phone: 617-535-2000
Internet: http://www.bu.edu

Brigham and Women's Hospital
75 Francis Street
Boston, MA 02115
Phone: 617-525-5500
TTY/TTD: 617-732-6458
Internet: http://
www.brighamandwomens.org

Minnesota

Mayo Foundation
200 First St., S.W.
Rochester, MN 5905
Toll Free: 800-297-1185
Phone: 507-284-2511
TDD: 507-284-9786
Internet: http://www.mayo.edu/
develop
E-Mail: development@mayo.edu

Missouri

Washington University School of Medicine
660 S. Euclid Ave.
St. Louis, MO 63110
Toll Free: 800-243-5864
Phone: 314-362-9047
Internet: http://
medicine.wustl.edu

New York

Mount Sinai School of Medicine
One Gustave L. Levy Place
New York, NY 10029
Phone: 212-241-8774
Internet: http://www.mssm.edu

Texas

University of Texas
301 University Boulevard
Galveston, TX 77555
Phone: 409-772-1011
Fax: 409-772-6216
Internet: http://www.utmb.edu
E-Mail: www@www.utmb.edu

Virginia

University of Virginia
P.O. Box 800395
Health Sciences Center
School of Medicine
Charlottesville, VA 22908-0395
Phone: 434-924-7236
Internet: http://
www.virginia.edu

Wisconsin

University of Wisconsin
1300 University Ave.
Madison, WI 52706
Phone: 608-263-4900
Internet: http://www.wisc.edu

Index

Index

Health Reference Series
COMPLETE CATALOG

AIDS Sourcebook, 1st Edition

Basic Information about AIDS and HIV Infection, Featuring Historical and Statistical Data, Current Research, Prevention, and Other Special Topics of Interest for Persons Living with AIDS

Along with Source Listings for Further Assistance

Edited by Karen Bellenir and Peter D. Dresser. 831 pages. 1995. 0-7808-0031-1. $78.

"One strength of this book is its practical emphasis. The intended audience is the lay reader . . . useful as an educational tool for health care providers who work with AIDS patients. Recommended for public libraries as well as hospital or academic libraries that collect consumer materials."
— *Bulletin of the Medical Library Association, Jan '96*

"This is the most comprehensive volume of its kind on an important medical topic. Highly recommended for all libraries." — *Reference Book Review, '96*

"Very useful reference for all libraries."
— *Choice, Association of College and Research Libraries, Oct '95*

"There is a wealth of information here that can provide much educational assistance. It is a must book for all libraries and should be on the desk of each and every congressional leader. Highly recommended."
— *AIDS Book Review Journal, Aug '95*

"Recommended for most collections."
— *Library Journal, Jul '95*

■

AIDS Sourcebook, 2nd Edition

Basic Consumer Health Information about Acquired Immune Deficiency Syndrome (AIDS) and Human Immunodeficiency Virus (HIV) Infection, Featuring Updated Statistical Data, Reports on Recent Research and Prevention Initiatives, and Other Special Topics of Interest for Persons Living with AIDS, Including New Antiretroviral Treatment Options, Strategies for Combating Opportunistic Infections, Information about Clinical Trials, and More

Along with a Glossary of Important Terms and Resource Listings for Further Help and Information

Edited by Karen Bellenir. 751 pages. 1999. 0-7808-0225-X. $78.

"Highly recommended."
— *American Reference Books Annual, 2000*

"Excellent sourcebook. This continues to be a highly recommended book. There is no other book that provides as much information as this book provides."
— *AIDS Book Review Journal, Dec-Jan 2000*

"Recommended reference source."
— *Booklist, American Library Association, Dec '99*

"A solid text for college-level health libraries."
— *The Bookwatch, Aug '99*

Cited in *Reference Sources for Small and Medium-Sized Libraries, American Library Association, 1999*

■

Alcoholism Sourcebook

Basic Consumer Health Information about the Physical and Mental Consequences of Alcohol Abuse, Including Liver Disease, Pancreatitis, Wernicke-Korsakoff Syndrome (Alcoholic Dementia), Fetal Alcohol Syndrome, Heart Disease, Kidney Disorders, Gastrointestinal Problems, and Immune System Compromise and Featuring Facts about Addiction, Detoxification, Alcohol Withdrawal, Recovery, and the Maintenance of Sobriety

Along with a Glossary and Directories of Resources for Further Help and Information

Edited by Karen Bellenir. 613 pages. 2000. 0-7808-0325-6. $78.

"This title is one of the few reference works on alcoholism for general readers. For some readers this will be a welcome complement to the many self-help books on the market. Recommended for collections serving general readers and consumer health collections."
— *E-Streams, Mar '01*

"This book is an excellent choice for public and academic libraries."
— *American Reference Books Annual, 2001*

"Recommended reference source."
— *Booklist, American Library Association, Dec '00*

"Presents a wealth of information on alcohol use and abuse and its effects on the body and mind, treatment, and prevention." — *SciTech Book News, Dec '00*

"Important new health guide which packs in the latest consumer information about the problems of alcoholism." — *Reviewer's Bookwatch, Nov '00*

SEE ALSO Drug Abuse Sourcebook, Substance Abuse Sourcebook

■

Allergies Sourcebook, 1st Edition

Basic Information about Major Forms and Mechanisms of Common Allergic Reactions, Sensitivities, and Intolerances, Including Anaphylaxis, Asthma, Hives and Other Dermatologic Symptoms, Rhinitis, and Sinusitis

Along with Their Usual Triggers Like Animal Fur, Chemicals, Drugs, Dust, Foods, Insects, Latex, Pollen, and Poison Ivy, Oak, and Sumac; Plus Information on Prevention, Identification, and Treatment

Edited by Allan R. Cook. 611 pages. 1997. 0-7808-0036-2. $78.

Allergies Sourcebook, 2nd Edition

Basic Consumer Health Information about Allergic Disorders, Triggers, Reactions, and Related Symptoms, Including Anaphylaxis, Rhinitis, Sinusitis, Asthma, Dermatitis, Conjunctivitis, and Multiple Chemical Sensitivity

Along with Tips on Diagnosis, Prevention, and Treatment, Statistical Data, a Glossary, and a Directory of Sources for Further Help and Information

Edited by Annemarie S. Muth. 598 pages. 2001. 0-7808-0376-0. $78.

Alternative Medicine Sourcebook

Basic Consumer Health Information about Alternatives to Conventional Medicine, Including Acupressure, Acupuncture, Aromatherapy, Ayurveda, Bioelectromagnetics, Environmental Medicine, Essence Therapy, Food and Nutrition Therapy, Herbal Therapy, Homeopathy, Imaging, Massage, Naturopathy, Reflexology, Relaxation and Meditation, Sound Therapy, Vitamin and Mineral Therapy, and Yoga, and More

Edited by Allan R. Cook. 737 pages. 1999. 0-7808-0200-4. $78.

"Recommended reference source."
 —Booklist, American Library Association, Feb '00

"A great addition to the reference collection of every type of library." *—American Reference Books Annual, 2000*

Alzheimer's, Stroke & 29 Other Neurological Disorders Sourcebook, 1st Edition

Basic Information for the Layperson on 31 Diseases or Disorders Affecting the Brain and Nervous System, First Describing the Illness, Then Listing Symptoms, Diagnostic Methods, and Treatment Options, and Including Statistics on Incidences and Causes

Edited by Frank E. Bair. 579 pages. 1993. 1-55888-748-2. $78.

"Nontechnical reference book that provides reader-friendly information."
 —Family Caregiver Alliance Update, Winter '96

"Should be included in any library's patient education section." *—American Reference Books Annual, 1994*

"Written in an approachable and accessible style. Recommended for patient education and consumer health collections in health science center and public libraries." *—Academic Library Book Review, Dec '93*

"It is very handy to have information on more than thirty neurological disorders under one cover, and there is no recent source like it." *—Reference Quarterly, American Library Association, Fall '93*

SEE ALSO *Brain Disorders Sourcebook*

Alzheimer's Disease Sourcebook, 2nd Edition

Basic Consumer Health Information about Alzheimer's Disease, Related Disorders, and Other Dementias, Including Multi-Infarct Dementia, AIDS-Related Dementia, Alcoholic Dementia, Huntington's Disease, Delirium, and Confusional States

Along with Reports Detailing Current Research Efforts in Prevention and Treatment, Long-Term Care Issues, and Listings of Sources for Additional Help and Information

Edited by Karen Bellenir. 524 pages. 1999. 0-7808-0223-3. $78.

"Provides a wealth of useful information not otherwise available in one place. This resource is recommended for all types of libraries."
 —American Reference Books Annual, 2000

"Recommended reference source."
 —Booklist, American Library Association, Oct '99

Arthritis Sourcebook

Basic Consumer Health Information about Specific Forms of Arthritis and Related Disorders, Including Rheumatoid Arthritis, Osteoarthritis, Gout, Polymyalgia Rheumatica, Psoriatic Arthritis, Spondyloarthropathies, Juvenile Rheumatoid Arthritis, and Juvenile Ankylosing Spondylitis

Along with Information about Medical, Surgical, and Alternative Treatment Options, and Including Strategies for Coping with Pain, Fatigue, and Stress

Edited by Allan R. Cook. 550 pages. 1998. 0-7808-0201-2. $78.

". . . accessible to the layperson."
 —Reference and Research Book News, Feb '99

Asthma Sourcebook

Basic Consumer Health Information about Asthma, Including Symptoms, Traditional and Nontraditional Remedies, Treatment Advances, Quality-of-Life Aids, Medical Research Updates, and the Role of Allergies, Exercise, Age, the Environment, and Genetics in the Development of Asthma

Along with Statistical Data, a Glossary, and Directories of Support Groups, and Other Resources for Further Information

Edited by Annemarie S. Muth. 628 pages. 2000. 0-7808-0381-7. $78.

"A worthwhile reference acquisition for public libraries and academic medical libraries whose readers desire a quick introduction to the wide range of asthma information." *—Choice, Association of College and Research Libraries, Jun '01*

"Recommended reference source."
 —Booklist, American Library Association, Feb '01

Back & Neck Disorders Sourcebook

Basic Information about Disorders and Injuries of the Spinal Cord and Vertebrae, Including Facts on Chiropractic Treatment, Surgical Interventions, Paralysis, and Rehabilitation

Along with Advice for Preventing Back Trouble

Edited by Karen Bellenir. 548 pages. 1997. 0-7808-0202-0. $78.

Blood & Circulatory Disorders Sourcebook

Basic Information about Blood and Its Components, Anemias, Leukemias, Bleeding Disorders, and Circulatory Disorders, Including Aplastic Anemia, Thalassemia, Sickle-Cell Disease, Hemochromatosis, Hemophilia, Von Willebrand Disease, and Vascular Diseases

Along with a Special Section on Blood Transfusions and Blood Supply Safety, a Glossary, and Source Listings for Further Help and Information

Edited by Karen Bellenir and Linda M. Shin. 554 pages. 1998. 0-7808-0203-9. $78.

Brain Disorders Sourcebook

Basic Consumer Health Information about Strokes, Epilepsy, Amyotrophic Lateral Sclerosis (ALS/Lou Gehrig's Disease), Parkinson's Disease, Brain Tumors, Cerebral Palsy, Headache, Tourette Syndrome, and More

Along with Statistical Data, Treatment and Rehabilitation Options, Coping Strategies, Reports on Current

Research Initiatives, a Glossary, and Resource Listings for Additional Help and Information

Edited by Karen Bellenir. 481 pages. 1999. 0-7808-0229-2. $78.

SEE ALSO Alzheimer's, Stroke & 29 Other Neurological Disorders Sourcebook, 1st Edition

Breast Cancer Sourcebook

Basic Consumer Health Information about Breast Cancer, Including Diagnostic Methods, Treatment Options, Alternative Therapies, Self-Help Information, Related Health Concerns, Statistical and Demographic Data, and Facts for Men with Breast Cancer

Along with Reports on Current Research Initiatives, a Glossary of Related Medical Terms, and a Directory of Sources for Further Help and Information

Edited by Edward J. Prucha and Karen Bellenir. 580 pages. 2001. 0-7808-0244-6. $78.

SEE ALSO Cancer Sourcebook for Women, 1st and 2nd Editions, Women's Health Concerns Sourcebook

Breastfeeding Sourcebook

Basic Consumer Health Information about the Benefits of Breastmilk, Preparing to Breastfeed, Breastfeeding as a Baby Grows, Nutrition, and More, Including Information on Special Situations and Concerns, Such as Mastitis, Illness, Medications, Allergies, Multiple Births, Prematurity, Special Needs, and Adoption

Along with a Glossary and Resources for Additional Help and Information

Edited by Jenni Lynn Colson. 350 pages. 2002. 0-7808-0332-9. $48.

SEE ALSO Pregnancy & Birth Sourcebook

Burns Sourcebook

Basic Consumer Health Information about Various Types of Burns and Scalds, Including Flame, Heat, Cold, Electrical, Chemical, and Sun Burns

Along with Information on Short-Term and Long-Term Treatments, Tissue Reconstruction, Plastic Surgery, Prevention Suggestions, and First Aid

Edited by Allan R. Cook. 604 pages. 1999. 0-7808-0204-7. $78.

"This is an exceptional addition to the series and is highly recommended for all consumer health collections, hospital libraries, and academic medical centers." — *E-Streams, Mar '00*

"Recommended reference source."

—*Booklist, American Library Association, Dec '99*

SEE ALSO *Skin Disorders Sourcebook*

■

Cancer Sourcebook, 1st Edition

Basic Information on Cancer Types, Symptoms, Diagnostic Methods, and Treatments, Including Statistics on Cancer Occurrences Worldwide and the Risks Associated with Known Carcinogens and Activities

Edited by Frank E. Bair. 932 pages. 1990. 1-55888-888-8. $78.

Cited in *Reference Sources for Small and Medium-Sized Libraries*, American Library Association, 1999

"Written in nontechnical language. Useful for patients, their families, medical professionals, and librarians." — *Guide to Reference Books, 1996*

"Designed with the non-medical professional in mind. Libraries and medical facilities interested in patient education should certainly consider adding the *Cancer Sourcebook* to their holdings. This compact collection of reliable information . . . is an invaluable tool for helping patients and patients' families and friends to take the first steps in coping with the many difficulties of cancer." — *Medical Reference Services Quarterly, Winter '91*

"Specifically created for the nontechnical reader . . . an important resource for the general reader trying to understand the complexities of cancer." — *American Reference Books Annual, 1991*

"This publication's nontechnical nature and very comprehensive format make it useful for both the general public and undergraduate students." — *Choice, Association of College and Research Libraries, Oct '90*

■

New Cancer Sourcebook, 2nd Edition

Basic Information about Major Forms and Stages of Cancer, Featuring Facts about Primary and Secondary Tumors of the Respiratory, Nervous, Lymphatic, Circulatory, Skeletal, and Gastrointestinal Systems, and Specific Organs; Statistical and Demographic Data; Treatment Options; and Strategies for Coping

Edited by Allan R. Cook. 1,313 pages. 1996. 0-7808-0041-9. $78.

"An excellent resource for patients with newly diagnosed cancer and their families. The dialogue is simple, direct, and comprehensive. Highly recommended for patients and families to aid in their understanding of cancer and its treatment." — *Booklist Health Sciences Supplement, American Library Association, Oct '97*

"The amount of factual and useful information is extensive. The writing is very clear, geared to general readers. Recommended for all levels." — *Choice, Association of College and Research Libraries, Jan '97*

■

Cancer Sourcebook, 3rd Edition

Basic Consumer Health Information about Major Forms and Stages of Cancer, Featuring Facts about Primary and Secondary Tumors of the Respiratory, Nervous, Lymphatic, Circulatory, Skeletal, and Gastrointestinal Systems, and Specific Organs

Along with Statistical and Demographic Data, Treatment Options, Strategies for Coping, a Glossary, and a Directory of Sources for Additional Help and Information

Edited by Edward J. Prucha. 1,069 pages. 2000. 0-7808-0227-6. $78.

"This title is recommended for health sciences and public libraries with consumer health collections." — *E-Streams, Feb '01*

". . . can be effectively used by cancer patients and their families who are looking for answers in a language they can understand. Public and hospital libraries should have it on their shelves." — *American Reference Books Annual, 2001*

"Recommended reference source." — *Booklist, American Library Association, Dec '00*

■

Cancer Sourcebook for Women, 1st Edition

Basic Information about Specific Forms of Cancer That Affect Women, Featuring Facts about Breast Cancer, Cervical Cancer, Ovarian Cancer, Cancer of the Uterus and Uterine Sarcoma, Cancer of the Vagina, and Cancer of the Vulva; Statistical and Demographic Data; Treatments, Self-Help Management Suggestions, and Current Research Initiatives

Edited by Allan R. Cook and Peter D. Dresser. 524 pages. 1996. 0-7808-0076-1. $78.

". . . written in easily understandable, non-technical language. Recommended for public libraries or hospital and academic libraries that collect patient education or consumer health materials." — *Medical Reference Services Quarterly, Spring '97*

"Would be of value in a consumer health library. . . . written with the health care consumer in mind. Medical jargon is at a minimum, and medical terms are explained in clear, understandable sentences." — *Bulletin of the Medical Library Association, Oct '96*

"The availability under one cover of all these pertinent publications, grouped under cohesive headings, makes this certainly a most useful sourcebook." — *Choice, Association of College and Research Libraries, Jun '96*

"Presents a comprehensive knowledge base for general readers. Men and women both benefit from the gold mine of information nestled between the two covers of this book. Recommended."
—*Academic Library Book Review, Summer '96*

"This timely book is highly recommended for consumer health and patient education collections in all libraries." — *Library Journal, Apr '96*

SEE ALSO Breast Cancer Sourcebook, Women's Health Concerns Sourcebook

∎

Cancer Sourcebook for Women, 2nd Edition

Basic Consumer Health Information about Gynecologic Cancers and Related Concerns, Including Cervical Cancer, Endometrial Cancer, Gestational Trophoblastic Tumor, Ovarian Cancer, Uterine Cancer, Vaginal Cancer, Vulvar Cancer, Breast Cancer, and Common Non-Cancerous Uterine Conditions, with Facts about Cancer Risk Factors, Screening and Prevention, Treatment Options, and Reports on Current Research Initiatives

Along with a Glossary of Cancer Terms and a Directory of Resources for Additional Help and Information

Edited by Karen Bellenir. 600 pages. 2002. 0-7808-0226-8. $78.

SEE ALSO Breast Cancer Sourcebook, Women's Health Concerns Sourcebook

∎

Cardiovascular Diseases & Disorders Sourcebook, 1st Edition

Basic Information about Cardiovascular Diseases and Disorders, Featuring Facts about the Cardiovascular System, Demographic and Statistical Data, Descriptions of Pharmacological and Surgical Interventions, Lifestyle Modifications, and a Special Section Focusing on Heart Disorders in Children

Edited by Karen Bellenir and Peter D. Dresser. 683 pages. 1995. 0-7808-0032-X. $78.

". . . comprehensive format provides an extensive overview on this subject."
—*Choice, Association of College and Research Libraries, Jun '96*

". . . an easily understood, complete, up-to-date resource. This well executed public health tool will make valuable information available to those that need it most, patients and their families. The typeface, sturdy non-reflective paper, and library binding add a feel of quality found wanting in other publications. Highly recommended for academic and general libraries. "
—*Academic Library Book Review, Summer '96*

SEE ALSO Healthy Heart Sourcebook for Women, Heart Diseases & Disorders Sourcebook, 2nd Edition

Caregiving Sourcebook

Basic Consumer Health Information for Caregivers, Including a Profile of Caregivers, Caregiving Responsibilities and Concerns, Tips for Specific Conditions, Care Environments, and the Effects of Caregiving

Along with Facts about Legal Issues, Financial Information, and Future Planning, a Glossary, and a Listing of Additional Resources

Edited by Joyce Brennfleck Shannon. 600 pages. 2001. 0-7808-0331-0. $78.

∎

Colds, Flu & Other Common Ailments Sourcebook

Basic Consumer Health Information about Common Ailments and Injuries, Including Colds, Coughs, the Flu, Sinus Problems, Headaches, Fever, Nausea and Vomiting, Menstrual Cramps, Diarrhea, Constipation, Hemorrhoids, Back Pain, Dandruff, Dry and Itchy Skin, Cuts, Scrapes, Sprains, Bruises, and More

Along with Information about Prevention, Self-Care, Choosing a Doctor, Over-the-Counter Medications, Folk Remedies, and Alternative Therapies, and Including a Glossary of Important Terms and a Directory of Resources for Further Help and Information

Edited by Chad T. Kimball. 638 pages. 2001. 0-7808-0435-X. $78.

∎

Communication Disorders Sourcebook

Basic Information about Deafness and Hearing Loss, Speech and Language Disorders, Voice Disorders, Balance and Vestibular Disorders, and Disorders of Smell, Taste, and Touch

Edited by Linda M. Ross. 533 pages. 1996. 0-7808-0077-X. $78.

"This is skillfully edited and is a welcome resource for the layperson. It should be found in every public and medical library." — *Booklist Health Sciences Supplement, American Library Association, Oct '97*

∎

Congenital Disorders Sourcebook

Basic Information about Disorders Acquired during Gestation, Including Spina Bifida, Hydrocephalus, Cerebral Palsy, Heart Defects, Craniofacial Abnormalities, Fetal Alcohol Syndrome, and More

Along with Current Treatment Options and Statistical Data

Edited by Karen Bellenir. 607 pages. 1997. 0-7808-0205-5. $78.

"Recommended reference source."
— *Booklist, American Library Association, Oct '97*

SEE ALSO Pregnancy & Birth Sourcebook

Consumer Issues in Health Care Sourcebook

Basic Information about Health Care Fundamentals and Related Consumer Issues, Including Exams and Ⓘⓐⓝⓝⓘⓝⓖ Ⓦⓔⓛⓛⓝ, Ⓤⓝⓘⓝⓢⓤⓡⓔⓓ Ⓟⓐⓣⓘⓔⓝⓣⓢ, Ⓒⓗⓞⓞⓢⓘⓝⓖ ⓐ Ⓓⓞⓒ *tor, Using Prescription and Over-the-Counter Medications Safely, Avoiding Health Scams, Managing Common Health Risks in the Home, Care Options for Chronically or Terminally Ill Patients, and a List of Resources for Obtaining Help and Further Information*

Edited by Karen Bellenir. 618 pages. 1998. 0-7808-0221-1. $78.

"Both public and academic libraries will want to have a copy in their collection for readers who are interested in self-education on health issues."
—American Reference Books Annual, 2000

"The editor has researched the literature from government agencies and others, saving readers the time and effort of having to do the research themselves. Recommended for public libraries."
—Reference and User Services Quarterly, American Library Association, Spring '99

"Recommended reference source."
—Booklist, American Library Association, Dec '98

∎

Contagious & Non-Contagious Infectious Diseases Sourcebook

Basic Information about Contagious Diseases like Measles, Polio, Hepatitis B, and Infectious Mononucleosis, and Non-Contagious Infectious Diseases like Tetanus and Toxic Shock Syndrome, and Diseases Occurring as Secondary Infections Such as Shingles and Reye Syndrome

Along with Vaccination, Prevention, and Treatment Information, and a Section Describing Emerging Infectious Disease Threats

Edited by Karen Bellenir and Peter D. Dresser. 566 pages. 1996. 0-7808-0075-3. $78.

∎

Death & Dying Sourcebook

Basic Consumer Health Information for the Layperson about End-of-Life Care and Related Ethical and Legal Issues, Including Chief Causes of Death, Autopsies, Pain Management for the Terminally Ill, Life Support Systems, Insurance, Euthanasia, Assisted Suicide, Hospice Programs, Living Wills, Funeral Planning, Counseling, Mourning, Organ Donation, and Physician Training

Along with Statistical Data, a Glossary, and Listings of Sources for Further Help and Information

Edited by Annemarie S. Muth. 641 pages. 1999. 0-7808-0230-6. $78.

"Public libraries, medical libraries, and academic libraries will all find this sourcebook a useful addition to their collections."
—American Reference Books Annual, 2001

"An extremely useful resource for those concerned with death and dying in the United States."
—Respiratory Care, Nov '00

"Recommended reference source."
—Booklist, American Library Association, Aug '00

"This book is a definite must for all those involved in end-of-life care." *—Doody's Review Service, 2000*

∎

Diabetes Sourcebook, 1st Edition

Ⓑⓐⓢⓘⓒ Ⓘⓝⓕⓞⓡⓜⓐⓣⓘⓞⓝ ⓐⓑⓞⓤⓣ Ⓘⓝⓢⓤⓛⓘⓝ Ⓓⓔⓟⓔⓝⓓⓔⓝⓣ ⓐⓝⓓ Ⓝⓞⓝ insulin-Dependent Diabetes Mellitus, Gestational Diabetes, and Diabetic Complications, Symptoms, Treatment, and Research Results, Including Statistics on Prevalence, Morbidity, and Mortality

Along with Source Listings for Further Help and Information

Edited by Karen Bellenir and Peter D. Dresser. 827 pages. 1994. 1-55888-751-2. $78.

". . . very informative and understandable for the layperson without being simplistic. It provides a comprehensive overview for laypersons who want a general understanding of the disease or who want to focus on various aspects of the disease."
—Bulletin of the Medical Library Association, Jan '96

∎

Diabetes Sourcebook, 2nd Edition

Basic Consumer Health Information about Type 1 Diabetes (Insulin-Dependent or Juvenile-Onset Diabetes), Type 2 (Noninsulin-Dependent or Adult-Onset Diabetes), Gestational Diabetes, and Related Disorders, Including Diabetes Prevalence Data, Management Issues, the Role of Diet and Exercise in Controlling Diabetes, Insulin and Other Diabetes Medicines, and Complications of Diabetes Such as Eye Diseases, Periodontal Disease, Amputation, and End-Stage Renal Disease

Along with Reports on Current Research Initiatives, a Glossary, and Resource Listings for Further Help and Information

Edited by Karen Bellenir. 688 pages. 1998. 0-7808-0224-1. $78.

"This comprehensive book is an excellent addition for high school, academic, medical, and public libraries. This volume is highly recommended."
—American Reference Books Annual, 2000

"An invaluable reference." *—Library Journal, May '00*

Selected as one of the 250 "Best Health Sciences Books of 1999." *—Doody's Rating Service, Mar-Apr 2000*

"Recommended reference source."
—Booklist, American Library Association, Feb '99

". . . provides reliable mainstream medical information . . . belongs on the shelves of any library with a consumer health collection." *—E-Streams, Sep '99*

"Provides useful information for the general public."
—Healthlines, University of Michigan Health Management Research Center, Sep/Oct '99

Diet & Nutrition Sourcebook, 1st Edition

Basic Information about Nutrition, Including the Dietary Guidelines for Americans, the Food Guide Pyramid, and Their Applications in Daily Diet, Nutritional Advice for Specific Age Groups, Current Nutritional Issues and Controversies, the New Food Label and How to Use It to Promote Healthy Eating, and Recent Developments in Nutritional Research

Edited by Dan R. Harris. 662 pages. 1996. 0-7808-0084-2. $78.

"Useful reference as a food and nutrition sourcebook for the general consumer." — *Booklist Health Sciences Supplement, American Library Association, Oct '97*

"Recommended for public libraries and medical libraries that receive general information requests on nutrition. It is readable and will appeal to those interested in learning more about healthy dietary practices." — *Medical Reference Services Quarterly, Fall '97*

"An abundance of medical and social statistics is translated into readable information geared toward the general reader." — *Bookwatch, Mar '97*

"With dozens of questionable diet books on the market, it is so refreshing to find a reliable and factual reference book. Recommended to aspiring professionals, librarians, and others seeking and giving reliable dietary advice. An excellent compilation." — *Choice, Association of College and Research Libraries, Feb '97*

SEE ALSO *Digestive Diseases & Disorders Sourcebook, Gastrointestinal Diseases & Disorders Sourcebook*

■

Diet & Nutrition Sourcebook, 2nd Edition

Basic Consumer Health Information about Dietary Guidelines, Recommended Daily Intake Values, Vitamins, Minerals, Fiber, Fat, Weight Control, Dietary Supplements, and Food Additives

Along with Special Sections on Nutrition Needs throughout Life and Nutrition for People with Such Specific Medical Concerns as Allergies, High Blood Cholesterol, Hypertension, Diabetes, Celiac Disease, Seizure Disorders, Phenylketonuria (PKU), Cancer, and Eating Disorders, and Including Reports on Current Nutrition Research and Source Listings for Additional Help and Information

Edited by Karen Bellenir. 650 pages. 1999. 0-7808-0228-4. $78.

"This book is an excellent source of basic diet and nutrition information." — *Booklist Health Sciences Supplement, American Library Association, Dec '00*

"This reference document should be in any public library, but it would be a very good guide for beginning students in the health sciences. If the other books in this publisher's series are as good as this, they should all be in the health sciences collections." — *American Reference Books Annual, 2000*

"This book is an excellent general nutrition reference for consumers who desire to take an active role in their health care for prevention. Consumers of all ages who select this book can feel confident they are receiving current and accurate information." — *Journal of Nutrition for the Elderly, Vol. 19, No. 4, '00*

"Recommended reference source." — *Booklist, American Library Association, Dec '99*

SEE ALSO *Digestive Diseases & Disorders Sourcebook, Gastrointestinal Diseases & Disorders Sourcebook*

■

Digestive Diseases & Disorders Sourcebook

Basic Consumer Health Information about Diseases and Disorders that Impact the Upper and Lower Digestive System, Including Celiac Disease, Constipation, Crohn's Disease, Cyclic Vomiting Syndrome, Diarrhea, Diverticulosis and Diverticulitis, Gallstones, Heartburn, Hemorrhoids, Hernias, Indigestion (Dyspepsia), Irritable Bowel Syndrome, Lactose Intolerance, Ulcers, and More

Along with Information about Medications and Other Treatments, Tips for Maintaining a Healthy Digestive Tract, a Glossary, and Directory of Digestive Diseases Organizations

Edited by Karen Bellenir. 335 pages. 1999. 0-7808-0327-2. $48.

"This title would be an excellent addition to all public or patient-research libraries." — *American Reference Books Annual, 2001*

"This title is recommended for public, hospital, and health sciences libraries with consumer health collections." — *E-Streams, Jul-Aug '00*

"Recommended reference source." — *Booklist, American Library Association, May '00*

SEE ALSO *Diet & Nutrition Sourcebook, 1st and 2nd Editions, Gastrointestinal Diseases & Disorders Sourcebook*

■

Disabilities Sourcebook

Basic Consumer Health Information about Physical and Psychiatric Disabilities, Including Descriptions of Major Causes of Disability, Assistive and Adaptive Aids, Workplace Issues, and Accessibility Concerns

Along with Information about the Americans with Disabilities Act, a Glossary, and Resources for Additional Help and Information

Edited by Dawn D. Matthews. 616 pages. 2000. 0-7808-0389-2. $78.

"A much needed addition to the Omnigraphics *Health Reference Series*. A current reference work to provide people with disabilities, their families, caregivers or those who work with them, a broad range of information in one volume, has not been available until now. . . . It is recommended for all public and academic library reference collections." — *E-Streams, May '01*

"An excellent source book in easy-to-read format covering many current topics; highly recommended for all libraries." — *Choice, Association of College and Research Libraries, Jan '01*

"Recommended reference source." — *Booklist, American Library Association, Jul '00*

"An involving, invaluable handbook." — *The Bookwatch, May '00*

Domestic Violence & Child Abuse Sourcebook

Basic Consumer Health Information about Spousal/ Partner, Child, Sibling, Parent, and Elder Abuse, Covering Physical, Emotional, and Sexual Abuse, Teen Dating Violence, and Stalking; Includes Information about Hotlines, Safe Houses, Safety Plans, and Other Resources for Support and Assistance, Community Initiatives, and Reports on Current Directions in Research and Treatment

Along with a Glossary, Sources for Further Reading, and Governmental and Non-Governmental Organizations Contact Information

Edited by Helene Henderson. 1,064 pages. 2000. 0-7808-0235-7. $78.

"Recommended reference source." — *Booklist, American Library Association, Apr '01*

"Important pick for college-level health reference libraries." — *The Bookwatch, Mar '01*

"Because this problem is so widespread and because this book includes a lot of issues within one volume, this work is recommended for all public libraries." — *American Reference Books Annual, 2001*

Drug Abuse Sourcebook

Basic Consumer Health Information about Illicit Substances of Abuse and the Diversion of Prescription Medications, Including Depressants, Hallucinogens, Inhalants, Marijuana, Narcotics, Stimulants, and Anabolic Steroids

Along with Facts about Related Health Risks, Treatment Issues, and Substance Abuse Prevention Programs, a Glossary of Terms, Statistical Data, and Directories of Hotline Services, Self-Help Groups, and Organizations Able to Provide Further Information

Edited by Karen Bellenir. 629 pages. 2000. 0-7808-0242-X. $78.

"Containing a wealth of information, this book will be useful to the college student just beginning to explore the topic of substance abuse. This resource belongs in libraries that serve a lower-division undergraduate or community college clientele as well as the general public." — *Choice, Association of College and Research Libraries, Jun '01*

"Recommended reference source." — *Booklist, American Library Association, Feb '01*

"Highly recommended." — *The Bookwatch, Jan '01*

"Even though there is a plethora of books on drug abuse, this volume is recommended for school, public, and college libraries." — *American Reference Books Annual, 2001*

SEE ALSO *Alcoholism Sourcebook, Substance Abuse Sourcebook*

Ear, Nose & Throat Disorders Sourcebook

Basic Information about Disorders of the Ears, Nose, Sinus Cavities, Pharynx, and Larynx, Including Ear Infections, Tinnitus, Vestibular Disorders, Allergic and Non-Allergic Rhinitis, Sore Throats, Tonsillitis, and Cancers That Affect the Ears, Nose, Sinuses, and Throat

Along with Reports on Current Research Initiatives, a Glossary of Related Medical Terms, and a Directory of Sources for Further Help and Information

Edited by Karen Bellenir and Linda M. Shin. 576 pages. 1998. 0-7808-0206-3. $78.

"Overall, this sourcebook is helpful for the consumer seeking information on ENT issues. It is recommended for public libraries." — *American Reference Books Annual, 1999*

"Recommended reference source." — *Booklist, American Library Association, Dec '98*

Eating Disorders Sourcebook

Basic Consumer Health Information about Eating Disorders, Including Information about Anorexia Nervosa, Bulimia Nervosa, Binge Eating, Body Dysmorphic Disorder, Pica, Laxative Abuse, and Night Eating Syndrome

Along with Information about Causes, Adverse Effects, and Treatment and Prevention Issues, and Featuring a Section on Concerns Specific to Children and Adolescents, a Glossary, and Resources for Further Help and Information

Edited by Dawn D. Matthews. 322 pages. 2001. 0-7808-0335-3. $78.

Endocrine & Metabolic Disorders Sourcebook

Basic Information for the Layperson about Pancreatic and Insulin-Related Disorders Such as Pancreatitis, Diabetes, and Hypoglycemia; Adrenal Gland Disorders Such as Cushing's Syndrome, Addison's Disease, and Congenital Adrenal Hyperplasia; Pituitary Gland Disorders Such as Growth Hormone Deficiency, Acromegaly, and Pituitary Tumors; Thyroid Disorders Such as Hypothyroidism, Graves' Disease, Hashimoto's Disease, and Goiter; Hyperparathyroidism; and Other Diseases and Syndromes of Hormone Imbalance or Metabolic Dysfunction

Along with Reports on Current Research Initiatives

Edited by Linda M. Shin. 574 pages. 1998. 0-7808-0207-1. $78.

Environmentally Induced Disorders Sourcebook

Basic Information about Diseases and Syndromes Linked to Exposure to Pollutants and Other Substances in Outdoor and Indoor Environments Such as Lead, Asbestos, Formaldehyde, Mercury, Emissions, Noise, and More

Edited by Allan R. Cook. 620 pages. 1997. 0-7808-0083-4. $78.

Ethnic Diseases Sourcebook

Basic Consumer Health Information for Ethnic and Racial Minority Groups in the United States, Including General Health Indicators and Behaviors, Ethnic Diseases, Genetic Testing, the Impact of Chronic Diseases, Women's Health, Mental Health Issues, and Preventive Health Care Services

Along with a Glossary and a Listing of Additional Resources

Edited by Joyce Brennfleck Shannon. 664 pages. 2001. 0-7808-0336-1. $78.

Family Planning Sourcebook

Basic Consumer Health Information about Planning for Pregnancy and Contraception, Including Traditional Methods, Barrier Methods, Hormonal Methods, Permanent Methods, Future Methods, Emergency Contraception, and Birth Control Choices for Women at Each Stage of Life

Along with Statistics, a Glossary, and Sources of Additional Information

Edited by Amy Marcaccio Keyzer. 520 pages. 2001. 0-7808-0379-5. $78.

SEE ALSO Pregnancy & Birth Sourcebook

Fitness & Exercise Sourcebook, 1st Edition

Basic Information on Fitness and Exercise, Including Fitness Activities for Specific Age Groups, Exercise for People with Specific Medical Conditions, How to Begin a Fitness Program in Running, Walking, Swimming, Cycling, and Other Athletic Activities, and Recent Research in Fitness and Exercise

Edited by Dan R. Harris. 663 pages. 1996. 0-7808-0186-5. $78.

Fitness & Exercise Sourcebook, 2nd Edition

Basic Consumer Health Information about the Fundamentals of Fitness and Exercise, Including How to Begin and Maintain a Fitness Program, Fitness as a Lifestyle, the Link between Fitness and Diet, Advice for Specific Groups of People, Exercise as It Relates to Specific Medical Conditions, and Recent Research in Fitness and Exercise

Along with a Glossary of Important Terms and Resources for Additional Help and Information

Edited by Kristen M. Gledhill. 646 pages. 2001. 0-7808-0334-5. $78.

Food & Animal Borne Diseases Sourcebook

Basic Information about Diseases That Can Be Spread to Humans through the Ingestion of Contaminated Food or Water or by Contact with Infected Animals and Insects, Such as Botulism, E. Coli, Hepatitis A, Trichinosis, Lyme Disease, and Rabies

Along with Information Regarding Prevention and Treatment Methods, and Including a Special Section for International Travelers Describing Diseases Such as Cholera, Malaria, Travelers' Diarrhea, and Yellow Fever, and Offering Recommendations for Avoiding Illness

Edited by Karen Bellenir and Peter D. Dresser. 535 pages. 1995. 0-7808-0033-8. $78.

589

Food Safety Sourcebook

Basic Consumer Health Information about the Safe Handling of Meat, Poultry, Seafood, Eggs, Fruit Juices, and Other Food Items, and Facts about Pesticides, Drinking Water, Food Safety Overseas, and the Onset, Duration, and Symptoms of Foodborne Illnesses, Including Types of Pathogenic Bacteria, Parasitic Protozoa, Worms, Viruses, and Natural Toxins

Along with the Role of the Consumer, the Food Handler, and the Government in Food Safety; a Glossary, and Resources for Additional Help and Information

Edited by Dawn D. Matthews. 339 pages. 1999. 0-7808-0326-4. $48.

"This book is recommended for public libraries and universities with home economic and food science programs." — *E-Streams, Nov '00*

"This book takes the complex issues of food safety and foodborne pathogens and presents them in an easily understood manner. [It does] an excellent job of covering a large and often confusing topic."
— *American Reference Books Annual, 2000*

"Recommended reference source."
— *Booklist, American Library Association, May '00*

■

Forensic Medicine Sourcebook

Basic Consumer Information for the Layperson about Forensic Medicine, Including Crime Scene Investigation, Evidence Collection and Analysis, Expert Testimony, Computer-Aided Criminal Identification, Digital Imaging in the Courtroom, DNA Profiling, Accident Reconstruction, Autopsies, Ballistics, Drugs and Explosives Detection, Latent Fingerprints, Product Tampering, and Questioned Document Examination

Along with Statistical Data, a Glossary of Forensics Terminology, and Listings of Sources for Further Help and Information

Edited by Annemarie S. Muth. 574 pages. 1999. 0-7808-0232-2. $78.

"Given the expected widespread interest in its content and its easy to read style, this book is recommended for most public and all college and university libraries."
— *E-Streams, Feb '01*

"There are several items that make this book attractive to consumers who are seeking certain forensic data. . . . This is a useful current source for those seeking general forensic medical answers."
— *American Reference Books Annual, 2000*

"Recommended for public libraries."
— *Reference & User Services Quarterly, American Library Association, Spring 2000*

"Recommended reference source."
— *Booklist, American Library Association, Feb '00*

"A wealth of information, useful statistics, references are up-to-date and extremely complete. This wonderful collection of data will help students who are interested in a career in any type of forensic field. It is a great

resource for attorneys who need information about types of expert witnesses needed in a particular case. It also offers useful information for fiction and nonfiction writers whose work involves a crime. A fascinating compilation. All levels." — *Choice, Association of College and Research Libraries, Jan 2000*

■

Gastrointestinal Diseases & Disorders Sourcebook

Basic Information about Gastroesophageal Reflux Disease (Heartburn), Ulcers, Diverticulosis, Irritable Bowel Syndrome, Crohn's Disease, Ulcerative Colitis, Diarrhea, Constipation, Lactose Intolerance, Hemorrhoids, Hepatitis, Cirrhosis, and Other Digestive Problems, Featuring Statistics, Descriptions of Symptoms, and Current Treatment Methods of Interest for Persons Living with Upper and Lower Gastrointestinal Maladies

Edited by Linda M. Ross. 413 pages. 1996. 0-7808-0078-8. $78.

". . . very readable form. The successful editorial work that brought this material together into a useful and understandable reference makes accessible to all readers information that can help them more effectively understand and obtain help for digestive tract problems."
— *Choice, Association of College and Research Libraries, Feb '97*

SEE ALSO *Diet & Nutrition Sourcebook, 1st and 2nd Editions, Digestive Diseases & Disorders Sourcebook*

■

Genetic Disorders Sourcebook, 1st Edition

Basic Information about Heritable Diseases and Disorders Such as Down Syndrome, PKU, Hemophilia, Von Willebrand Disease, Gaucher Disease, Tay-Sachs Disease, and Sickle-Cell Disease, Along with Information about Genetic Screening, Gene Therapy, Home Care, and Including Source Listings for Further Help and Information on More Than 300 Disorders

Edited by Karen Bellenir. 642 pages. 1996. 0-7808-0034-6. $78.

"Recommended for undergraduate libraries or libraries that serve the public."
— *Science & Technology Libraries, Vol. 18, No. 1, '99*

"Provides essential medical information to both the general public and those diagnosed with a serious or fatal genetic disease or disorder."
— *Choice, Association of College and Research Libraries, Jan '97*

"Geared toward the lay public. It would be well placed in all public libraries and in those hospital and medical libraries in which access to genetic references is limited." — *Doody's Health Sciences Book Review, Oct '96*

Genetic Disorders Sourcebook, 2nd Edition

Basic Consumer Health Information about Hereditary Diseases and Disorders, Including Cystic Fibrosis, Down Syndrome, Hemophilia, Huntington's Disease, Sickle Cell Anemia, and More; Facts about Genes, Gene Research and Therapy, Genetic Screening, Ethics of Gene Testing, Genetic Counseling, and Advice on Coping and Caring

Along with a Glossary of Genetic Terminology and a Resource List for Help, Support, and Further Information

Edited by Kathy Massimini. 768 pages. 2001. 0-7808-0241-1. $78.

"Recommended for public libraries and medical and hospital libraries with consumer health collections."
— *E-Streams, May '01*

"Recommended reference source."
— *Booklist, American Library Association, Apr '01*

"Important pick for college-level health reference libraries." — *The Bookwatch, Mar '01*

Head Trauma Sourcebook

Basic Information for the Layperson about Open-Head and Closed-Head Injuries, Treatment Advances, Recovery, and Rehabilitation

Along with Reports on Current Research Initiatives

Edited by Karen Bellenir. 414 pages. 1997. 0-7808-0208-X. $78.

Health Insurance Sourcebook

Basic Information about Managed Care Organizations, Traditional Fee-for-Service Insurance, Insurance Portability and Pre-Existing Conditions Clauses, Medicare, Medicaid, Social Security, and Military Health Care

Along with Information about Insurance Fraud

Edited by Wendy Wilcox. 530 pages. 1997. 0-7808-0222-5. $78.

"Particularly useful because it brings much of this information together in one volume. This book will be a handy reference source in the health sciences library, hospital library, college and university library, and medium to large public library."
— *Medical Reference Services Quarterly, Fall '98*

Awarded "Books of the Year Award"
— *American Journal of Nursing, 1997*

"The layout of the book is particularly helpful as it provides easy access to reference material. A most useful addition to the vast amount of information about health insurance. The use of data from U.S. government agencies is most commendable. Useful in a library or learning center for healthcare professional students."
— *Doody's Health Sciences Book Reviews, Nov '97*

Health Reference Series Cumulative Index 1999

A Comprehensive Index to the Individual Volumes of the Health Reference Series, Including a Subject Index, Name Index, Organization Index, and Publication Index

Along with a Master List of Acronyms and Abbreviations

Edited by Edward J. Prucha, Anne Holmes, and Robert Rudnick. 990 pages. 2000. 0-7808-0382-5. $78.

"This volume will be most helpful in libraries that have a relatively complete collection of the Health Reference Series."
— *American Reference Books Annual, 2001*

"Essential for collections that hold any of the numerous *Health Reference Series* titles."
— *Choice, Association of College and Research Libraries, Nov '00*

Healthy Aging Sourcebook

Basic Consumer Health Information about Maintaining Health through the Aging Process, Including Advice on Nutrition, Exercise, and Sleep, Help in Making Decisions about Midlife Issues and Retirement, and Guidance Concerning Practical and Informed Choices in Health Consumerism

Along with Data Concerning the Theories of Aging, Different Experiences in Aging by Minority Groups, and Facts about Aging Now and Aging in the Future; and Featuring a Glossary, a Guide to Consumer Help, Additional Suggested Reading, and Practical Resource Directory

Edited by Jenifer Swanson. 536 pages. 1999. 0-7808-0390-6. $78.

"Recommended reference source."
— *Booklist, American Library Association, Feb '00*

SEE ALSO *Physical & Mental Issues in Aging Sourcebook*

Healthy Heart Sourcebook for Women

Basic Consumer Health Information about Cardiac Issues Specific to Women, Including Facts about Major Risk Factors and Prevention, Treatment and Control Strategies, and Important Dietary Issues

Along with a Special Section Regarding the Pros and Cons of Hormone Replacement Therapy and Its Impact on Heart Health, and Additional Help, Including Recipes, a Glossary, and a Directory of Resources

Edited by Dawn D. Matthews. 336 pages. 2000. 0-7808-0329-9. $48.

"A good reference source and recommended for all public, academic, medical, and hospital libraries."
— *Medical Reference Services Quarterly, Summer '01*

"Because of the lack of information specific to women on this topic, this book is recommended for public libraries and consumer libraries."
—American Reference Books Annual, 2001

"Contains very important information about coronary artery disease that all women should know. The information is current and presented in an easy-to-read format. The book will make a good addition to any library."
— American Medical Writers Association Journal, Summer '00

"Important, basic reference."
Environs's Book and In Jul '00

SEE ALSO Cardiovascular Diseases & Disorders Sourcebook, 1st Edition, Heart Diseases & Disorders Sourcebook, 2nd Edition, Women's Health Concerns Sourcebook

■

Heart Diseases & Disorders Sourcebook, 2nd Edition

Basic Consumer Health Information about Heart Attacks, Angina, Rhythm Disorders, Heart Failure, Valve Disease, Congenital Heart Disorders, and More, Including Descriptions of Surgical Procedures and Other Interventions, Medications, Cardiac Rehabilitation, Risk Identification, and Prevention Tips

Along with Statistical Data, Reports on Current Research Initiatives, a Glossary of Cardiovascular Terms, and Resource Directory

Edited by Karen Bellenir. 612 pages. 2000. 0-7808-0238-1. $78.

"This work stands out as an imminently accessible resource for the general public. It is recommended for the reference and circulating shelves of school, public, and academic libraries."
—American Reference Books Annual, 2001

"Recommended reference source."
—Booklist, American Library Association, Dec '00

"Provides comprehensive coverage of matters related to the heart. This title is recommended for health sciences and public libraries with consumer health collections."
— E-Streams, Oct '00

SEE ALSO Cardiovascular Diseases & Disorders Sourcebook, 1st Edition, Healthy Heart Sourcebook for Women

■

Household Safety Sourcebook

Basic Consumer Health Information about Household Safety, Including Information about Poisons, Chemicals, Fire, and Water Hazards in the Home

Along with Advice about the Safe Use of Home Maintenance Equipment, Choosing Toys and Nursery Furniture, Holiday and Recreation Safety, a Glossary, and Resources for Further Help and Information

Edited by Dawn D. Matthews. 606 pages. 2001. 0-7808-0338-8. $78.

Immune System Disorders Sourcebook

Basic Information about Lupus, Multiple Sclerosis, Guillain-Barré Syndrome, Chronic Granulomatous Disease, and More

Along with Statistical and Demographic Data and Reports on Current Research Initiatives

Edited by Allan R. Cook. 608 pages. 1997. 0-7808-0209-8. $78.

■

Infant & Toddler Health Sourcebook

Basic Consumer Health Information about the Physical and Mental Development of Newborns, Infants, and Toddlers, Including Neonatal Concerns, Nutrition Recommendations, Immunization Schedules, Common Pediatric Disorders, Assessments and Milestones, Safety Tips, and Advice for Parents and Other Caregivers

Along with a Glossary of Terms and Resource Listings for Additional Help

Edited by Jenifer Swanson. 585 pages. 2000. 0-7808-0246-2. $78.

"As a reference for the general public, this would be useful in any library."
— E-Streams, May '01

"Recommended reference source."
— Booklist, American Library Association, Feb '01

"This is a good source for general use."
—American Reference Books Annual, 2001

■

Kidney & Urinary Tract Diseases & Disorders Sourcebook

Basic Information about Kidney Stones, Urinary Incontinence, Bladder Disease, End Stage Renal Disease, Dialysis, and More

Along with Statistical and Demographic Data and Reports on Current Research Initiatives

Edited by Linda M. Ross. 602 pages. 1997. 0-7808-0079-6. $78.

■

Learning Disabilities Sourcebook

Basic Information about Disorders Such as Dyslexia, Visual and Auditory Processing Deficits, Attention Deficit/Hyperactivity Disorder, and Autism

Along with Statistical and Demographic Data, Reports on Current Research Initiatives, an Explanation of the Assessment Process, and a Special Section for Adults with Learning Disabilities

Edited by Linda M. Shin. 579 pages. 1998. 0-7808-0210-1. $78.

Named "Outstanding Reference Book of 1999."
— *New York Public Library, Feb 2000*

"An excellent candidate for inclusion in a public library reference section. It's a great source of information. Teachers will also find the book useful. Definitely worth reading."
— *Journal of Adolescent & Adult Literacy, Feb 2000*

"Readable . . . provides a solid base of information regarding successful techniques used with individuals who have learning disabilities, as well as practical suggestions for educators and family members. Clear language, concise descriptions, and pertinent information for contacting multiple resources add to the strength of this book as a useful tool." — *Choice, Association of College and Research Libraries, Feb '99*

"Recommended reference source."
— *Booklist, American Library Association, Sep '98*

"A useful resource for libraries and for those who don't have the time to identify and locate the individual publications." — *Disability Resources Monthly, Sep '98*

![]

Liver Disorders Sourcebook

Basic Consumer Health Information about the Liver and How It Works; Liver Diseases, Including Cancer, Cirrhosis, Hepatitis, and Toxic and Drug Related Diseases; Tips for Maintaining a Healthy Liver; Laboratory Tests, Radiology Tests, and Facts about Liver Transplantation

Along with a Section on Support Groups, a Glossary, and Resource Listings

Edited by Joyce Brennfleck Shannon. 591 pages. 2000. 0-7808-0383-3. $78.

"A valuable resource."
— *American Reference Books Annual, 2001*

"This title is recommended for health sciences and public libraries with consumer health collections."
— *E-Streams, Oct '00*

"Recommended reference source."
— *Booklist, American Library Association, Jun '00*

![]

Medical Tests Sourcebook

Basic Consumer Health Information about Medical Tests, Including Periodic Health Exams, General Screening Tests, Tests You Can Do at Home, Findings of the U.S. Preventive Services Task Force, X-ray and Radiology Tests, Electrical Tests, Tests of Blood and Other Body Fluids and Tissues, Scope Tests, Lung Tests, Genetic Tests, Pregnancy Tests, Newborn Screening Tests, Sexually Transmitted Disease Tests, and Computer Aided Diagnoses

Along with a Section on Paying for Medical Tests, a Glossary, and Resource Listings

Edited by Joyce Brennfleck Shannon. 691 pages. 1999. 0-7808-0243-8. $78.

"A valuable reference guide."
— *American Reference Books Annual, 2000*

"Recommended for hospital and health sciences libraries with consumer health collections."
— *E-Streams, Mar '00*

"This is an overall excellent reference with a wealth of general knowledge that may aid those who are reluctant to get vital tests performed."
— *Today's Librarian, Jan 2000*

![]

Men's Health Concerns Sourcebook

Basic Information about Health Issues That Affect Men, Featuring Facts about the Top Causes of Death in Men, Including Heart Disease, Stroke, Cancers, Prostate Disorders, Chronic Obstructive Pulmonary Disease, Pneumonia and Influenza, Human Immunodeficiency Virus and Acquired Immune Deficiency Syndrome, Diabetes Mellitus, Stress, Suicide, Accidents and Homicides; and Facts about Common Concerns for Men, Including Impotence, Contraception, Circumcision, Sleep Disorders, Snoring, Hair Loss, Diet, Nutrition, Exercise, Kidney and Urological Disorders, and Backaches

Edited by Allan R. Cook. 738 pages. 1998. 0-7808-0212-8. $78.

"This comprehensive resource and the series are highly recommended."
— *American Reference Books Annual, 2000*

"Recommended reference source."
— *Booklist, American Library Association, Dec '98*

![]

Mental Health Disorders Sourcebook, 1st Edition

Basic Information about Schizophrenia, Depression, Bipolar Disorder, Panic Disorder, Obsessive-Compulsive Disorder, Phobias and Other Anxiety Disorders, Paranoia and Other Personality Disorders, Eating Disorders, and Sleep Disorders

Along with Information about Treatment and Therapies

Edited by Karen Bellenir. 548 pages. 1995. 0-7808-0040-0. $78.

"This is an excellent new book . . . written in easy-to-understand language."
— *Booklist Health Sciences Supplement, American Library Association, Oct '97*

". . . useful for public and academic libraries and consumer health collections."
— *Medical Reference Services Quarterly, Spring '97*

"The great strengths of the book are its readability and its inclusion of places to find more information. Especially recommended." — *Reference Quarterly, American Library Association, Winter '96*

". . . a good resource for a consumer health library."
— *Bulletin of the Medical Library Association, Oct '96*

"The information is data-based and couched in brief, concise language that avoids jargon. . . . a useful reference source." — *Readings, Sep '96*

"The text is well organized and adequately written for its target audience." — *Choice, Association of College and Research Libraries, Jun '96*

". . . provides information on a wide range of mental disorders, presented in nontechnical language." — *Exceptional Child Education Resources, Spring '96*

"Recommended for public and academic libraries." — *Reference Book Review, 1996*

Mental Health Disorders Sourcebook, 2nd Edition

Basic Consumer Health Information about Anxiety Disorders, Depression and Other Mood Disorders, Eating Disorders, Personality Disorders, Schizophrenia, and More, Including Disease Descriptions, Treatment Options, and Reports on Current Research Initiatives

Along with Statistical Data, Tips for Maintaining Mental Health, a Glossary, and Directory of Sources for Additional Help and Information

Edited by Karen Bellenir. 605 pages. 2000. 0-7808-0240-3. $78.

"Well organized and well written." — *American Reference Books Annual, 2001*

"Recommended reference source." — *Booklist, American Library Association, Jun '00*

Mental Retardation Sourcebook

Basic Consumer Health Information about Mental Retardation and Its Causes, Including Down Syndrome, Fetal Alcohol Syndrome, Fragile X Syndrome, Genetic Conditions, Injury, and Environmental Sources

Along with Preventive Strategies, Parenting Issues, Educational Implications, Health Care Needs, Employment and Economic Matters, Legal Issues, a Glossary, and a Resource Listing for Additional Help and Information

Edited by Joyce Brennfleck Shannon. 642 pages. 2000. 0-7808-0377-9. $78.

"Public libraries will find the book useful for reference and as a beginning research point for students, parents, and caregivers." — *American Reference Books Annual, 2001*

"The strength of this work is that it compiles many basic fact sheets and addresses for further information in one volume. It is intended and suitable for the general public. The sourcebook is relevant to any collection providing health information to the general public." — *E-Streams, Nov '00*

"From preventing retardation to parenting and family challenges, this covers health, social and legal issues and will prove an invaluable overview." — *Reviewer's Bookwatch, Jul '00*

Obesity Sourcebook

Basic Consumer Health Information about Diseases and Other Problems Associated with Obesity, and Including Facts about Risk Factors, Prevention Issues, and Management Approaches

Along with Statistical and Demographic Data, Information about Special Populations, Research Updates, a Glossary, and Source Listings for Further Help and Information

Edited by Wilma Caldwell and Chad T. Kimball. 376 pages. 2001. 0-7808-0333-7. $48.

" Recommended pick both for specialty health library collections and any general consumer health reference collection." — *The Bookwatch, Apr '01*

"Recommended reference source." — *Booklist, American Library Association, Apr '01*

Ophthalmic Disorders Sourcebook

Basic Information about Glaucoma, Cataracts, Macular Degeneration, Strabismus, Refractive Disorders, and More

Along with Statistical and Demographic Data and Reports on Current Research Initiatives

Edited by Linda M. Ross. 631 pages. 1996. 0-7808-0081-8. $78.

Oral Health Sourcebook

Basic Information about Diseases and Conditions Affecting Oral Health, Including Cavities, Gum Disease, Dry Mouth, Oral Cancers, Fever Blisters, Canker Sores, Oral Thrush, Bad Breath, Temporomandibular Disorders, and other Craniofacial Syndromes

Along with Statistical Data on the Oral Health of Americans, Oral Hygiene, Emergency First Aid, Information on Treatment Procedures and Methods of Replacing Lost Teeth

Edited by Allan R. Cook. 558 pages. 1997. 0-7808-0082-6. $78.

"Unique source which will fill a gap in dental sources for patients and the lay public. A valuable reference tool even in a library with thousands of books on dentistry. Comprehensive, clear, inexpensive, and easy to read and use. It fills an enormous gap in the health care literature." — *Reference and User Services Quarterly, American Library Association, Summer '98*

"Recommended reference source." — *Booklist, American Library Association, Dec '97*

Osteoporosis Sourcebook

Basic Consumer Health Information about Primary and Secondary Osteoporosis and Juvenile Osteoporosis and Related Conditions, Including Fibrous Dysplasia, Gaucher Disease, Hyperthyroidism, Hypophosphatasia, Myeloma, Osteopetrosis, Osteogenesis Imperfecta, and Paget's Disease

Along with Information about Risk Factors, Treatments, Traditional and Non-Traditional Pain Management, a Glossary of Related Terms, and a Directory of Resources

Edited by Allan R. Cook. 584 pages. 2001. 0-7808-0239-X. $78.

SEE ALSO Women's Health Concerns Sourcebook

■

Pain Sourcebook

Basic Information about Specific Forms of Acute and Chronic Pain, Including Headaches, Back Pain, Muscular Pain, Neuralgia, Surgical Pain, and Cancer Pain

Along with Pain Relief Options Such as Analgesics, Narcotics, Nerve Blocks, Transcutaneous Nerve Stimulation, and Alternative Forms of Pain Control, Including Biofeedback, Imaging, Behavior Modification, and Relaxation Techniques

Edited by Allan R. Cook. 667 pages. 1997. 0-7808-0213-6. $78.

"The text is readable, easily understood, and well indexed. This excellent volume belongs in all patient education libraries, consumer health sections of public libraries, and many personal collections."
—American Reference Books Annual, 1999

"A beneficial reference." —Booklist Health Sciences Supplement, American Library Association, Oct '98

"The information is basic in terms of scholarship and is appropriate for general readers. Written in journalistic style . . . intended for non-professionals. Quite thorough in its coverage of different pain conditions and summarizes the latest clinical information regarding pain treatment." —Choice, Association of College and Research Libraries, Jun '98

"Recommended reference source."
—Booklist, American Library Association, Mar '98

■

Pediatric Cancer Sourcebook

Basic Consumer Health Information about Leukemias, Brain Tumors, Sarcomas, Lymphomas, and Other Cancers in Infants, Children, and Adolescents, Including Descriptions of Cancers, Treatments, and Coping Strategies

Along with Suggestions for Parents, Caregivers, and Concerned Relatives, a Glossary of Cancer Terms, and Resource Listings

Edited by Edward J. Prucha. 587 pages. 1999. 0-7808-0245-4. $78.

"A valuable addition to all libraries specializing in health services and many public libraries."
—American Reference Books Annual, 2000

"Recommended reference source."
—Booklist, American Library Association, Feb '00

"An excellent source of information. Recommended for public, hospital, and health science libraries with consumer health collections." —E-Streams, Jun '00

Physical & Mental Issues in Aging Sourcebook

Basic Consumer Health Information on Physical and Mental Disorders Associated with the Aging Process, Including Concerns about Cardiovascular Disease, Pulmonary Disease, Oral Health, Digestive Disorders, Musculoskeletal and Skin Disorders, Metabolic Changes, Sexual and Reproductive Issues, and Changes in Vision, Hearing, and Other Senses

Along with Data about Longevity and Causes of Death, Information on Acute and Chronic Pain, Descriptions of Mental Concerns, a Glossary of Terms, and Resource Listings for Additional Help

Edited by Jenifer Swanson. 660 pages. 1999. 0-7808-0233-0. $78.

"Recommended for public libraries."
—American Reference Books Annual, 2000

"This is a treasure of health information for the layperson." — Choice Health Sciences Supplement, Association of College & Research Libraries, May 2000

"Recommended reference source."
—Booklist, American Library Association, Oct '99

SEE ALSO Healthy Aging Sourcebook

■

Podiatry Sourcebook

Basic Consumer Health Information about Foot Conditions, Diseases, and Injuries, Including Bunions, Corns, Calluses, Athlete's Foot, Plantar Warts, Hammertoes and Clawtoes, Clubfoot, Heel Pain, Gout, and More

Along with Facts about Foot Care, Disease Prevention, Foot Safety, Choosing a Foot Care Specialist, a Glossary of Terms, and Resource Listings for Additional Information

Edited by M. Lisa Weatherford. 380 pages. 2001. 0-7808-0215-2. $78.

■

Pregnancy & Birth Sourcebook

Basic Information about Planning for Pregnancy, Maternal Health, Fetal Growth and Development, Labor and Delivery, Postpartum and Perinatal Care, Pregnancy in Mothers with Special Concerns, and Disorders of Pregnancy, Including Genetic Counseling, Nutrition and Exercise, Obstetrical Tests, Pregnancy Discomfort, Multiple Births, Cesarean Sections, Medical Testing of Newborns, Breastfeeding, Gestational Diabetes, and Ectopic Pregnancy

Edited by Heather E. Aldred. 737 pages. 1997. 0-7808-0216-0. $78.

"A well-organized handbook. Recommended."
— Choice, Association of College and Research Libraries, Apr '98

"Recommended reference source."
—Booklist, American Library Association, Mar '98

SEE ALSO *Congenital Disorders Sourcebook, Family Planning Sourcebook*

Prostate Cancer Sourcebook

Basic Consumer Health Information about Prostate Cancer, Including Information about the Associated Risk Factors, Detection, Diagnosis, and Treatment of Prostate Cancer

Along with Information on Non-Malignant Prostate Conditions, and Featuring a Section Listing Support and Treatment Centers and a Glossary of Related Terms

Edited by Dawn D. Matthews. 358 pages. 2001. 0-7808-0324-8. $78.

Public Health Sourcebook

Basic Information about Government Health Agencies, Including National Health Statistics and Trends, Healthy People 2000 Program Goals and Objectives, the Centers for Disease Control and Prevention, the Food and Drug Administration, and the National Institutes of Health

Along with Full Contact Information for Each Agency

Edited by Wendy Wilcox. 698 pages. 1998. 0-7808-0220-9. $78.

Reconstructive & Cosmetic Surgery Sourcebook

Basic Consumer Health Information on Cosmetic and Reconstructive Plastic Surgery, Including Statistical Information about Different Surgical Procedures, Things to Consider Prior to Surgery, Plastic Surgery Techniques and Tools, Emotional and Psychological Considerations, and Procedure-Specific Information

Along with a Glossary of Terms and a Listing of Resources for Additional Help and Information

Edited by M. Lisa Weatherford. 374 pages. 2001. 0-7808-0214-4. $48.

Rehabilitation Sourcebook

*Basic Consumer Health Information about Rehabilitation for People Recovering from Heart Surgery, Spinal Cord Injury, Stroke, Orthopedic Impairments, Amputation, Pulmonary Impairments, Traumatic In-*jury, and More, Including Physical Therapy, Occupational Therapy, Speech/ Language Therapy, Massage Therapy, Dance Therapy, Art Therapy, and Recreational Therapy

Along with Information on Assistive and Adaptive Devices, a Glossary, and Resources for Additional Help and Information

Edited by Dawn D. Matthews. 531 pages. 1999. 0-7808-0236-5. $78.

Respiratory Diseases & Disorders Sourcebook

Basic Information about Respiratory Diseases and Disorders, Including Asthma, Cystic Fibrosis, Pneumonia, the Common Cold, Influenza, and Others, Featuring Facts about the Respiratory System, Statistical and Demographic Data, Treatments, Self-Help Management Suggestions, and Current Research Initiatives

Edited by Allan R. Cook and Peter D. Dresser. 771 pages. 1995. 0-7808-0037-0. $78.

Sexually Transmitted Diseases Sourcebook, 1st Edition

Basic Information about Herpes, Chlamydia, Gonorrhea, Hepatitis, Nongonoccocal Urethritis, Pelvic Inflammatory Disease, Syphilis, AIDS, and More

Along with Current Data on Treatments and Preventions

Edited by Linda M. Ross. 550 pages. 1997. 0-7808-0217-9. $78.

Sexually Transmitted Diseases Sourcebook, 2nd Edition

Basic Consumer Health Information about Sexually Transmitted Diseases, Including Information on the Diagnosis and Treatment of Chlamydia, Gonorrhea, Hepatitis, Herpes, HIV, Mononucleosis, Syphilis, and Others

Along with Information on Prevention, Such as Condom Use, Vaccines, and STD Education; And Featuring a Section on Issues Related to Youth and Adolescents, a Glossary, and Resources for Additional Help and Information

Edited by Dawn D. Matthews. 538 pages. 2001. 0-7808-0249-7. $78.

"Recommended pick both for specialty health library collections and any general consumer health reference collection." *— The Bookwatch, Apr '01*

"Recommended reference source."
—Booklist, American Library Association, Apr '01

Skin Disorders Sourcebook

Basic Information about Common Skin and Scalp Conditions Caused by Aging, Allergies, Immune Reactions, Sun Exposure, Infectious Organisms, Parasites, Cosmetics, and Skin Traumas, Including Abrasions, Cuts, and Pressure Sores

Along with Information on Prevention and Treatment

Edited by Allan R. Cook. 647 pages. 1997. 0-7808-0080-X. $78.

". . . comprehensive, easily read reference book."
—Doody's Health Sciences Book Reviews, Oct '97

SEE ALSO Burns Sourcebook

Sleep Disorders Sourcebook

Basic Consumer Health Information about Sleep and Its Disorders, Including Insomnia, Sleepwalking, Sleep Apnea, Restless Leg Syndrome, and Narcolepsy

Along with Data about Shiftwork and Its Effects, Information on the Societal Costs of Sleep Deprivation, Descriptions of Treatment Options, a Glossary of Terms, and Resource Listings for Additional Help

Edited by Jenifer Swanson. 439 pages. 1998. 0-7808-0234-9. $78.

"This text will complement any home or medical library. It is user-friendly and ideal for the adult reader."
—American Reference Books Annual, 2000

"Recommended reference source."
—Booklist, American Library Association, Feb '99

"A useful resource that provides accurate, relevant, and accessible information on sleep to the general public. Health care providers who deal with sleep disorders patients may also find it helpful in being prepared to answer some of the questions patients ask."
—Respiratory Care, Jul '99

Sports Injuries Sourcebook

Basic Consumer Health Information about Common Sports Injuries, Prevention of Injury in Specific Sports, Tips for Training, and Rehabilitation from Injury

Along with Information about Special Concerns for Children, Young Girls in Athletic Training Programs, Senior Athletes, and Women Athletes, and a Directory of Resources for Further Help and Information

Edited by Heather E. Aldred. 624 pages. 1999. 0-7808-0218-7. $78.

"Public libraries and undergraduate academic libraries will find this book useful for its nontechnical language." *—American Reference Books Annual, 2000*

"While this easy-to-read book is recommended for all libraries, it should prove to be especially useful for public, high school, and academic libraries; certainly it should be on the bookshelf of every school gymnasium." *—E-Streams, Mar '00*

Substance Abuse Sourcebook

Basic Health-Related Information about the Abuse of Legal and Illegal Substances Such as Alcohol, Tobacco, Prescription Drugs, Marijuana, Cocaine, and Heroin; and Including Facts about Substance Abuse Prevention Strategies, Intervention Methods, Treatment and Recovery Programs, and a Section Addressing the Special Problems Related to Substance Abuse during Pregnancy

Edited by Karen Bellenir. 573 pages. 1996. 0-7808-0038-9. $78.

"A valuable addition to any health reference section. Highly recommended."
—The Book Report, Mar/Apr '97

". . . a comprehensive collection of substance abuse information that's both highly readable and compact. Families and caregivers of substance abusers will find the information enlightening and helpful, while teachers, social workers and journalists should benefit from the concise format. Recommended."
—Drug Abuse Update, Winter '96/'97

SEE ALSO Alcoholism Sourcebook, Drug Abuse Sourcebook

Transplantation Sourcebook

Basic Consumer Health Information about Organ and Tissue Transplantation, Including Physical and Financial Preparations, Procedures and Issues Relating to Specific Solid Organ and Tissue Transplants, Rehabilitation, Pediatric Transplant Information, the Future of Transplantation, and Organ and Tissue Donation

Along with a Glossary and Listings of Additional Resources

Edited by Joyce Brennfleck Shannon. 600 pages. 2002. 0-7808-0322-1. $78.

Traveler's Health Sourcebook

Basic Consumer Health Information for Travelers, Including Physical and Medical Preparations, Transportation Health and Safety, Essential Information about Food and Water, Sun Exposure, Insect and Snake Bites, Camping and Wilderness Medicine, and Travel with Physical or Medical Disabilities

Along with International Travel Tips, Vaccination Recommendations, Geographical Health Issues, Disease Risks, a Glossary, and a Listing of Additional Resources

Edited by Joyce Brennfleck Shannon. 613 pages. 2000. 0-7808-0384-1. $78.

"Recommended reference source."
   —Booklist, American Library Association, Feb '01

"This book is recommended for any public library, any travel collection, and especially any collection for the physically disabled."
   —American Reference Books Annual, 2001

■

Women's Health Concerns Sourcebook

Basic Information about Health Issues That Affect Women, Featuring Facts about Menstruation and Other Gynecological Concerns, Including Endometriosis, Fibroids, Menopause, and Vaginitis; Reproductive Concerns, Including Birth Control, Infertility, and Abortion; and Facts about Additional Physical, Emotional, and Mental Health Concerns Prevalent among Women Such as Osteoporosis, Urinary Tract Disorders, Eating Disorders, and Depression

Along with Tips for Maintaining a Healthy Lifestyle

Edited by Heather E. Aldred. 567 pages. 1997. 0-7808-0219-5. $78.

"Handy compilation. There is an impressive range of diseases, devices, disorders, procedures, and other physical and emotional issues covered . . . well organized, illustrated, and indexed." *—Choice, Association of College and Research Libraries, Jan '98*

SEE ALSO *Breast Cancer Sourcebook, Cancer Sourcebook for Women, 1st and 2nd Editions, Healthy Heart Sourcebook for Women, Osteoporosis Sourcebook*

Workplace Health & Safety Sourcebook

Basic Consumer Health Information about Workplace Health and Safety, Including the Effect of Workplace Hazards on the Lungs, Skin, Heart, Ears, Eyes, Brain, Reproductive Organs, Musculoskeletal System, and Other Organs and Body Parts

Along with Information about Occupational Cancer, Personal Protective Equipment, Toxic and Hazardous Chemicals, Child Labor, Stress, and Workplace Violence

Edited by Chad T. Kimball. 626 pages. 2000. 0-7808-0231-4. $78.

"Provides helpful information for primary care physicians and other caregivers interested in occupational medicine. . . . General readers; professionals."
   — Choice, Association of College and Research Libraries, May '01

"Recommended reference source."
   —Booklist, American Library Association, Feb '01

"Highly recommended."   *—The Bookwatch, Jan '01*

■

Worldwide Health Sourcebook

Basic Information about Global Health Issues, Including Malnutrition, Reproductive Health, Disease Dispersion and Prevention, Emerging Diseases, Risky Health Behaviors, and the Leading Causes of Death

Along with Global Health Concerns for Children, Women, and the Elderly, Mental Health Issues, Research and Technology Advancements, and Economic, Environmental, and Political Health Implications, a Glossary, and a Resource Listing for Additional Help and Information

Edited by Joyce Brennfleck Shannon. 614 pages. 2001. 0-7808-0330-2. $78.